Advances in Knee Surgery

Advances in Knee Surgery

Editors

Yong In
In Jun Koh

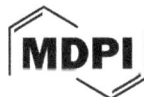

Basel • Beijing • Wuhan • Barcelona • Belgrade • Novi Sad • Cluj • Manchester

Editors
Yong In
The Catholic University of Korea
Seoul, Republic of Korea

In Jun Koh
The Catholic University of Korea
Seoul, Republic of Korea

Editorial Office
MDPI
St. Alban-Anlage 66
4052 Basel, Switzerland

This is a reprint of articles from the Special Issue published online in the open access journal *Medicina* (ISSN 1648-9144) (available at: https://www.mdpi.com/journal/medicina/special_issues/Knee_Surgery_).

For citation purposes, cite each article independently as indicated on the article page online and as indicated below:

Lastname, A.A.; Lastname, B.B. Article Title. *Journal Name* **Year**, *Volume Number*, Page Range.

ISBN 978-3-0365-9608-2 (Hbk)
ISBN 978-3-0365-9609-9 (PDF)
doi.org/10.3390/books978-3-0365-9609-9

© 2023 by the authors. Articles in this book are Open Access and distributed under the Creative Commons Attribution (CC BY) license. The book as a whole is distributed by MDPI under the terms and conditions of the Creative Commons Attribution-NonCommercial-NoDerivs (CC BY-NC-ND) license.

Contents

About the Editors ix

Dojoon Park, Youn Ho Choi, Se Hyun Kang, Hae Seok Koh and Yong In
Bone Marrow Aspirate Concentrate versus Human Umbilical Cord Blood-Derived Mesenchymal Stem Cells for Combined Cartilage Regeneration Procedure in Patients Undergoing High Tibial Osteotomy: A Systematic Review and Meta-Analysis
Reprinted from: *Medicina* **2023**, *59*, 634, doi:10.3390/medicina59030634 1

Dong Hwan Lee, Seon Ae Kim, Jun-Seob Song, Asode Ananthram Shetty, Bo-Hyoung Kim and Seok Jung Kim
Cartilage Regeneration Using Human Umbilical Cord Blood Derived Mesenchymal Stem Cells: A Systematic Review and Meta Analysis
Reprinted from: *Medicina* **2022**, *58*, 1801, doi:10.3390/medicina58121801 17

You Seung Chun, Seon Ae Kim, Yun Hwan Kim, Joong Hoon Lee, Asode Ananthram Shetty and Seok Jung Kim
Autologous Collagen-Induced Chondrogenesis: From Bench to Clinical Development
Reprinted from: *Medicina* **2023**, *59*, 530, doi:10.3390/medicina59030530 33

Yong-Beom Park, Han-Jun Lee, Hyun-Cheul Nam and Jung-Gwan Park
Allogeneic Umbilical Cord-Blood-Derived Mesenchymal Stem Cells and Hyaluronate Composite Combined with High Tibial Osteotomy for Medial Knee Osteoarthritis with Full-Thickness Cartilage Defects
Reprinted from: *Medicina* **2023**, *59*, 148, doi:10.3390/medicina59010148 45

Dominik Sieroń, Izabella Jabłońska, Paweł Niemiec, Dawid Lukoszek, Karol Szyluk, Ivan Platzek, et al.
Relationship between Outerbridge Scale and Chondropathy Femorotibial Joint in Relation to Gender and Age—The Use of 1.5T and 3.0T MRI Scanners
Reprinted from: *Medicina* **2022**, *58*, 1634, doi:10.3390/medicina58111634 55

Elias Primetis, Dionysios Drakopoulos, Dominik Sieron, Hugo Meusburger, Karol Szyluk, Paweł Niemiec, et al.
Knee Diameter and Cross-Sectional Area as Biomarkers for Cartilage Knee Degeneration on Magnetic Resonance Images
Reprinted from: *Medicina* **2023**, *59*, 27, doi:10.3390/medicina59010027 67

Tae-Jin Lee, Ki-Mo Jang, Tae-Jin Kim, Sang-Min Lee and Ji-Hoon Bae
Adjustable-Loop Cortical Suspensory Fixation Results in Greater Tibial Tunnel Widening Compared to Interference Screw Fixation in Primary Anterior Cruciate Ligament Reconstruction
Reprinted from: *Medicina* **2022**, *58*, 1193, doi:10.3390/medicina58091193 79

O-Sung Lee, Joong Il Kim, Seok Hyeon Han and Joon Kyu Lee
Beneficial Effect of Curved Dilator System for Femoral Tunnel Creation in Preventing Femoral Tunnel Widening after Anterior Cruciate Ligament Reconstruction
Reprinted from: *Medicina* **2023**, *59*, 1437, doi:10.3390/medicina59081437 89

Kyu Sung Chung, Jeong Ku Ha, Jin Seong Kim and Jin Goo Kim
Changes in Bone Marrow Lesions Following Root Repair Surgery Using Modified Mason–Allen Stitches in Medial Meniscus Posterior Root Tears
Reprinted from: *Medicina* **2022**, *58*, 1601, doi:10.3390/medicina58111601 99

Hyun-Soo Moon, Chong-Hyuk Choi, Min Jung, Kwangho Chung, Se-Han Jung, Yun-Hyeok Kim and Sung-Hwan Kim
Medial Meniscus Posterior Root Tear: How Far Have We Come and What Remains?
Reprinted from: *Medicina* **2023**, *59*, 1181, doi:10.3390/medicina59071181 111

Tae Woo Kim and June Seok Won
Anatomical Study of the Lateral Tibial Spine as a Landmark for Weight Bearing Line Assessment during High Tibial Osteotomy
Reprinted from: *Medicina* **2023**, *59*, 1571, doi:10.3390/medicina59091571 129

Sung-Sahn Lee, Jaesung Park and Dae-Hee Lee
Comparison of Anatomical Conformity between TomoFix Anatomical Plate and TomoFix Conventional Plate in Open-Wedge High Tibial Osteotomy
Reprinted from: *Medicina* **2022**, *58*, 1045, doi:10.3390/medicina58081045 139

Jae-Jung Kim, In-Jun Koh, Man-Soo Kim, Keun-Young Choi, Ki-Ho Kang and Yong In
Central Sensitization Is Associated with Inferior Patient-Reported Outcomes and Increased Osteotomy Site Pain in Patients Undergoing Medial Opening-Wedge High Tibial Osteotomy
Reprinted from: *Medicina* **2022**, *58*, 1752, doi:10.3390/medicina58121752 147

Back Kim, Do Weon Lee, Sanggyu Lee, Sunho Ko, Changwung Jo, Jaeseok Park, et al.
Automated Detection of Surgical Implants on Plain Knee Radiographs Using a Deep Learning Algorithm
Reprinted from: *Medicina* **2022**, *58*, 1677, doi:10.3390/medicina58111677 157

Keun Young Choi, Sheen-Woo Lee, Yong In, Man Soo Kim, Yong Deok Kim, Seung-yeol Lee, et al.
Dual-Energy CT-Based Bone Mineral Density Has Practical Value for Osteoporosis Screening around the Knee
Reprinted from: *Medicina* **2022**, *58*, 1085, doi:10.3390/medicina58081085 169

Dai-Soon Kwak, Yong Deok Kim, Nicole Cho, Ho-Jung Cho, Jaeryong Ko, Minji Kim, et al.
Guided-Motion Bicruciate-Stabilized Total Knee Arthroplasty Reproduces Native Medial Collateral Ligament Strain
Reprinted from: *Medicina* **2022**, *58*, 1751, doi:10.3390/medicina58121751 181

Jin-Ho Cho, Jun Young Choi and Sung-Sahn Lee
Accuracy of the Tibial Component Alignment by Extramedullary System Using Simple Radiographic References in Total Knee Arthroplasty
Reprinted from: *Medicina* **2022**, *58*, 1212, doi:10.3390/medicina58091212 191

Yong Bum Joo, Young Mo Kim, Byung Kuk An, Cheol Won Lee, Soon Tae Kwon and Ju-Ho Song
Topical Tranexamic Acid Can Be Used Safely Even in High Risk Patients: Deep Vein Thrombosis Examination Using Routine Ultrasonography of 510 Patients
Reprinted from: *Medicina* **2022**, *58*, 1750, doi:10.3390/medicina58121750 201

Michele Coviello, Antonella Abate, Francesco Ippolito, Vittorio Nappi, Roberto Maddalena, Giuseppe Maccagnano, et al.
Continuous Cold Flow Device Following Total Knee Arthroplasty: Myths and Reality
Reprinted from: *Medicina* **2022**, *58*, 1537, doi:10.3390/medicina58111537 209

Myung-Ku Kim, Sang-Hyun Ko, Yoon-Cheol Nam, Yoon-Sang Jeon, Dae-Gyu Kwon and Dong-Jin Ryu
Optimal Release Timing of Drain Clamping to Reduce Postoperative Bleeding after Total Knee Arthroplasty with Intraarticular Injection of Tranexamic Acid
Reprinted from: *Medicina* **2022**, *58*, 1226, doi:10.3390/medicina58091226 221

Lorenzo Moretti, Michele Coviello, Federica Rosso, Giuseppe Calafiore, Edoardo Monaco, Massimo Berruto and Giuseppe Solarino
Current Trends in Knee Arthroplasty: Are Italian Surgeons Doing What Is Expected?
Reprinted from: *Medicina* **2022**, *58*, 1164, doi:10.3390/medicina58091164 229

O-Sung Lee, Myung Chul Lee, Chung Yeob Shin and Hyuk-Soo Han
Spacer Block Technique Was Superior to Intramedullary Guide Technique in Coronal Alignment of Femoral Component after Fixed-Bearing Medial Unicompartmental Knee Arthroplasty: A Case–Control Study
Reprinted from: *Medicina* **2023**, *59*, 89, doi:10.3390/medicina59010089 243

Ki Ho Kang, Man Soo Kim, Jae Jung Kim and Yong In
Risk Factors and Preventive Strategies for Perioperative Distal Femoral Fracture in Patients Undergoing Total Knee Arthroplasty
Reprinted from: *Medicina* **2023**, *59*, 369, doi:10.3390/medicina59020369 255

Man-Soo Kim, Jae-Jung Kim, Ki-Ho Kang, Jeong-Han Lee and Yong In
Detection of Prosthetic Loosening in Hip and Knee Arthroplasty Using Machine Learning: A Systematic Review and Meta-Analysis
Reprinted from: *Medicina* **2023**, *59*, 782, doi:10.3390/medicina59040782 265

About the Editors

Yong In

Yong In, MD, Ph.D., is a professor at the Orthopedic Surgery Department of the College of Medicine at the Catholic University of Korea, Seoul, Republic of Korea. He is currently a chief knee surgeon and the former president of the Orthopedic Surgery Department of Seoul St. Mary's Hospital, Seoul, Republic of Korea. He is a member of multiple national and international orthopedic societies including ISAKOS, AAHKS, the Korean Knee Society, and the Korean Orthopaedic Association and an editorial board member of the *Journal of Arthroplasty* and *Clinics in Orthopedic Surgery*. In addition, he is a member and trustee of multiple Korean societies related to orthopedics and stem cells. He has authored or co-authored numerous orthopedic journal articles and consulted multiple international knee arthroplasty companies.

In Jun Koh

In Jun Koh, MD, Ph.D., is currently the Director of the Joint Reconstruction Center and a chief surgeon in the Knee Surgery and Sports Medicine Division at Eunpyeong St. Mary's Hospital. In addition, he is currently a professor and teaches with the affiliated Orthopedic Surgery Department at the College of Medicine, Catholic University of Korea, Seoul, Republic of Korea. He is currently a member of multiple committees of the Korean Orthopaedic Association, the Korean Knee Society, and the Korean Arthroscopy Society. Moreover, he is a member of multiple advisory boards of national healthcare agencies and an editorial board member of *Clinics in Orthopedic Surgery*, *Knee Surgery & Related Research*, and *Medicina*. He is the author or co-author of more than 100 peer-reviewed, highly-ranked orthopedic journal articles and has received numerous awards.

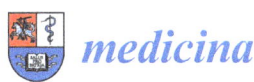

Systematic Review

Bone Marrow Aspirate Concentrate versus Human Umbilical Cord Blood-Derived Mesenchymal Stem Cells for Combined Cartilage Regeneration Procedure in Patients Undergoing High Tibial Osteotomy: A Systematic Review and Meta-Analysis

Dojoon Park [1], Youn Ho Choi [1], Se Hyun Kang [1], Hae Seok Koh [1] and Yong In [2,*]

[1] Department of Orthopedic Surgery, St. Vincent Hospital, College of Medicine, 93, Jungbu-daero, Paldal-gu, Suwon-si 16247, Republic of Korea
[2] Department of Orthopaedic Surgery, Seoul St. Mary's Hospital, College of Medicine, The Catholic University of Korea, 222, Banpo-daero, Seocho-gu, Seoul 06591, Republic of Korea
* Correspondence: iy1000@catholic.ac.kr

Abstract: *Background and objectives:* Cartilage regeneration using mesenchymal stem cells (MSCs) has been attempted to improve articular cartilage regeneration in varus knee osteoarthritis (OA) patients undergoing high tibial osteotomy (HTO). Bone marrow aspirate concentrate (BMAC) and human umbilical cord blood-derived MSCs (hUCB-MSCs) have been reported to be effective. However, whether BMAC is superior to hUCB-MSCs remains unclear. This systematic review and meta-analysis aimed to determine the clinical efficacy of cartilage repair procedures with BMAC or hUCB-MSCs in patients undergoing HTO. *Materials and Methods:* A systematic search was conducted using three global databases, PubMed, EMBASE, and the Cochrane Library, for studies in which the clinical outcomes after BMAC or hUCB-MSCs were used in patients undergoing HTO for varus knee OA. Data extraction, quality control, and meta-analysis were performed. To compare the clinical efficacy of BMAC and hUCB-MSCs, reported clinical outcome assessments and second-look arthroscopic findings were analyzed using standardized mean differences (SMDs) with 95% confidence intervals (CIs). *Results:* The present review included seven studies of 499 patients who received either BMAC (BMAC group, n = 169) or hUCB-MSCs (hUCB-MSC group, n = 330). Improved clinical outcomes were found in both BMAC and hUCB-MSC groups; however, a significant difference was not observed between procedures (International Knee Documentation Committee score; p = 0.91, Western Ontario and McMaster Universities OA Index; p = 0.05, Knee Society Score (KSS) Pain; p = 0.85, KSS Function; p = 0.37). On second-look arthroscopy, the hUCB-MSC group showed better International Cartilage Repair Society Cartilage Repair Assessment grade compared with the BMAC group (p < 0.001). *Conclusions:* Both BMAC and hUCB-MSCs with HTO improved clinical outcomes in varus knee OA patients, and there was no difference in clinical outcomes between them. However, hUCB-MSCs were more effective in articular cartilage regeneration than BMAC augmentation.

Keywords: high tibial osteotomy; bone marrow aspirate concentrate; human umbilical cord blood-derived mesenchymal stem cells; knee osteoarthritis

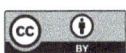

1. Introduction

High tibial osteotomy (HTO) is a reliable surgical method for physically active or young patients with medial compartment knee osteoarthritis (OA) with varus deformity [1–3]. The HTO procedure reduces the weight loading of the medial compartment through alteration of the weight-bearing axis, and healing of the damaged cartilage can be expected due to reduced stress [4,5]. Satisfactory clinical and radiological improvement after HTO at short-term and mid-term follow-up have been reported in several studies [6,7]; however, long-term follow-up data revealed a troubling trend of deteriorating outcomes in some patients, necessitating revision total knee arthroplasty (TKA) due to unsatisfactory results [8,9]. Therefore, a combination of additional cartilage regeneration procedures with HTO has been attempted to improve articular cartilage regeneration and surgical outcomes [10]. Among additional procedures, mesenchymal stem cell (MSC) enhancement is an emerging option for cartilage regeneration procedures for OA [11,12], and its effectiveness has been demonstrated in several clinical trials [13–15].

Bone marrow aspirate concentrate (BMAC) and human umbilical cord blood-derived mesenchymal stem cells (hUCB-MSCs) are representative stem cell-based orthobiologics [16]. BMAC augmentation relies on the inclusion of many growth factors and pluripotent stromal cells that induce MSC differentiation into chondrocytes, potentially leading to the production of native, hyaline-like cartilage [17,18]. hUCB-MSCs have low immunogenicity and can be collected using a noninvasive method. In addition, hUCB-MSCs have a good expansion capacity to provide sufficient cells for treatment [19,20].

The superior results of the combination of HTO and cartilage regeneration procedures compared with HTO alone have been reported in several studies [21,22]. Despite promising results regarding cartilage regeneration procedures using MSC-based orthobiologics, the optimal cartilage regeneration procedure that can be performed with HTO remains unclear. Direct comparison of the efficacy of BMAC or hUCB-MSCs combined with HTO has been conducted in few studies to date [23,24].

The purpose of this meta-analysis was to identify available studies on the clinical efficacy of HTO with cartilage regeneration procedure using BMAC or hUCB-MSCs in varus knee OA patients, and to compare the efficacy of the two procedures for clinical improvement and cartilage regeneration. To the best of our knowledge, this is the first meta-analysis in which this topic was investigated. We hypothesized equivalent clinical effects of BMAC and hUCB-MSCs with HTO in varus knee OA patients.

2. Materials and Methods

2.1. Meta-Analyses Principles

This analysis was conducted under the Preferred Reporting Items for Systematic Reviews and Meta-Analysis (PRISMA) principle [25]. Studies in which the clinical effects of BMAC and hUCB-MSCs in patients undergoing HTO for varus knee OA were systematically reviewed. Ethical approval was unnecessary because all analyses were conducted using existing literature.

2.2. Search Strategy

A systematic search was conducted by two reviewers using three global online databases (PubMed, EMBASE, and Cochrane Library) for studies published by 22 September 2022, in which clinical effects after the use of BMAC or hUCB-MSCs in patients undergoing HTO for varus knee OA were investigated. The publication language was restricted to English.

A search for relevant articles was conducted using various combinations of the following keywords: "osteoarthritis", "knee", "high tibial osteotomy", "bone marrow aspirate concentrate", and "umbilical cord blood-derived mesenchymal stem cells." Details of the search terms and strategy are presented in Supplemental Table S1.

A secondary manual search was performed on the related reviews and meta-analyses and their reference lists to retrieve relevant articles that were not identified using the databases.

2.3. Study Criteria and Screening Process

Two independent reviewers evaluated the eligibility of potentially relevant articles retrieved after removing duplicates based on the predefined criteria. The review was conducted on the title and abstract of the study and, in cases of uncertainty, was performed on the entire text. Discrepancies were discussed with a third reviewer.

The inclusion criteria were as follows: (1) studies using BMAC or hUCB-MSCs with HTO for treatment of varus knee OA, (2) studies investigating the clinical effects of BMAC or hUCB-MSCs with HTO on postoperative outcome, and (3) studies with a mean follow-up period >18 months. The exclusion criteria were as follows: (1) reviews, meta-analyses, case reports, and letters; (2) duplicates of previously published articles.

2.4. Data Extraction and Quality Control

Data extraction was performed using standardized protocols. The following variables of the included studies were collected: first author, publication year, study design, level of evidence, type of osteotomy, type of intervention, sex, age, body mass index (BMI), sample size, preoperative Kellgren–Lawrence grade [26], preoperative International Cartilage Repair Society (ICRS) grade [27], cartilage defect size, mean follow-up duration, preoperative hip-knee-ankle (HKA) angle, clinical assessment, postoperative ICRS-Cartilage Repair Assessment (CRA) grade [28], postoperative Koshino stage [29], a brief description of the preparation method of intervention, postoperative rehabilitation protocol, and reported adverse events.

Because the final eligible studies did not include randomized controlled trials, two independent reviewers evaluated the bias and risk of all eligible observational studies using the Methodological Item for Non-Randomized Studies (MINORS) [30], with 12 categories for comparative studies and 8 categories for noncomparative studies. Each category was rated 0 (not reported), 1 (reported but inadequate), or 2 (reported and adequate).

2.5. Statistical Analyses

Descriptive statistics including the mean and standard deviation for any numerical variable were recorded. Any missing standard deviation was estimated using pre-established methodologies [31]. The 95% confidence interval (CI) of the appropriate variable was reported. Heterogeneity was determined using the I^2 statistic; if $I^2 < 50\%$ (low heterogeneity), a fixed-effects model was used; otherwise, a random-effects model was used, and a funnel plot was used to assess the existence of publication bias (Supplemental Figure S1). A p-value < 0.05 was considered statistically significant.

Clinical outcome was evaluated using the mean International Knee Documentation Committee (IKDC) score [32], Western Ontario and McMaster Universities OA Index (WOMAC) score [33], and other clinical outcome measures performed before and after surgery. The quality of articular cartilage regeneration was determined using the ICRS-CRA on second-look arthroscopy. Clinical efficacy based on the type of treatment was estimated using the standardized mean difference (SMD) and was analyzed to compare the clinical effects between patients who received BMAC (BMAC group, $n = 169$) or hUCB-MSCs (hUCB-MSC group, $n = 330$). Statistical significance was set at $p < 0.05$. All statistical analyses were conducted using Review Manager software (version 5.3; The Nordic Cochrane Centre, Copenhagen, Denmark).

3. Results

3.1. Study Characteristics

Details of the search process, including literature identification and verification, are presented in Figure 1. A total of 33 potentially relevant studies were retrieved from 3 databases, of which 23 remained after 10 duplicate articles were removed. During the review process, the titles and abstracts of the studies were reviewed, and for three uncertain cases, the review was extended to include full texts for identification. One article was added after a related review article search. After comprehensive screening, 7 studies involving 499 patients were included in this systematic review.

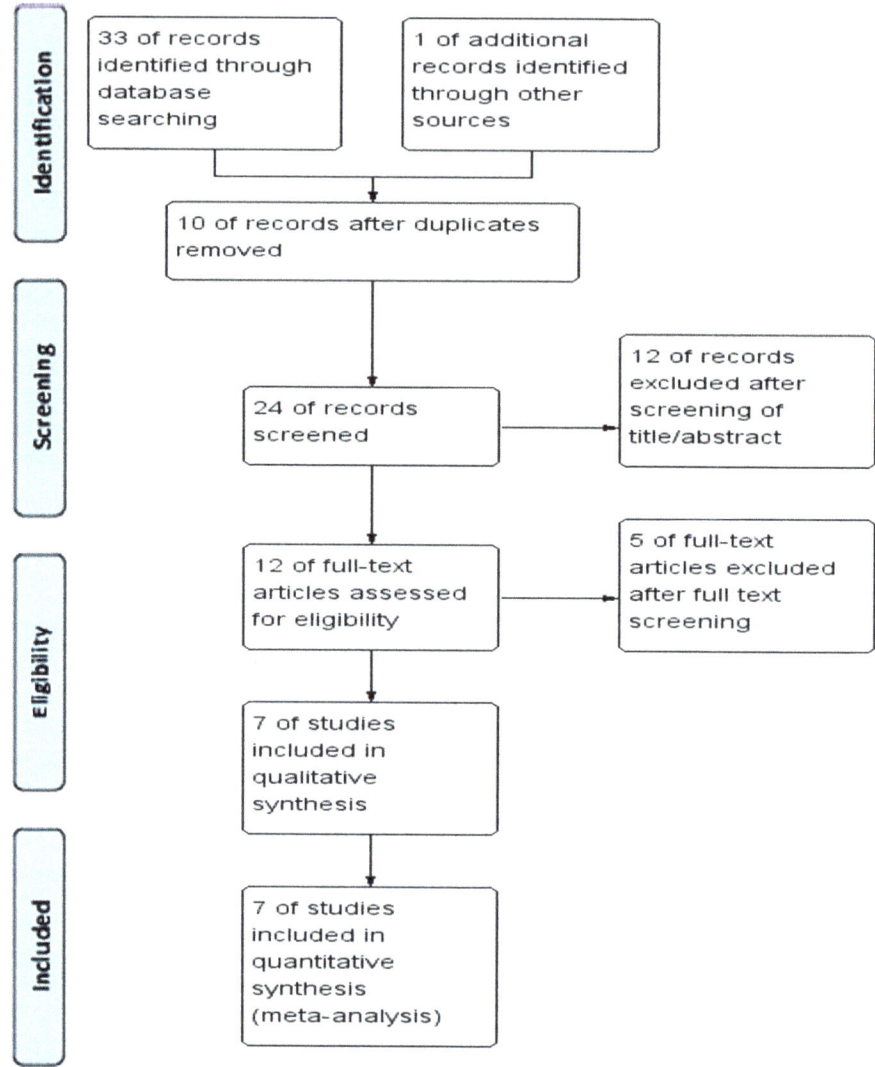

Figure 1. PRISMA flow diagram for the systematic review.

The outcomes of HTO with BMAC were reported in two studies, the outcomes of HTO with hUCB-MSCs were reported in three studies, and comparative outcomes between HTO with BMAC and HTO with hUCB-MSCs were reported in two studies. The baseline characteristics of the studies are summarized in Tables 1–3.

3.2. Methodological Quality

The level of evidence was 3 in three studies [23,24,34] (42.9%) and 4 in four studies [35–38] (57.1%). The mean MINORS score for comparative studies (three studies, maximum of 24 points) was 14.7 ± 2.4 (range 13–18), and noncomparative studies (four studies, maximum of 16 points) had a mean MINORS score of 9 ± 1.5 (range, 6–11; Supplemental Table S3).

Table 1. Characteristics of the included studies.

Study	Level of Evidence	Design	Type of Osteotomy	Intervention	Gender (M, F)	Age (Years)	BMI (kg/m^2)	Number of Patients in Intervention Group
Cavallo, 2018 [35]	IV	retrospective case series study	HTO (medial opening-wedge)	bone marrow-derived cells + PRF	BMAC (15, 9)	47.9 ± 12.3	Not reported	24
Song, 2020 [36]	IV	retrospective case series study	HTO	hUCB-MSC + multiple holes	hUCB-MSC (2, 23)	64.9 ± 4.4	24.9 ± 3.1	25
Song, 2020 [37]	IV	retrospective case series study	HTO (uniplanar osteotomy)	hUCB-MSC + multiple holes	hUCB-MSC (30, 95)	58.3 ± 6.8	25.6 ± 2.7	125
Jin, 2021 [34]	III	retrospective comparative study	HTO (biplanar opening wedge osteotomy)	BMAC + MFx vs. MFx	BMAC (11, 37)	56.9 ± 6.1	25.8 ± 3.1 (range, 18.1–33.2)	48
Chung, 2021 [38]	IV	retrospective case series study	HTO (biplanar opening wedge osteotomy)	hUCB-MSC + multiple drill holes	Not reported	56.6 (range, 43–65)	25.3 (range, 20.9–33.2)	93
Lee, 2021 [24]	III	retrospective comparative study	HTO (biplanar opening wedge osteotomy)	BMAC + MFx vs. hUCB-MSC + MFx	BMAC (6, 36); hUCB-MSC (6, 26)	BMAC, 60.7 ± 4.1; hUCB-MSC, 58.1 ± 3.6	BMAC, 26.1 ± 2.8; hUCB-MSC, 26.6 ± 3	BMAC (42), hUCB-MSC (32)
Yang, 2022 [23]	III	retrospective cohort study	HTO (biplanar opening wedge osteotomy)	BMAC + MFx vs. hUCB-MSC + MFx	BMAC (17, 38); hUCB-MSC (13, 42)	BMAC, 55.0 ± 7.3; hUCB-MSC, 56.4 ± 5.3	BMAC, 27.2 ± 3.9 hUCB-MSC, 26.8 ± 3.2	BMAC (55), hUCB-MSC (55)

BMI, body mass index; Pre-OP, preoperative; K-L, Kellgren–Lawrence; HTO, high tibial osteotomy; PRF, platelet-rich fibrin; hUCB-MSCs, human umbilical cord blood-derived mesenchymal stem cells; BMAC, bone marrow aspirate concentrate; MFx, microfracture.

Table 2. Preoperative status and outcomes of interventions of the included studies.

Study	Pre-OP K-L Grade	Pre-OP ICRS Grade	Defect Size (MFC, cm²)	Mean Follow-Up (Months)	HKA Angle (Pre-OP vs. Post-OP)	Clinical Assessment	Number of Patients Undergoing 2nd-Look Arthroscopy	Post-OP ICRS-CRA Grade	Post-OP Koshino Staging
Cavallo, 2018 [35]	IV or less	Not reported	Not reported	44.4 ± 17.7	Pre-OP, varus 1–15°; Post-OP, Not reported	IKDC, KOOS, VAS, Tegner	NA	Not reported	Not reported
Song, 2020 [36]	Not reported	Not reported	7.2 ± 1.9	26.7 ± 1.8	Pre-OP, ≥3°; Post-OP, Not reported	IKDC, VAS, WOMAC	14	I (6), II (8), III (0), IV (0)	Not reported
Song, 2020 [37]	III or less	IV (125)	6.9 ± 2.0	Not reported	Pre-OP, 7.6 ± 2.4; Post-OP, Not reported	IKDC, WOMAC, VAS	125	I (73), II (37), III (15), IV (0)	Not reported
Jin, 2021 [34]	III (36), IV (12)	III (41), IV (7)	2.3 ± 0.9	33.6 ± 6.6	7.5 ± 3.4 vs. −2.9 ± 2.5	IKDC, WOMAC, KSS-pain, KSS-function	33	I (1), II (18), III (11), IV (3)	A (2), B (15), C (16)
Chung, 2021 [38]	III	III or IV	6.5 (range, 2.0–12.8)	20.4 (range, 12–42)	Pre-OP, >3°; Post-OP, Not reported	IKDC, WOMAC, KSS-pain, KSS-function, HSS	49	I (4), II (34), III (11), IV (0)	A (0), B (12), C (37)
Lee, 2021 [24]	Not reported	BMAC, MFC 3.9 ± 0.3, MTC 3.9 ± 0.3; hUCB-MSC, MFC 3.9 ± 0.3, MTC 3.9 ± 0.3	BMAC, 6.5 ± 2.9; hUCB-MSC, 7 ± 1.9	BMAC, 20.7 ± 6.1; hUCB-MSC, 15.6 ± 2.8	BMAC, 8.6 ± 3.1 vs. −2.8 ± 3.2; hUCB-MSC, 7.4 ± 2.6 vs. −2.9 ± 1.6	HSS, WOMAC, KSS-pain, KSS-function	BMAC (42), hUCB-MSC (32)	BMAC (42), I (1), II (18), III (12), IV (11); hUCB-MSC (32), I (6), II (20), III (6), IV (0)	Not reported
Yang, 2022 [23]	III	BMAC (55), III (5), IV (50); hUCB-MSC (55), III (3), IV (52)	BMAC, 6.4 ± 3.1; hUCB-MSC, 6.2 ± 2.4	BMAC, 34.2 ± 8.4; hUCB-MSC, 31.0 ± 6.0	BMAC, 7.6 ± 2.9 vs. −1.5 ± 2.3; hUCB-MSC, 7.5 ± 2.7 vs. −1.6 ± 2.2	IKDC, KOOS, SF-36, Tegner	BMAC (37), hUCB-MSC (44)	BMAC (37), I (1), II (20), III (11), IV (5); hUCB-MSC (44), I (4), II (30), III (10), IV (0)	BMAC (37), A (4), B (12), C (21); hUCB-MSC (44), A (0), B (12), C (32)

Pre-OP, preoperative; K-L, Kellgren–Lawrence; hUCB-MSCs, human umbilical cord blood-derived mesenchymal stem cells; BMAC, bone marrow aspirate concentrate; MFC, medial femoral condyle; HKA, hip-knee-ankle; IKDC, International Knee Documentation Committee; KOOS, Knee injury and Osteoarthritis Outcome Score; VAS, Visual Analog Scale; WOMAC, Western Ontario and McMaster Universities Arthritis index; KSS, Knee Society Score; ICRS-CRA, International Cartilage Repair Society Cartilage Repair Assessment; SF-36, Short Form 36 Health Survey.

Table 3. Preoperative preservation, rehabilitation and complications of the included studies.

Study	Pre-OP BMAC or hUCB-MSC Preservation	Rehabilitation	Complication	Number of Patients in Control Group
Cavallo, 2018 [35]	60 mL of bone marrow from the posterior iliac crest, 15 min centrifugation cycles, a collagen scaffold	Partial weight-bearing was after six weeks; full weight-bearing at eight weeks after evaluation of bone consolidation	Knee swelling due to hemarthrosis in three cases; two cases of infrapatellar nerve injury; one case of delayed union of the osteotomy	NA
Song, 2020 [36]	hUCB-MSCs were used as a stem cell drug (CARTISTEM, MEDIPost-OP), mixed with sodium hyaluronate, therapeutic dosage 500 μL/cm² of the defect area with a cell concentration of 0.5×10^7 cells/mL	Non-weight-bearing for eight weeks, full weight-bearing after twelve weeks	Not reported	NA
Song, 2020 [37]	CARTISTEM® (MediPost-OP, Seongnam-si, Gyeonggi-do, Republic of Korea), 1.5 mL hUCB-MSCs (7.5×10^6 cells/vial) and 4% hyaluronic acid (HA) hydrogel, therapeutic dose 500 mL/cm²	Partial weight-bearing after four weeks; full weight-bearing at six weeks	Not reported	NA
Jin, 2021 [34]	contralateral anterior superior iliac spine, at least 40 mL of bone marrow, centrifuged for 4 min at 2500 rpm	Non-weight-bearing to partial weight-bearing after six weeks; full weight-bearing after twelve weeks considering bone healing	Not reported	MFx (43)
Chung, 2021 [38]	Cartistem, 1.5 mL of cord blood-derived MSCs (7.5×10^6) and 4% HA, 500 mL/cm² of defect with a cell concentration of 0.5×10^7 cells/mL.	Non-weight-bearing walking after six weeks; full weight-bearing after twelve weeks based on the level of bone healing	Some patients, knee swelling for up to one month	NA
Lee, 2021 [24]	BMAC, contralateral anterior superior iliac spine, at least 40 mL of bone marrow, centrifuge for 4 min at 2500 rpm; Cartistem, hUCB-MSCs-HA hydrogel composites	Non-weight-bearing to partial weight-bearing after six weeks; full weight-bearing after twelve weeks depending on the level of bone healing	Not reported	NA
Yang, 2022 [23]	BMAC, contralateral anterior superior iliac spine, at least 40 mL of bone marrow, centrifuged for 4 min at 2500 rpm; Cartistem, 1.5 mL of cord blood-derived MSCs (7.5×10^6) and 4% HA, 500 mL/cm2 of defect with a cell concentration of 0.5×10^7 cells/mL	Partial weight-bearing after six weeks; full weight-bearing after twelve weeks.	BMAC: one patient complained of postoperative stiffness	NA

Pre-OP, preoperative; HTO, hUCB-MSCs, human umbilical cord blood-derived mesenchymal stem cells; BMAC, bone marrow aspirate concentrate; HA, hyaluronic acid; NA, not applicable.

3.3. Meta-Analysis Results

The study population consisted of 499 patients treated with HTO and either BMAC (169 patients) or hUCB-MSCs (330 patients). The mean age of subjects was not significantly different between the BMAC and hUCB-MSC groups (57.7 ± 7.3 and 57.8 ± 5.4 years, respectively; $p = 0.86$). In all studies except one (6/7; 85.7%), preoperative BMI was reported. Based on the available data, the BMAC group had a higher BMI than the hUCB-MSC group (26.3 ± 3.4 vs. 25.9 ± 2.7 kg/m^2, $p = 0.02$).

3.3.1. Clinical Outcomes

- **IKDC**: In six [23,34–38] of the seven studies, the IKDC score used to evaluate the clinical effects of BMAC or hUCB-MSCs with HTO in patients with varus knee OA was reported. The IKDC subgroup consisted of 127 patients treated using BMAC, and 298 patients treated using hUCB-MSCs. Significant heterogeneity was found ($p < 0.001$, $I^2 = 94\%$), and the random effects model was used. Patients treated with BMAC had significantly improved IKDC scores (SMD, 4.13; 95% CI, 1.23–7.00), as did those in the hUCB-MSC group (SMD, 3.92; 95% CI, 3.65–4.20). However, based on IKDC score, the clinical effects of BMAC vs. hUCB-MSCs for combined cartilage regeneration in patients undergoing HTO were equivalent ($p = 0.91$; Figure 2).

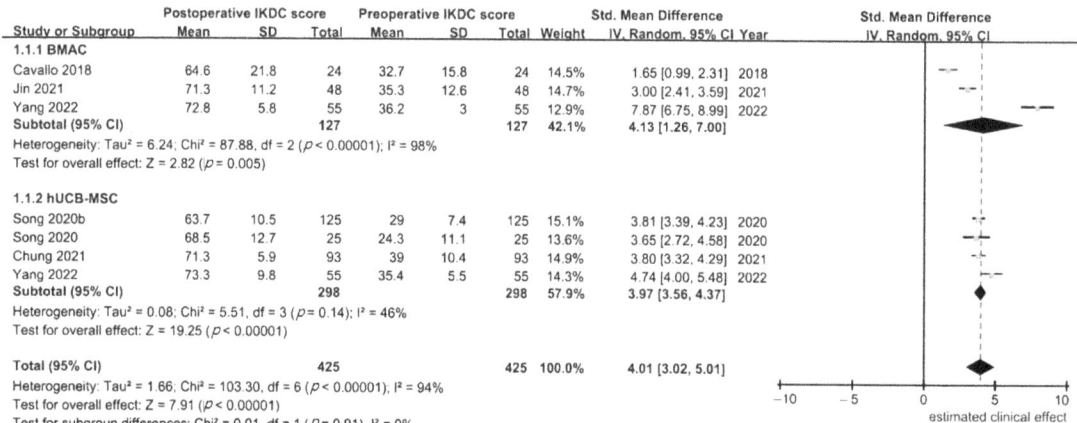

Figure 2. Estimated clinical effects of bone marrow aspirate concentrate (BMAC) and human umbilical cord blood-derived mesenchymal stem cells (hUCB-MSCs) in knee osteoarthritis (OA) patients treated with high tibial osteotomy (HTO) based on the International Knee Documentation Committee (IKDC) score [23,34–38].

- **WOMAC**: In 5 studies [24,34,36–38], the WOMAC score was reported, and 90 and 275 participants were included in the BMAC and hUCB-MSC groups, respectively. Since only one [38] of five studies reported WOMAC subscales, while the other four reported only a total WOMAC score, and only the total WOMAC score was compared. Significant heterogeneity was found ($p < 0.001$; $I^2 = 93\%$), and a random effects model was used. Based on the WOMAC index, both BMAC and hUCB-MSCs had a significant clinical effect compared with the preoperative status (SMD 2.09, 95% CI, 1.25–2.93 for BMAC and 3.39, 95% CI, 2.39–4.397 for hUCB-MSCs). However, the difference between groups did not reach statistical significance ($p = 0.05$; Figure 3).

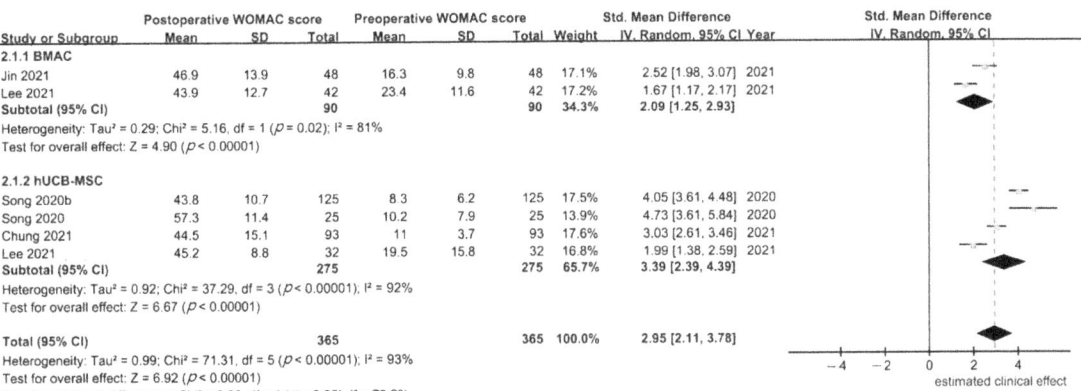

Figure 3. Estimated clinical effects of bone marrow aspirate concentrate (BMAC) and human umbilical cord blood-derived mesenchymal stem cells (hUCB-MSCs) in knee osteoarthritis (OA) patients treated with high tibial osteotomy (HTO) based on the Western Ontario and McMaster Universities OA Index (WOMAC) [24,34,36–38].

- **Other reported clinical outcomes**: Other reported outcomes were KSS score (three studies), VAS (three studies), KOOS (two studies), HSS (two studies), SF-36 (one study), and Tegner activity score (two studies). The mean preoperative and postoperative values for the outcome scales are shown in Table 4. KSS was the only measure used in more than one study to evaluate BMAC and hUCB-MSCs; it was used in three studies [24,34,38]. Mean KSS subscale (pain and function) values were reported in all studies; statistically significant heterogeneity was detected (KSS pain, $p = 0.01$, $I^2 = 73\%$; KSS function, $p < 0.001$, $I^2 = 84\%$). In a random effects model, patients treated with BMAC or hUCB-MSCs showed improved clinical outcome after surgery (KSS pain SMD, 1.51, 95% CI, 0.43–2.59 for BMAC and 1.40; 95% CI, 1.12–1.68 for hUCB-MSCs; KSS function SMD, 1.99, 95% CI, 0.63–3.34 for BMAC and 1.35; 95% CI, 1.08–1.63 for hUCB-MSCs). However, differences in KSS pain and function scores were not found between the two treatment groups ($p = 0.85$ and $p = 0.37$, respectively; Figure 4).

3.3.2. Second-Look Arthroscopic Findings

In six studies [23,24,34,36–38], second-look findings were reported, and four studies [23,24,34,37] compared preoperative ICRS grade with postoperative ICRS-CRA grade. Significant heterogeneity was found, and a random effects model was used. Greater improvement in articular cartilage regeneration was observed in patients treated with hUCB-MSCs (SMD, 4.18; 95% CI, 3.61–4.75) than in patients treated with BMAC (SMD, 1.81; 95% CI, 1.10–2.53; $p < 0.001$, Figure 5).

Table 4. Reported clinical outcome measures of the included studies.

Study	Reported Outcomes	IKDC	WOMAC	KSS-Pain	KSS-Function	KOOS	VAS	HSS	SF-36	Tegner
Cavallo, 2018 [35]	IKDC, KOOS, VAS, Tegner	BMAC, 32.7 ± 15.8 vs. 64.6 ± 21.8	-	-	-	BMAC, 30.46 ± 11.67 vs. 72.38 ± 20.1	BMAC, 7.50 ± 1.24 vs. 3.00 ± 2.08	-	-	BMAC, 1.21 ± 1.02 vs. 2.12 ± 1.39
Song, 2020 [36]	IKDC, VAS, WOMAC	hUCB-MSC, 24.3 ± 11.1 vs. 68.5 ± 12.7	hUCB-MSC, 57.3 ± 11.4 vs. 10.2 ± 7.9	-	-	-	hUCB-MSC, 76.4 ± 16.6 vs. 12.8 ± 11.7	-	-	-
Song, 2020 [37]	IKDC, WOMAC, VAS	hUCB-MSC, 29 ± 7.4 vs. 63.7 ± 10.5	hUCB-MSC, 43.8 ± 10.7 vs. 8.3 ± 6.2	-	-	-	hUCB-MSC, 7.6 ± 1.36 vs. 1.7 ± 1.4	-	-	-
Jin, 2021 [34]	IKDC, WOMAC, KSS-pain, KSS-function	BMAC, 35.3 ± 12.6 vs. 71.3 ± 11.2	BMAC, 46.9 ± 13.9 vs. 16.3 ± 9.8	BMAC, 27.2 ± 7.6 vs. 42.6 ± 7.2	BMAC, 58.9 ± 13.3 vs. 91.0 ± 10.2	-	-	-	-	-
Chung, 2021 [38]	IKDC, WOMAC, KSS-pain, KSS-function, HSS	hUCB-MSC, 39.0 ± 10.4 vs. 71.3 ± 5.9	hUCB-MSC, 44.5 ± 15.1 vs. 11.0 ± 3.7	hUCB-MSC, 29.8 ± 11.8 vs. 43.2 ± 5.0	hUCB-MSC, 61.0 ± 16.3 vs. 81.2 ± 13.7	-	-	hUCB-MSC, 61.6 ± 12.9 vs. 82.7 ± 13.5	-	-
Lee, 2021 [24]	HSS, WOMAC, KSS-pain, KSS-function	-	BMAC, 43.9 ± 12.7 vs. 23.4 ± 11.6; hUCB-MSC, 45.2 ± 8.8 vs. 19.5 ± 15.8	BMAC, 30.8 ± 11.0 vs. 40.6 ± 6.1; hUCB-MSC, 31.6 ± 10.4 vs. 42.8 ± 7.9	BMAC, 62.3 ± 11.9 vs. 80.1 ± 15.0; hUCB-MSC, 63.1 ± 11.2 vs. 82.4 ± 15.5	-	-	BMAC, 57.9 ± 12.9 vs. 79.2 ± 11.5; hUCB-MSC, 56.1 ± 10.6 vs. 84.6 ± 15.5	-	-
Yang, 2022 [23]	IKDC, KOOS, SF-36, Tegner	BMAC, 43.9 ± 12.7 vs. 23.4 ± 11.6; hUCB-MSC, 45.2 ± 8.8 vs. 19.5 ± 15.8	-	-	-	BMAC, 37.7 ± 2.7 vs. 78.2 ± 7.9; hUCB-MSC, 36.8 ± 7.1 vs. 78.4 ± 8.6	-	-	BMAC, 43.6 ± 10.4 vs. 64.0 ± 11.6; hUCB-MSC, 45.8 ± 12.3 vs. 64.5 ± 11.9	BMAC, 2.3 ± 0.9 vs. 4.0 ± 0.5; hUCB-MSC, 2.2 ± 0.8 vs. 4.1 ± 0.5

IKDC, International Knee Documentation Committee; KOOS, Knee injury and Osteoarthritis Outcome Score; VAS, Visual Analog Scale; WOMAC, Western Ontario and McMaster Universities Arthritis index; KSS, Knee Society Score; HSS, Hospital for Special Surgery; SF-36, Short Form 36 Health Survey.

(a)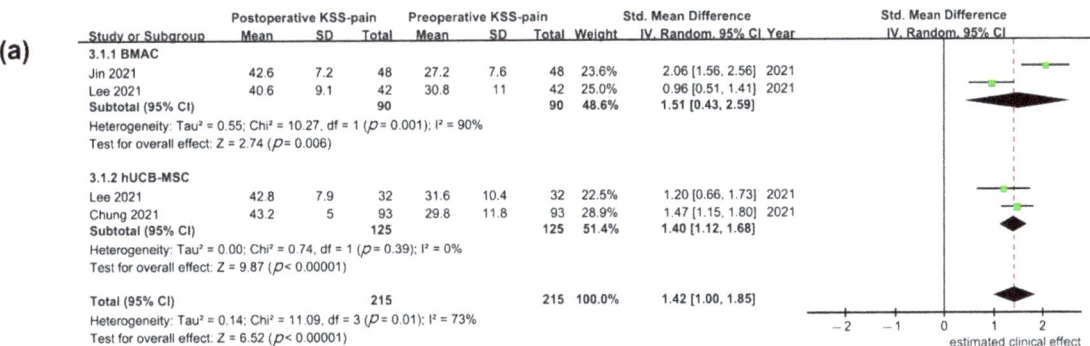

(b)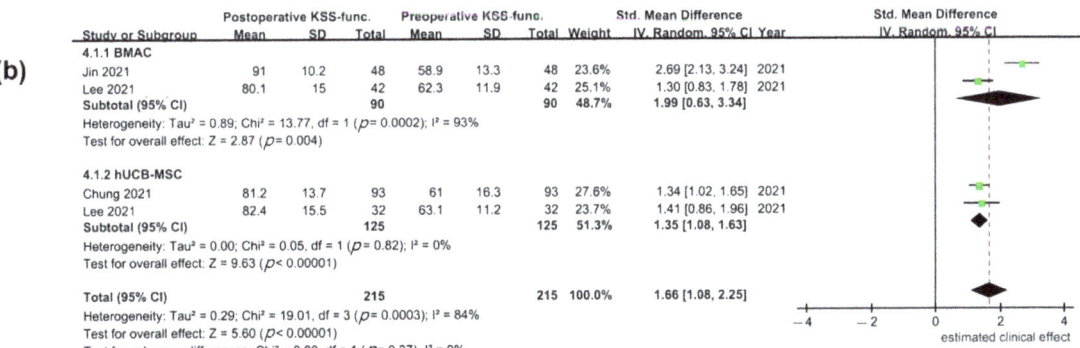

Figure 4. Estimated clinical effects of bone marrow aspirate concentrate (BMAC) and human umbilical cord blood-derived mesenchymal stem cells (hUCB-MSCs) in knee osteoarthritis (OA) patients treated with high tibial osteotomy (HTO) based on Knee Society Scores of (**a**) pain (KSS-pain) and (**b**) function (KSS-function) [24,34,38].

Figure 5. Estimated clinical effects of bone marrow aspirate concentrate (BMAC) and human umbilical cord blood-derived mesenchymal stem cells (hUCB-MSCs) in knee osteoarthritis (OA) patients treated with high tibial osteotomy (HTO) based on second-look arthroscopic articular cartilage status [23,24,34,37].

4. Discussion

The main finding of this study was that patients who underwent HTO for varus knee OA had improved clinical outcomes regardless of whether BMAC or hUCB-MSCs were used for cartilage regeneration. Postoperative clinical outcomes were significantly improved in both groups compared with preoperative baseline measurements, and both treatments provided reliable results in terms of functional score improvement and pain relief, without group differences. However, in comparison of second-look arthroscopic findings, hUCB-MSCs were more effective in articular cartilage regeneration than BMAC.

HTO provides a mechanical environment that can prevent the progression of degenerative changes by correcting the axis in which the weight is focused on the medial side of the knee of OA patients. Several studies have reported successful short- and medium-term outcomes after HTO [6,7]. However, with long-term follow-up, a trend for worsening outcomes was observed, with some patients requiring revision TKA due to poor outcomes [8,9]. It is unclear if deterioration of HTO results over time is associated with inappropriate cartilage regeneration of medial osteoarthritic cartilage [4,39].

Therefore, many attempts have been made to combine HTO with several types of cartilage regeneration procedures to improve long-term outcomes. Among such procedures, augmentation using MSCs that can differentiate into chondrocytes and produce extracellular matrix molecules important for cartilage regeneration is a promising option for managing cartilage defects [40]. Because the etiology of knee OA involves both biomechanical and biochemical changes in knee articular cartilage, combining HTO and MSC augmentation procedures appears promising.

MSCs concentrated after extraction from autologous bone marrow were introduced as a next-generation therapy for cartilage disease [34]. This procedure has the advantage of obtaining MSCs quickly and easily, and all processes from harvesting to transplantation can be performed in a single operation [41]. Considering the cell concentration, the most commonly used method for collecting BMAC is to collect aspirate from the iliac crest [42], but BMAC can also be collected from other sites, such as the proximal tibia [43]. Because only approximately 0.001% of MSCs of nucleated cells are obtained from aspirate, they are concentrated using density-gradient centrifugation to increase the number [44]. The concentrated BMAC is then injected directly into the affected joint or used in combination with other surgical procedures, such as proximal tibial osteotomy, to promote cartilage regeneration. Various growth factors included in BMAC induce cartilage regeneration and provide a favorable environment for MSC adhesion [45]. The immune control and anti-inflammatory effects of BMAC also help restore cartilage [40]. In patients receiving HTO, microfractures treated with BMAC were reported to have better arthroscopic findings regarding cartilage recovery than microfractures not treated with BMAC [34]; however, limitations exist. Because of the systems used in the field, including centrifuges, obtaining uniform cell numbers and concentrations is difficult. In addition, the amount of ideal BMAC required per unit defect size has not been established [46].

hUCB-MSCs are mesenchymal stem cells that are derived from human umbilical cord blood. Recently, hUCB-MSCs have been selected as a new treatment option for cartilage regeneration, and improved clinical results of knee OA with application of hUCB-MSCs have been reported in several studies [47,48]. These cells have been shown to have a high potential for cartilage regeneration, as well as anti-inflammatory and immunomodulatory properties [36,49]. hUCB-MSCs can be obtained from a donor, and they are typically expanded in culture before being injected directly into the affected joint or used in combination with other surgical procedures. hUCB-MSCs have several advantages over BMAC. First, hUCB-MSC showed higher proliferation rates and more than 1000-fold greater expansion capacity [49]. Second, because hUCB-MSCs are easy to obtain through cord blood banks, donor site morbidity is not a concern. However, the average additional cost of approximately $5300 or more compared with BMAC is a major obstacle to hUCB-MSC treatment.

The specific surgical method for using BMAC or hUCB-MSCs in combination with proximal tibial osteotomy will depend on the individual patient's condition and the surgeon's preferences. However, in general, these procedures involve the transplantation of stem cells with cartilage preparations such as microfracture before or after osteotomy [10].

Various treatment options that can be combined with HTO for cartilage regeneration have been reviewed; however, direct comparisons between BMAC and hUCB-MSCs are limited. To the best of our knowledge, this study is the first meta-analysis of the clinical outcome of HTO combined with BMAC or hUCB-MSCs. In the present study, both groups showed significantly improved postoperative clinical outcomes compared with preoperative baseline measurements. Basically, HTO results in clinical improvement because the joint reaction force is transferred to the lateral side of the knee via mechanical axis transfer, which is located lateral to the intercondylar eminence or at least to the center of the knee [50]. In a meta-analysis of seven studies to confirm the effectiveness of concurrent procedures during HTO [10], the combined cartilage regeneration procedure reportedly had a slightly beneficial effect on clinical outcome. However, in subgroup analysis of that meta-analysis, similar to the results obtained in the present study, the clinical results were significantly improved in the MSC subgroup. These positive synergistic effects are likely a result of the more effective cartilage regeneration potential and pain-reducing anti-inflammatory properties of MSCs due to paracrine effects. Magnetic resonance imaging (MRI) and histological examinations have been used to evaluate the improvement in cartilage status. MRI or histological examination was not used in any of the seven studies reviewed in the present systematic analysis. However, improvements in cartilage condition were observed in four studies [23,24,34,37,38] in which comparable preoperative and postoperative ICRS grades were reported, and hUCB-MSCs were significantly superior to BMAC in the meta-analysis performed.

The potential side effects associated with MSC-based treatments include local reactions, such as pain and swelling, as well as the potential for cells to differentiate into inappropriate cell types and the risk of tumor growth [51]. However, tumor growth is not a common side effect of MSC-based treatments [52]. Among the studies included in this analysis, swelling was the most common adverse event, and no adverse events met the criteria for being classified as serious according to the individual study protocols. However, the follow-up period in these studies was not sufficiently long to assess the risk of tumorigenicity.

The current review is the first systematic review and meta-analysis comparing the results of HTO combined with BMAC or hUCB-MSCs. However, the present review had several limitations. First, the studies included in the review were of a retrospective nature with levels of evidence of 3 or 4. Due to the absence of randomized controlled trials and prospective comparative studies, further studies with higher power are needed to control for possible confounding factors and to strengthen or refute current conclusions. However, due to the inherent strength of meta-analyses, an analysis including the single-arm study was conducted to provide useful information to clinicians. Second, sensitivity analysis confirmed high heterogeneity between studies, for which a random effects model was adopted when integrating the results. In addition, an independent analysis on various scoring scales used to evaluate clinical results was performed to accommodate the diversity of outcome variables. Third, the follow-up period of the reviewed studies was not sufficiently long to evaluate long-term clinical outcomes and survival rates. The follow-up period is an important factor in evaluating the stability of orthobiologics, so the results of this study should be interpreted carefully. In addition, the healing and maturation processes of articular cartilage may vary depending on the timing of second-look arthroscopy, resulting in potential bias. Finally, the absence of a control group that underwent HTO alone may bias the interpretation of the results.

In future studies, it is recommended to consider standardized outcome measures for assessing clinical improvement, as well as imaging techniques such as MRI or histological examination to evaluate the quality and quantity of cartilage regeneration.

5. Conclusions

Clinical outcomes were improved for both BMAC and hUCB-MSCs combined with HTO in varus knee OA patients, and postoperative outcomes did not differ between the two groups. However, hUCB-MSCs showed better articular cartilage regeneration in ICRS-CRA grade compared with BMAC. Further verification of the results requires larger, well-designed randomized controlled trials that include assessments of long-term follow-up.

Supplementary Materials: The following supporting information can be downloaded at https://www.mdpi.com/article/10.3390/medicina59030634/s1, Supplemental Table S1: Keywords and search details; Supplemental Figure S1: Funnel plot of comparison: BMAC and hUCB-MSC, outcome: IKDC score; Supplemental Table S2: Risk-of-bias assessment performed using the MINORS score.

Author Contributions: Conceptualization, Y.I. and D.P.; methodology, Y.I., D.P. and Y.H.C.; software, D.P.; validation, Y.I., D.P., Y.H.C. and H.S.K.; formal analysis, Y.I., D.P., Y.H.C., S.H.K. and H.S.K.; investigation, Y.I., D.P. and H.S.K.; resources, Y.I., D.P. and H.S.K.; data curation, D.P., Y.H.C., S.H.K. and H.S.K.; writing—original draft, D.P.; writing—review and editing, Y.I.; visualization, Y.I. and D.P.; supervision, Y.I.; project administration, Y.I. All authors have read and agreed to the published version of the manuscript.

Funding: This research received no external funding.

Institutional Review Board Statement: Ethical review and approval were waived for this study due to the nature of the systematic review article.

Informed Consent Statement: Patient consent was waived due to the nature of the systematic review article.

Data Availability Statement: The data published in this research are available on request from the first author (D.P.).

Conflicts of Interest: The authors declare no conflict of interest.

References

1. Biant, L.C.; McNicholas, M.J.; Sprowson, A.P.; Spalding, T. The surgical management of symptomatic articular cartilage defects of the knee: Consensus statements from United Kingdom knee surgeons. *Knee* **2015**, *22*, 446–449. [CrossRef] [PubMed]
2. Akizuki, S.; Shibakawa, A.; Takizawa, T.; Yamazaki, I.; Horiuchi, H. The long-term outcome of high tibial osteotomy: A ten- to 20-year follow-up. *J. Bone Joint. Surg. Br.* **2008**, *90*, 592–596. [CrossRef] [PubMed]
3. Amendola, A.; Bonasia, D.E. Results of high tibial osteotomy: Review of the literature. *Int. Orthop.* **2010**, *34*, 155–160. [CrossRef] [PubMed]
4. Matsunaga, D.; Akizuki, S.; Takizawa, T.; Yamazaki, I.; Kuraishi, J. Repair of articular cartilage and clinical outcome after osteotomy with microfracture or abrasion arthroplasty for medial gonarthrosis. *Knee* **2007**, *14*, 465–471. [CrossRef] [PubMed]
5. Kanamiya, T.; Naito, M.; Hara, M.; Yoshimura, I. The influences of biomechanical factors on cartilage regeneration after high tibial osteotomy for knees with medial compartment osteoarthritis: Clinical and arthroscopic observations. *Arthroscopy* **2002**, *18*, 725–729. [CrossRef] [PubMed]
6. Niemeyer, P.; Stöhr, A.; Köhne, M.; Hochrein, A. Medial opening wedge high tibial osteotomy. *Oper. Orthop. Traumatol.* **2017**, *29*, 294–305. [CrossRef] [PubMed]
7. Jung, W.-H.; Takeuchi, R.; Chun, C.-W.; Lee, J.-S.; Ha, J.-H.; Kim, J.-H.; Jeong, J.-H. Second-look arthroscopic assessment of cartilage regeneration after medial opening-wedge high tibial osteotomy. *Arthroscopy* **2014**, *30*, 72–79. [CrossRef] [PubMed]
8. Hui, C.; Salmon, L.J.; Kok, A.; Williams, H.A.; Hockers, N.; van der Tempel, W.M.; Chana, R.; Pinczewski, L.A. Long-term survival of high tibial osteotomy for medial compartment osteoarthritis of the knee. *Am. J. Sports Med.* **2011**, *39*, 64–70. [CrossRef]
9. Wu, L.-D.; Hahne, H.J.; Hassenpflug, T. A long-term follow-up study of high tibial osteotomy for medial compartment osteoarthrosis. *Chin. J. Traumatol.* **2004**, *7*, 348–353.
10. Lee, O.-S.; Ahn, S.; Ahn, J.H.; Teo, S.H.; Lee, Y.S. Effectiveness of concurrent procedures during high tibial osteotomy for medial compartment osteoarthritis: A systematic review and meta-analysis. *Arch. Orthop. Trauma Surg.* **2018**, *138*, 227–236. [CrossRef]
11. Ha, C.-W.; Park, Y.-B.; Kim, S.H.; Lee, H.-J. Intra-articular Mesenchymal Stem Cells in Osteoarthritis of the Knee: A Systematic Review of Clinical Outcomes and Evidence of Cartilage Repair. *Arthroscopy* **2019**, *35*, 277–288.e2. [CrossRef] [PubMed]
12. Kim, S.H.; Djaja, Y.P.; Park, Y.-B.; Park, J.-G.; Ko, Y.-B.; Ha, C.-W. Intra-articular Injection of Culture-Expanded Mesenchymal Stem Cells Without Adjuvant Surgery in Knee Osteoarthritis: A Systematic Review and Meta-analysis. *Am. J. Sports Med.* **2020**, *48*, 2839–2849. [CrossRef] [PubMed]

13. Kim, Y.S.; Koh, Y.G. Comparative Matched-Pair Analysis of Open-Wedge High Tibial Osteotomy With Versus Without an Injection of Adipose-Derived Mesenchymal Stem Cells for Varus Knee Osteoarthritis: Clinical and Second-Look Arthroscopic Results. *Am. J. Sports Med.* **2018**, *46*, 2669–2677. [CrossRef] [PubMed]
14. Koh, Y.-G.; Kwon, O.-R.; Kim, Y.-S.; Choi, Y.-J. Comparative outcomes of open-wedge high tibial osteotomy with platelet-rich plasma alone or in combination with mesenchymal stem cell treatment: A prospective study. *Arthroscopy* **2014**, *30*, 1453–1460. [CrossRef] [PubMed]
15. Wong, K.L.; Lee, K.B.; Tai, B.C.; Law, P.; Lee, E.H.; Hui, J.H. Injectable cultured bone marrow-derived mesenchymal stem cells in varus knees with cartilage defects undergoing high tibial osteotomy: A prospective, randomized controlled clinical trial with 2 years' follow-up. *Arthroscopy* **2013**, *29*, 2020–2028. [CrossRef]
16. Park, Y.-B.; Ha, C.-W.; Rhim, J.H.; Lee, H.-J. Stem Cell Therapy for Articular Cartilage Repair: Review of the Entity of Cell Populations Used and the Result of the Clinical Application of Each Entity. *Am. J. Sports Med.* **2018**, *46*, 2540–2552. [CrossRef]
17. Scharstuhl, A.; Schewe, B.; Benz, K.; Gaissmaier, C.; Bühring, H.-J.; Stoop, R. Chondrogenic potential of human adult mesenchymal stem cells is independent of age or osteoarthritis etiology. *Stem Cells* **2007**, *25*, 3244–3251. [CrossRef]
18. Ando, W.; Tateishi, K.; Katakai, D.; Hart, D.A.; Higuchi, C.; Nakata, K.; Hashimoto, J.; Fujie, H.; Shino, K.; Yoshikawa, H.; et al. In vitro generation of a scaffold-free tissue-engineered construct (TEC) derived from human synovial mesenchymal stem cells: Biological and mechanical properties and further chondrogenic potential. *Tissue Eng. Part A* **2008**, *14*, 2041–2049. [CrossRef]
19. Kern, S.; Eichler, H.; Stoeve, J.; Klüter, H.; Bieback, K. Comparative analysis of mesenchymal stem cells from bone marrow, umbilical cord blood, or adipose tissue. *Stem Cells* **2006**, *24*, 1294–1301. [CrossRef]
20. Flynn, A.; Barry, F.; O'Brien, T. UC blood-derived mesenchymal stromal cells: An overview. *Cytotherapy* **2007**, *9*, 717–726. [CrossRef]
21. Kahlenberg, C.A.; Nwachukwu, B.U.; Hamid, K.S.; Steinhaus, M.E.; Williams, R.J., 3rd. Analysis of Outcomes for High Tibial Osteotomies Performed With Cartilage Restoration Techniques. *Arthroscopy* **2017**, *33*, 486–492. [CrossRef] [PubMed]
22. Wen, H.-J.; Yuan, L.-B.; Tan, H.-B.; Xu, Y.-Q. Microfracture versus Enhanced Microfracture Techniques in Knee Cartilage Restoration: A Systematic Review and Meta-Analysis. *J. Knee Surg.* **2022**, *35*, 707–717. [CrossRef] [PubMed]
23. Yang, H.-Y.; Song, E.-K.; Kang, S.-J.; Kwak, W.-K.; Kang, J.-K.; Seon, J.-K. Allogenic umbilical cord blood-derived mesenchymal stromal cell implantation was superior to bone marrow aspirate concentrate augmentation for cartilage regeneration despite similar clinical outcomes. *Knee Surg. Sports Traumatol. Arthrosc.* **2022**, *30*, 208–218. [CrossRef] [PubMed]
24. Lee, N.-H.; Na, S.-M.; Ahn, H.-W.; Kang, J.-K.; Seon, J.-K.; Song, E.-K. Allogenic Human Umbilical Cord Blood-Derived Mesenchymal Stem Cells Are More Effective Than Bone Marrow Aspiration Concentrate for Cartilage Regeneration After High Tibial Osteotomy in Medial Unicompartmental Osteoarthritis of Knee. *Arthroscopy* **2021**, *37*, 2521–2530. [CrossRef]
25. Moher, D.; Liberati, A.; Tetzlaff, J.; Altman, D.G. Preferred reporting items for systematic reviews and meta-analyses: The PRISMA statement. *PLoS Med.* **2009**, *6*, e1000097. [CrossRef] [PubMed]
26. Kohn, M.D.; Sassoon, A.A.; Fernando, N.D. Classifications in Brief: Kellgren-Lawrence Classification of Osteoarthritis. *Clin. Orthop. Relat. Res.* **2016**, *474*, 1886–1893. [CrossRef] [PubMed]
27. van den Borne, M.P.; Raijmakers, N.J.; Vanlauwe, J.; Victor, J.; de Jong, S.N.; Bellemans, J.; Saris, D.B. International Cartilage Repair Society (ICRS) and Oswestry macroscopic cartilage evaluation scores validated for use in Autologous Chondrocyte Implantation (ACI) and microfracture. *Osteoarthr. Cartil.* **2007**, *15*, 1397–1402. [CrossRef]
28. Sumida, Y.; Nakamura, K.; Feil, S.; Siebold, M.; Kirsch, J.; Siebold, R. Good healing potential of patellar chondral defects after all-arthroscopic autologous chondrocyte implantation with spheroids: A second-look arthroscopic assessment. *Knee Surg. Sports Traumatol. Arthrosc.* **2022**, *30*, 1535–1542. [CrossRef] [PubMed]
29. Koshino, T.; Wada, S.; Ara, Y.; Saito, T. Regeneration of degenerated articular cartilage after high tibial valgus osteotomy for medial compartmental osteoarthritis of the knee. *Knee* **2003**, *10*, 229–236. [CrossRef]
30. Slim, K.; Nini, E.; Forestier, D.; Kwiatkowski, F.; Panis, Y.; Chipponi, J. Methodological index for non-randomized studies (minors): Development and validation of a new instrument. *ANZ J. Surg.* **2003**, *73*, 712–716. [CrossRef]
31. Weir, C.J.; Butcher, I.; Assi, V.; Lewis, S.C.; Murray, G.D.; Langhorne, P.; Brady, M.C. Dealing with missing standard deviation and mean values in meta-analysis of continuous outcomes: A systematic review. *BMC Med. Res. Methodol.* **2018**, *18*, 25. [CrossRef]
32. Higgins, L.D.; Taylor, M.K.; Park, D.; Ghodadra, N.; Marchant, M.; Pietrobon, R.; Cook, C. Reliability and validity of the International Knee Documentation Committee (IKDC) Subjective Knee Form. *Jt. Bone Spine* **2007**, *74*, 594–599. [CrossRef] [PubMed]
33. Thumboo, J.; Chew, L.H.; Soh, C.H. Validation of the Western Ontario and Mcmaster University osteoarthritis index in Asians with osteoarthritis in Singapore. *Osteoarthr. Cartil.* **2001**, *9*, 440–446. [CrossRef] [PubMed]
34. Jin, Q.-H.; Chung, Y.-W.; Na, S.-M.; Ahn, H.-W.; Jung, D.-M.; Seon, J.-K. Bone marrow aspirate concentration provided better results in cartilage regeneration to microfracture in knee of osteoarthritic patients. *Knee Surg. Sports Traumatol. Arthrosc.* **2021**, *29*, 1090–1097. [CrossRef] [PubMed]
35. Cavallo, M.; Sayyed-Hosseinian, S.-H.; Parma, A.; Buda, R.; Mosca, M.; Giannini, S. Combination of High Tibial Osteotomy and Autologous Bone Marrow Derived Cell Implantation in Early Osteoarthritis of Knee: A Preliminary Study. *Arch. Bone Jt. Surg.* **2018**, *6*, 112–118. [PubMed]
36. Song, J.-S.; Hong, K.-T.; Kim, N.-M.; Park, H.-S.; Choi, N.-H. Human umbilical cord blood-derived mesenchymal stem cell implantation for osteoarthritis of the knee. *Arch. Orthop. Trauma Surg.* **2020**, *140*, 503–509. [CrossRef] [PubMed]

37. Song, J.-S.; Hong, K.-T.; Kong, C.-G.; Kim, N.-M.; Jung, J.-Y.; Park, H.-S.; Kim, Y.J.; Chang, K.B.; Kim, S.J. High tibial osteotomy with human umbilical cord blood-derived mesenchymal stem cells implantation for knee cartilage regeneration. *World J. Stem Cells* **2020**, *12*, 514–526. [CrossRef]
38. Chung, Y.-W.; Yang, H.-Y.; Kang, S.-J.; Song, E.-K.; Seon, J.-K. Allogeneic umbilical cord blood-derived mesenchymal stem cells combined with high tibial osteotomy: A retrospective study on safety and early results. *Int. Orthop.* **2021**, *45*, 481–488. [CrossRef]
39. Sterett, W.I.; Steadman, J.R.; Huang, M.J.; Matheny, L.M.; Briggs, K.K. Chondral resurfacing and high tibial osteotomy in the varus knee: Survivorship analysis. *Am. J. Sports Med.* **2010**, *38*, 1420–1424. [CrossRef]
40. Betzler, B.K.; Chew, A.H.B.M.R.; Razak, H.R.B.A. Intra-articular injection of orthobiologics in patients undergoing high tibial osteotomy for knee osteoarthritis is safe and effective—A systematic review. *J. Exp. Orthop.* **2021**, *8*, 83. [CrossRef]
41. Turner, L.G. Federal Regulatory Oversight of US Clinics Marketing Adipose-Derived Autologous Stem Cell Interventions: Insights From 3 New FDA Draft Guidance Documents. *Mayo Clin. Proc.* **2015**, *90*, 567–571. [CrossRef] [PubMed]
42. Jäger, M.; Hernigou, P.; Zilkens, C.; Herten, M.; Li, X.; Fischer, J.; Krauspe, R. Cell therapy in bone healing disorders. *Orthop. Rev.* **2010**, *2*, e20.
43. Cavallo, C.; Boffa, A.; de Girolamo, L.; Merli, G.; Kon, E.; Cattini, L.; Santo, E.; Grigolo, B.; Filardo, G. Bone marrow aspirate concentrate quality is affected by age and harvest site. *Knee Surg. Sports Traumatol. Arthrosc.* **2022**. [CrossRef] [PubMed]
44. Chahla, J.; Mannava, S.; Cinque, M.E.; Geeslin, A.G.; Codina, D.; LaPrade, R.F. Bone Marrow Aspirate Concentrate Harvesting and Processing Technique. *Arthrosc. Tech.* **2017**, *6*, e441–e445. [CrossRef] [PubMed]
45. Steinert, A.F.; Rackwitz, L.; Gilbert, F.; Nöth, U.; Tuan, R.S. Concise review: The clinical application of mesenchymal stem cells for musculoskeletal regeneration: Current status and perspectives. *Stem. Cells Transl. Med.* **2012**, *1*, 237–247. [CrossRef]
46. Madry, H.; Gao, L.; Eichler, H.; Orth, P.; Cucchiarini, M. Bone Marrow Aspirate Concentrate-Enhanced Marrow Stimulation of Chondral Defects. *Stem Cells Int.* **2017**, *2017*, 1609685. [CrossRef] [PubMed]
47. Park, Y.-B.; Ha, C.-W.; Lee, C.-H.; Yoon, Y.C.; Park, Y. Cartilage Regeneration in Osteoarthritic Patients by a Composite of Allogeneic Umbilical Cord Blood-Derived Mesenchymal Stem Cells and Hyaluronate Hydrogel: Results from a Clinical Trial for Safety and Proof-of-Concept with 7 Years of Extended Follow-Up. *Stem Cells Transl. Med.* **2017**, *6*, 613–621. [CrossRef] [PubMed]
48. Song, J.-S.; Hong, K.-T.; Kim, N.-M.; Jung, J.-Y.; Park, H.-S.; Lee, S.H.; Cho, Y.J.; Kim, S.J. Implantation of allogenic umbilical cord blood-derived mesenchymal stem cells improves knee osteoarthritis outcomes: Two-year follow-up. *Regen. Ther.* **2020**, *14*, 32–39. [CrossRef]
49. Yang, S.-E.; Ha, C.-W.; Jung, M.; Jin, H.-J.; Lee, M.; Song, H.; Choi, S.; Oh, W.; Yang, Y.-S. Mesenchymal stem/progenitor cells developed in cultures from UC blood. *Cytotherapy* **2004**, *6*, 476–486. [CrossRef]
50. Agneskirchner, J.D.; Hurschler, C.; Wrann, C.D.; Lobenhoffer, P. The effects of valgus medial opening wedge high tibial osteotomy on articular cartilage pressure of the knee: A biomechanical study. *Arthroscopy* **2007**, *23*, 852–861. [CrossRef]
51. Bagno, L.; Hatzistergos, K.E.; Balkan, W.; Hare, J.M. Mesenchymal Stem Cell-Based Therapy for Cardiovascular Disease: Progress and Challenges. *Mol. Ther.* **2018**, *26*, 1610–1623. [CrossRef] [PubMed]
52. Galipeau, J.; Sensébé, L. Mesenchymal Stromal Cells: Clinical Challenges and Therapeutic Opportunities. *Cell Stem Cell* **2018**, *22*, 824–833. [CrossRef] [PubMed]

Disclaimer/Publisher's Note: The statements, opinions and data contained in all publications are solely those of the individual author(s) and contributor(s) and not of MDPI and/or the editor(s). MDPI and/or the editor(s) disclaim responsibility for any injury to people or property resulting from any ideas, methods, instructions or products referred to in the content.

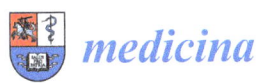

Systematic Review

Cartilage Regeneration Using Human Umbilical Cord Blood Derived Mesenchymal Stem Cells: A Systematic Review and Meta-Analysis

Dong Hwan Lee [1], Seon Ae Kim [2], Jun-Seob Song [3], Asode Ananthram Shetty [4], Bo-Hyoung Kim [1] and Seok Jung Kim [2,*]

1. Department of Orthopedic Surgery, Yeouido St. Mary's Hospital, College of Medicine, The Catholic University of Korea, 10, 63-ro, Seoul 07345, Republic of Korea
2. Department of Orthopaedic Surgery, Uijeongbu St. Mary's Hospital, College of Medicine, The Catholic University of Korea, 271, Cheonbo-Ro, Uijeongbu-si 11765, Republic of Korea
3. Department of Orthopaedic Surgery, Gangnam JS Hospital, Seoul 06259, Republic of Korea
4. Institute of Medical Sciences, Faculty of Health and Wellbeing, Chatham Maritime, Canterbury Christ Church University, Kent ME4 4UF, UK
* Correspondence: peter@catholic.ac.kr; Tel.: +82-31-820-3654; Fax: +82-31-847-3671

Citation: Lee, D.H.; Kim, S.A.; Song, J.-S.; Shetty, A.A.; Kim, B.-H.; Kim, S.J. Cartilage Regeneration Using Human Umbilical Cord Blood Derived Mesenchymal Stem Cells: A Systematic Review and Meta-Analysis. *Medicina* 2022, 58, 1801. https://doi.org/10.3390/medicina58121801

Academic Editor: Yong In

Received: 29 October 2022
Accepted: 5 December 2022
Published: 6 December 2022

Publisher's Note: MDPI stays neutral with regard to jurisdictional claims in published maps and institutional affiliations.

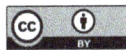

Copyright: © 2022 by the authors. Licensee MDPI, Basel, Switzerland. This article is an open access article distributed under the terms and conditions of the Creative Commons Attribution (CC BY) license (https://creativecommons.org/licenses/by/4.0/).

Abstract: *Background and Objectives:* Human umbilical-cord-blood-derived mesenchymal stem cells (hUCB-MSCs) have recently been used in clinical cartilage regeneration procedures with the expectation of improved regeneration capacity. However, the number of studies using hUCB-MSCs is still insufficient, and long-term follow-up results after use are insufficient, indicating the need for additional data and research. We have attempted to prove the efficacy and safety of hUCB-MSC treatment in a comprehensive analysis by including all subjects with knee articular cartilage defect or osteoarthritis who have undergone cartilage repair surgery using hUCB-MSCs. We conducted a meta-analysis and demonstrated efficacy and safety based on a systematic review. *Materials and Methods:* This systematic review was conducted following the Preferred Reporting Items for Systematic Reviews and Meta-Analysis (PRISMA) guidelines. For this study, we searched the PubMed, Embase, Web of Science, Scopus, and Cochrane Library literature databases up to June 2022. A total of seven studies were included, and quality assessment was performed for each included study using the Newcastle–Ottawa Quality Assessment Scale. Statistical analysis was performed on the extracted pooled clinical outcome data, and subgroup analyses were completed. *Results:* A total of 570 patients were included in the analysis. In pooled analysis, the final follow-up International Knee Documentation Committee (IKDC) score showed a significant increase (mean difference (MD), −32.82; 95% confidence interval (CI), −38.32 to −27.32; $p < 0.00001$) with significant heterogeneity ($I^2 = 93\%$, $p < 0.00001$) compared to the preoperative score. The Western Ontario and McMaster Universities Osteoarthritis Index (WOMAC) scores at final follow-up were significantly decreased (MD, 30.73; 95% CI, 24.10–37.36; $p < 0.00001$) compared to the preoperative scores, with significant heterogeneity ($I^2 = 95\%$, $p < 0.00001$). The visual analog scale (VAS) score at final follow-up was significantly decreased (MD, 4.81; 95% CI, 3.17–6.46; $p < 0.00001$) compared to the preoperative score, with significant heterogeneity ($I^2 = 98\%$, $p < 0.00001$). Two studies evaluated the modified Magnetic Resonance Observation of Cartilage Repair Tissue (M-MOCART) score and confirmed sufficient improvement. In a study analyzing a group treated with bone marrow aspiration concentrate (BMAC), there was no significant difference in clinical outcome or M-MOCART score, and the post-treatment International Cartilage Repair Society (ICRS) grade increased. *Conclusion:* This analysis demonstrated the safety, efficacy, and quality of repaired cartilage following hUCB-MSC therapy. However, there was no clear difference in the comparison with BMAC. In the future, comparative studies with other stem cell therapies or cartilage repair procedures should be published to support the superior effect of hUCB-MSC therapy to improve treatment of cartilage defect or osteoarthritis.

Keywords: human umbilical cord blood derived mesenchymal stem cells; cartilage regeneration; cartilage repair; osteoarthritis treatment; stem cell therapy

1. Introduction

Osteoarthritis is one of the main diseases of the modern aging population, and available methods for its treatment are gradually expanding with the development of arthroplasty, oral medications, and physiotherapy [1]. Recently, with improvements in quality of life, the target and favored treatment methods of osteoarthritis have changed. Patient needs for early diagnosis and treatment of osteoarthritis are gradually increasing, and many studies are being conducted on joint-preserving surgery. With the introduction of magnetic resonance imaging (MRI), it became possible to evaluate the condition of articular cartilage more precisely before surgery [2], and treatments for articular cartilage defects have advanced. However, due to the limited regenerative capacity of cartilage, no treatment method has achieved a dramatic effect. As cartilage regeneration through microfracture surgery is regenerated by fibrocartilage, its limitations are already well known [3,4]. Accordingly, various methods such as autologous matrix-induced chondrogenesis, autologous chondrocyte implantation, and osteochondral autograft transfer system surgery have been tested for hyaline-like cartilage regeneration [5]. However, problems such as donor site morbidity and the need for multiple operations remain, and problems also persist postoperatively in the long term due to limited cartilage regeneration [6]. In addition to surgical treatment, studies using small-molecule drugs to enhance cell regeneration are also active, which are used not only in cartilage but also in various tissues [7,8].

Basic and clinical research efforts on various types of stem cell therapy are now active. Mesenchymal stem cells (MSCs) have a high regeneration capacity and are most suitable for cartilage repair, and many associated studies have been conducted. MSCs can be obtained from various sources, such as bone marrow, adipose tissue, placenta, and umbilical cords. Methods for extracting MSCs from bone marrow or adipose tissue, such as bone marrow aspiration concentrate (BMAC), adipose-tissue-derived MSCs (Ad-MSCs), and adipose-tissue-derived stromal vascular fraction (ADSVF), have been studied, and their efficacy has been demonstrated [9,10]. However, this treatment approach also involves the need for invasive collection of stem cells, and there are issues with the quantity or quality of stem cells that can be obtained [10]. In contrast, there are fewer problems with the human umbilical cord blood derived MSC (hUCB-MSC) collection process, there are fewer ethical concerns that may arise when using embryonic stem cells, and these cells have a superior differentiation capacity compared to adult stem cells. Accordingly, researchers in various medical fields are increasingly focusing in this direction [11–13]. The usage for cartilage repair has also been analyzed in many animal studies [14], and it has been approved as a medical product and is used in clinical practice. Cartistem® (Medipost Inc., Sungnam, Gyeonggi-do, South Korea) was approved by the Korea Food and Drug Administration and is being used in practice, and clinical studies on this product are currently underway in the United States [9]. However, Cartistem® has not yet been used in countries other than Korea, and long-term follow-up results after use are insufficient, indicating the need for additional data and research. Therefore, we aimed to support the efficacy of the cartilage regeneration procedure using hUCB-MSCs as a treatment for cartilage defects through this systematic review. The objective of this systematic review was to prove the efficacy and safety of hUCB-MSCs treatment in a comprehensive analysis by including all subjects with knee articular cartilage defect or osteoarthritis who have undergone cartilage repair surgery using hUCB-MSCs. We included all cartilage repair surgeries without dividing them into arthroscopic assist and open procedure and excluded subjects with injection and other treatments. A meta-analysis synthesizing the clinical outcomes of studies published thus far and an analysis of the collective results were conducted. In some of the included studies, BMAC and microfracture procedures were used as comparison targets for the treatment of cartilage defects, and the results were analyzed. It is expected that the reliability of hUCB-MSC therapy will increase, and more studies will be conducted to achieve more effective treatment methods.

2. Materials and Methods

This systematic review was conducted following the Preferred Reporting Items for Systematic Reviews and Meta-Analysis (PRISMA) guidelines [15].

2.1. Search Strategy

Two reviewers independently conducted an electronic literature search on the treatment of knee cartilage defects and osteoarthritis using umbilical-cord-blood-derived stem cells. The PubMed, Embase, Web of Science, Scopus, and Cochrane Library databases were searched by two reviewers up to June 2022. The main search keywords were (MeSH term "Cartilage, Articular" or "knee joint" or "Osteoarthritis, knee") AND ("Umbilical cord blood-derived mesenchymal stem cell" or the MeSH term "Cord Blood Stem Cell Transplantation"), and the search was conducted including additional keywords related to these terms. After the initial search, duplicates were deleted, and each reviewer verified that there were no missing articles from the electronic search (Supplementary Materials File S1).

2.2. Study Selection with Eligibility Criteria

The inclusion and exclusion criteria are shown in Table 1. We searched all studies using hUCB-MSCs as a treatment for knee cartilage defects and osteoarthritis. Due to the small number of studies, randomized controlled trials (RCTs), prospective cohort studies, retrospective cohort studies, and case–control studies were all included. Only cases reporting on direct surgical treatment of cartilage lesions using hUCB-MSCs were included, and those involving intra-articular injection were excluded. Animal studies, phase I/II clinical trials, case reports, technical notes, review articles, and articles without accessible full-text versions were excluded, and when two or more studies were published by a single center, any with overlapping patient groups were excluded.

Table 1. Inclusion and exclusion criteria.

Inclusion criteria
a. Using hUCB-MSCs as a treatment for knee cartilage defects and osteoarthritis.
b. Only direct surgical treatment of cartilage lesions using hUCB-MSCs.
c. Randomized controlled trials (RCTs), prospective cohort studies, retrospective cohort studies, and case–control studies.
d. Full text available, written in English.
Exclusion criteria
a. Using hUCB-MSCs for intra-articular injection therapy.
b. If there is no clinical outcome comparison between before and after surgery.
c. If there is a risk of overlapping patient groups.
d. Animal studies, phase I/II clinical trials, case reports, technical notes, review articles, and articles without accessible full-text versions.

2.3. Data Extraction and Quality Assessment

Two reviewers extracted the following data from the included studies: first author, publication year, inclusion criteria, number of participants, age, body mass index, defect size, follow-up duration, outcome, concomitant intervention, and study design. Each extracted data point was verified by the rest of the reviewers. If additional information was needed from the included studies, the author of the study was contacted, and information was obtained.

Quality assessment of the included studies was conducted independently by two reviewers using the Newcastle–Ottawa scale [16]. The study by Lim et al. [17] was evaluated using the Newcastle–Ottawa scale because of the analysis of the clinical outcome during extended follow-up after their RCT. Three quality parameters of the Newcastle–Ottawa scale were evaluated, selection, comparability, and outcome. When the opinions of the reviewers differed, the final decision was achieved through discussion. The final evaluation was divided by the number of stars, and a score ≥ 7 points was indicative of high quality, that of 5–6 points was indicative of moderate quality, and that of four or fewer points was indicative of low quality.

2.4. Data and Statistical Analyses

In the included studies, statistical analysis was performed by extracting information on the preoperative clinical outcome and clinical outcome at final follow-up in all cases where hUCB-MSCs were used for treatment. Meta-analysis was performed on the measurement method used simultaneously in three or more studies among the clinical outcome scoring methods. In the study by Lim et al. [17], extended follow-up was performed up to 5 years after the RCT, but the analysis was conducted using the outcome measured at the 3-year follow-up, in line with the follow-up period of other included studies. In the study by Song et al. [18], analysis was performed by dividing the participants into two groups according to the presence or absence of trochlea lesions. Six studies evaluating participants using the International Knee Documentation Committee (IKDC) score, six studies evaluating participants using the Western Ontario and McMaster Universities Osteoarthritis Index (WOMAC), and five studies evaluating participants using the visual analog scale (VAS) were assessed with each measurement method. Each outcome was a continuous variable and was measured as the mean difference (MD) with 95% confidence interval (CI). Heterogeneity was assessed using the I^2 test. When $I^2 < 50\%$, a fixed-effects model was used; in other cases, a random-effects model was used. All statistical analyses were performed using RevMan version 5.4 (The Cochrane Collaboration, London, UK).

3. Results

3.1. Identification of Studies

Figure 1 presents the search information and shows a PRISMA flow diagram of the study selection process. An electronic literature search found 202 articles, and 53 duplicate articles were removed. After checking the titles/abstracts of the remaining 149 articles, those that met the exclusion criteria were removed, and the full-text versions of the remaining articles (n = 14) were analyzed. Among them, seven articles were additionally removed based on the inclusion/exclusion criteria, and seven articles were finally reviewed and meta-analyzed.

3.2. Characteristics of Included Studies

Table 2 summarizes the characteristics of the seven studies included in this review, including inclusion criteria, number of participants, age, body mass index, defect size, follow-up duration, outcome, concomitant intervention (performance of high tibial osteotomy (HTO)), and study design. In four studies, HTO was performed concomitantly [18–21], HTO was not performed in two studies [17,19], and one study did not consider HTO [20]. In two studies, only kissing lesions in the medial compartment were used as inclusion criteria [21,22]. In two studies, the results were evaluated using a modified Magnetic Resonance Observation of Cartilage Repair Tissue (M-MOCART) score generated with MRI [19,20]. All seven studies included in the analysis scored ≥ 6 points when evaluated using the Newcastle–Ottawa scale. Four studies scored 6 points (moderate quality), two studies scored 7 points, and one study scored 8 points (high quality) (Table 3).

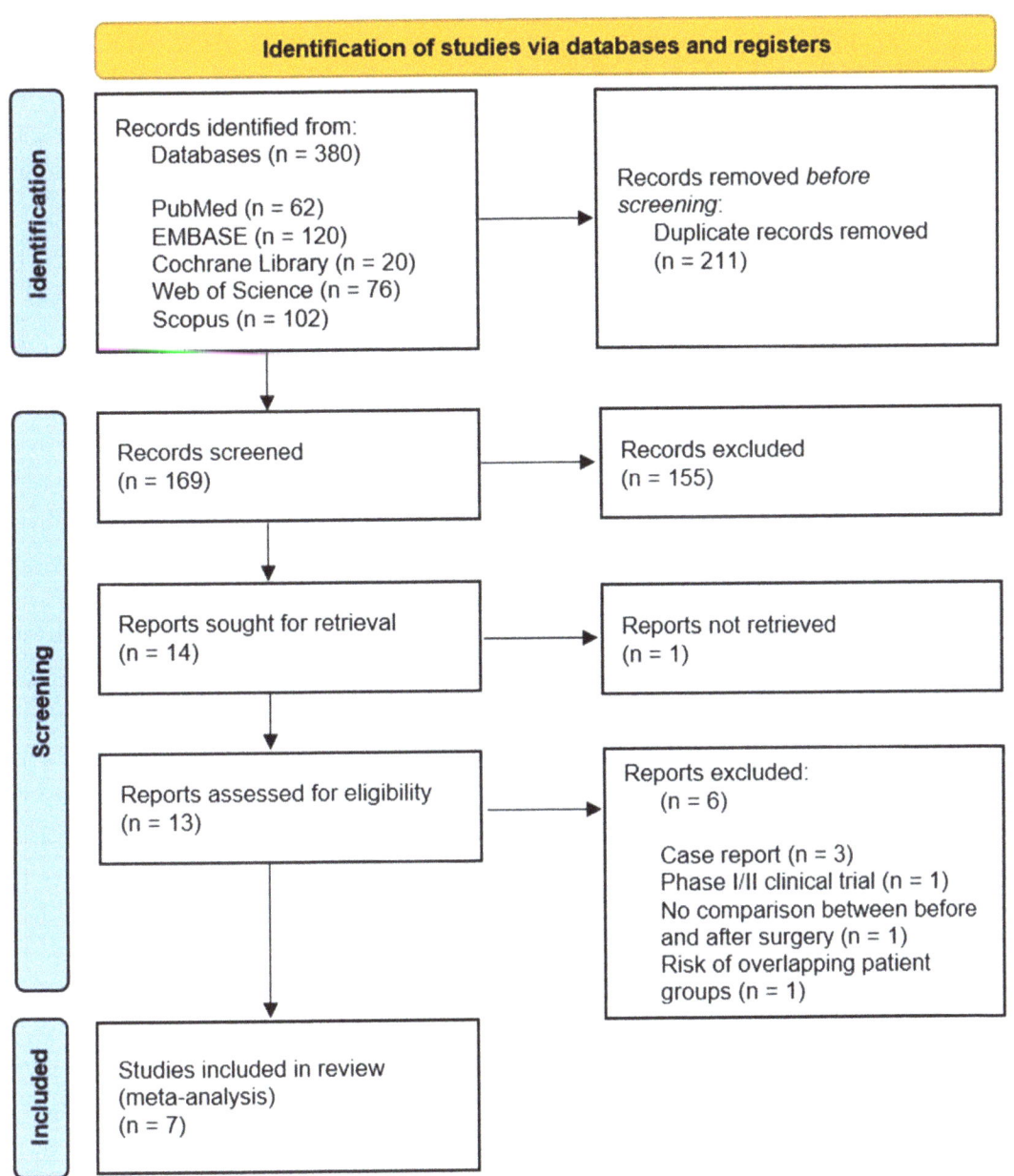

Figure 1. PRISMA flow diagram for the systematic review.

Table 2. Characteristics of included studies.

Study	Inclusion Criteria	Number of Patients Total	Number of Patients Each Group	Age, Mean ± SD	BMI, kg/m², Mean ± SD	Defect, cm², Mean ± SD	Follow-Up	Outcome	Concomitant Intervention (HTO)	Study Design	etc.
chung 2021 [23]	younger than 65 years, ICRS grade III or IV cartilage defects (>2 cm²), mechanical femorotibial varus angles > 3°, and KL grade 3	93	N/A	56.6 years (43–65)	25.8 kg/m² (20.9–33.2)	median 6.5 cm² (2.0–12.8)	mean 1.7 Y (1.0–3.5 Y)	IKDC, WOMAC, KSS, HSS, and ICRS	with HTO	retrospective cohort	N/A
song 2020 (1) [19]	older than 40 years, ICRS IV (>2 cm²), KL grade 1–3, and femorotibial angle (varus or valgus) < 8°	128	N/A	56.5 ± 7.9 (40–78)	24.6 ± 3.6 kg/m² (17–45.8)	one/two/three, 67 (4.5 ± 1.3)/49 (7.3 ± 2.9)/12 (9.8 ± 3.6)	36.1 ± 6.4 M (25–47 M)	VAS, WOMAC, IKDC, and MOCART (for 34 pts)	without HTO	retrospective cohort	subgroup analysis: trochlea lesion, age, and lesion size
song 2020 (2) [18]	older than 40 years, ICRS IV (>4 cm²) in medial compartment, KL grade 1–3, and femorotibial angle varus > 5°	125	with trochlea lesion: 73 without trochlea lesion: 52	58.3 ± 6.8 (43–74)	25.6 ± 2.7 kg/m² (19.2–35.5)	6.9 ± 2 cm²	3 Y	VAS, WOMAC, IKDC, and ICRS	with HTO	retrospective cohort	subgroup analysis: age, obesity, lesion size, location, and number of lesions
song 2020 (3) [21]	older than 60 years with a kissing lesion of the medial compartment, full-thickness chondral defect ≥ 4 cm² of MFC, and varus deformity ≥3°	25	N/A	64.9 ± 4.4 (60–76)	24.9 ± 3.1 kg/m² (19.2–34.2)	total: 9.4 ± 3.1 cm² (5.3–18.9 cm²), MFC: 7.2 ± 1.9 cm² (4.2–12.8 cm²), and MTC: 2.2 ± 1.1 cm² (0.2–6.1 cm²)	26.7 ± 1.8 M (24–31 M)	VAS, WOMAC, IKDC, and ICRS	with HTO	retrospective cohort	with kissing lesion
Lee 2021 [22]	ICRS ≥ 3B with kissing lesion in medial compartment	74	BMAC: 42 hUCB-MSC: 32	60.7 ± 4.1 58.1 ± 3.6	26.1 ± 2.8 26.6 ± 3.0 kg/m²	6.5 ± 2.9 cm² 7.0 ± 1.9 cm²	20.7 ± 6.1 M 15.6 ± 2.8 M	HSS, WOMAC, KSS, and ICRS	with HTO	retrospective cohort	with kissing lesion
Ryu 2022 [20]	KL grade ≤ 2, ICRS IV, older than 15 years, and lesion size 2–10 cm² (BMAC 15–50 yrs)	52	BMAC: 25 hUCB-MSC: 27	39.64 ± 9.83 53.93 ± 8.6	26.19 ± 3.74 kg/m² 26.38 ± 3.54 kg/m²	4.33 ± 1.66 cm² 4.77 ± 1.81 cm²	2 Y	VAS, IKDC, KOOS, and MOCART	5 pts with HTO 8 pts with HTO	retrospective cohort	subgroup analysis based on age (45 yrs)

Table 2. Cont.

Study	Inclusion Criteria	Number of Patients		Age, Mean ± SD	BMI, kg/m², Mean ± SD	Defect, cm², Mean ± SD	Follow-Up	Outcome	Concomitant Intervention (HTO)	Study Design	etc.
		Total	Each Group								
	aged > 18 years, full-thickness chondral defect 2–9 cm², ICRS 4, and KL grade 1–3	89	hUCB-MSC: 43	55.3 ± 8.9	25.7 ± 2.8 kg/m²	4.9 ± 2.0 cm²	2 Y				
			microfracture: 46	54.4 ± 10.8	26.7 ± 3.9 kg/m²	4.0 ± 1.8 cm²	2 Y				
Lim 2021 [17]	numbers of patients (extended follow-up data after RCT)	73	hUCB-MSC: 36	36 M: 33 (3 loss)	48 M: 28 (4 loss, 3 withdrew consent, and 1 AE)	60 M: 29 (3 loss, 3 withdrew consent, and 1 AE)	5 Y	VAS, IKDC, WOMAC, and ICRS	without HTO	extended study after RCT	subgroup analysis: age, lesion size
			microfracture: 37	36 M: 36 (1 loss)	48 M: 30 (6 withdrew consent, 1 reintervention)	60 M: 28 (7 withdrew consent, 2 reintervention)	5 Y				

BMI = body mass index, SD = standard deviation, HTO = high tibial osteotomy, ICRS = International Cartilage Repair Society, KL = Kellgren Lawrence, MFC = medial femoral condyle, RCT = randomized controlled trial, Y = year, M = month, hUCB-MSC = human umbilical cord blood derived mesenchymal stem cell, BMAC = bone marrow aspiration concentrate, IKDC = International Knee Documentation Committee score, WOMAC = Western Ontario and McMaster Universities Osteoarthritis Index, VAS = visual analogue scale, KSS = Knee Society score, HSS = Hospital for Special Surgery, KOOS = Knee Osteoarthritis Outcome score, MOCART = Magnetic Resonance Observation of Cartilage Repair Tissue.

Table 3. Newcastle–Ottawa Scale Quality Assessment of included studies.

Study	Selection				Comparability		Outcome			Total	Quality
	Representativeness of the Exposed Cohort	Selection of Non-exposed Cohort	Ascertainment of Exposure	Outcome of Interest	Cohorts	Control for Additional Factor	Assessment of Outcome	Sufficient Follow-Up	Adequacy of Follow-Up		
chung 2021 [23]	*	0	*	*	*	0	*	*	0	6	moderate
song 2020 (1) [19]	*	0	*	*	*	0	*	*	0	6	moderate
song 2020 (2) [18]	*	0	*	*	*	0	*	*	0	6	moderate
song 2020 (3) [21]	*	0	*	*	*	0	*	*	0	6	moderate
Lee 2021 [22]	*	*	*	*	*	0	*	*	0	7	high
Ryu 2022 [20]	*	0	*	*	*	0	*	*	*	7	high
Lim 2021 [17]	*	*	*	*	*	0	*	*	*	8	high

* means the subject gets points in that area

3.3. Subgroup Analysis of Included Studies

Subgroup analysis was performed in five studies, which are described in Table 2. Analysis of these studies showed that age had no effect on outcome [17–20], except in one study [21]. In addition, subgroup analysis of lesion size revealed that it did not affect the outcome in three studies [17–19] but did so in one study [21]. Unlike in other studies, subgroup analysis revealed that a younger age and a larger lesion size led to significantly greater improvements in the 2-year outcome in the study by Song et al. [21]. However, as the inclusion criteria of this study included age >60 years and kissing lesions in the medial compartment, the age cutoff for dividing the younger/older age groups was 65 years. As the regenerative ability of those > 65 years of age is significantly reduced, this result should be considered separately from the results of the other four studies. In addition, the number of patients included in this study was rather small (n = 25 participants). Therefore, it would be reasonable to conclude that age and lesion size have little effect on outcome based on the collected research results. In two studies [18,19], subgroup analyses were performed on other factors, such as lesion location and number, and neither the presence of trochlear lesions nor the number of lesions had a significant effect on the outcome. However, medial femoral condyle (MFC) lesions led to a significantly worse outcome than trochlear lesions [19]. In addition, subgroup analysis was performed considering obesity in two studies [18,21], showing that obesity did not have a significant effect on the outcome.

3.4. Study Outcome

The outcomes of each included study are summarized in Table 4. Publication bias was evaluated using a funnel plot, which showed a symmetrical appearance, suggesting low possibility of bias (Supplementary Materials File S2).

3.4.1. IKDC Score

The preoperative and final follow-up scores were extracted from six studies evaluating IKDC scores and analyzed. Totals of 441 patients with preoperative scores and 431 patients with final follow-up scores were included. The shortest final follow-up period was a mean of 1.7 years, and most studies presented 2–3 years of follow-up data (Table 2). However, in the study by Lim et al. [17], 3-year follow-up data were extracted and used for analysis. In the study by Song et al. [18], the divided groups were evaluated according to the presence or absence of trochlear lesions. In pooled analysis, the final follow-up IKDC score was significantly increased (MD, -32.82; 95% CI, -38.32 to -27.32; $p < 0.00001$) compared to the preoperative score, with significant heterogeneity ($I^2 = 93\%$, $p < 0.00001$) (Figure 2).

3.4.2. WOMAC Score

The preoperative and final follow-up WOMAC scores were extracted from six studies and analyzed. For this, 446 patients with preoperative scores and 436 patients with final follow-up scores were included. The shortest final follow-up period was a mean of 15.6 months, and most studies presented 2–3 years of data (Table 2). As before, 3-year follow-up data were used from the study by Lim et al. [17], and the data of Song et al. [18] were divided into two groups and analyzed. In pooled analysis, WOMAC final follow-up scores were significantly decreased (MD, 30.73; 95% CI, 24.10–37.36; $p < 0.00001$) compared to preoperative scores, with significant heterogeneity ($I^2 = 95\%$, $p < 0.00001$) (Figure 3).

Table 4. Clinical outcomes of included studies.

Study	Follow-Up	Treatment and Subgroup	IKDC					WOMAC					VAS				
chung 2021 [23]	mean 1.7 Y (1.0–3.5)	hUCB-MSC	pre 39.0 ± 10.4	final 71.3 ± 5.9				pre 44.5 ± 15.1	final 11.0 ± 3.7				N/A				
song (1) 2020 [19]	36.1 ± 6.4 M (25–47)	hUCB-MSC	pre 32.5 ± 8.3	1 Y 55.8 ± 14.3	final 61.2 ± 17.2			pre 39.3 ± 12.2	1 Y 17.2 ± 12.7	final 13.9 ± 14.1			pre 7.0 ± 1.6	1 Y 2.5 ± 1.7	final 2.0 ± 2.1		
song (2) 2021 [18]	3 Y	hUCB-MSC trochlear lesion	pre 29.3 ± 7.3	1 Y 56.7 ± 9.7	2 Y 61.6 ± 10.7	3 Y 64.7 ± 11		pre 44.8 ± 10.3	1 Y 13.8 ± 7.5	2 Y 10.7 ± 6.9	3 Y 8.4 ± 6.4		pre 7.8 ± 1.2	1 Y 2.6 ± 1.7	2 Y 2.1 ± 1.5	3 Y 1.6 ± 1.4	
		no trochlear lesion	pre 28.5 ± 7.6	1 Y 56.7 ± 9.7	2 Y 61.4 ± 9.5	3 Y 65.3 ± 11.4		pre 43.1 ± 11.1	1 Y 13.2 ± 8.2	2 Y 11.3 ± 8.5	3 Y 8.4 ± 6.8		pre 7.3 ± 1.3	1 Y 2.3 ± 1.6	2 Y 2.0 ± 1.7	3 Y 1.4 ± 1.6	
song (3) 2020 [21]	26.7 ± 1.8 M	hUCB-MSC	pre 24.3 ± 11.1	1 Y 58.9 ± 10.3	2 Y 68.5 ± 12.7			pre 57.3 ± 11.4	1 Y 15.6 ± 9.6	2 Y 10.2 ± 7.9			pre 76.4 ± 16.6	1 Y 20.4 ± 15.1	2 Y 12.8 ± 11.7		
Lee 2021 [22]	20.7 ± 6.1 M / 15.6 ± 2.8 M	BMAC	N/A					pre 43.9 ± 12.7	48 weeks 23.4 ± 11.6	final			N/A				
		hUCB-MSC	N/A					pre 45.2 ± 8.8	48 weeks 19.5 ± 15.8				N/A				
Ryu 2022 [20]	2 Y	BMAC	pre 44.17 ± 12.5	final 80.27 ± 9.48				N/A					pre 5.2 ± 1.1	final 0.92 ± 0.98			
		hUCB-MSC	pre 42.02 ± 13.63	final 81.35 ± 11.07				N/A					pre 5.0 ± 1.2	final 0.85 ± 0.86			

Study	Follow-up	Treatment and Subgroup	IKDC					WOMAC					VAS				
Lim 2021 [17]	5 Y	microfracture	pre 41.8 ± 13.4	48 weeks 53.5 (48.5 to 58.5)	3 Y 49.0 (43.3 to 54.7)	4 Y 48.9 (42.1 to 55.7)	5 Y 47.1 (41.1 to 53.2)	pre 40.4 ± 14.8	48 weeks 26.2 (21.1 to 31.2)	3 Y 34.5 (27.2 to 41.8)	4 Y 35.8 (27.6 to 44.1)	5 Y 36.2 (28.6 to 43.8)	pre 44.6 ± 12.9	48 weeks 24.1 (18.3 to 29.9)	3 Y 41.1 (32.2 to 50.0)	4 Y 43.3 (34.7 to 51.8)	5 Y 43.5 (35.3 to 51.6)
		hUCB-MSC	pre 42.7 ± 13.9	48 weeks 53.4 (49.0 to 57.8)	3 Y 57.4 (50.8 to 64.1)	4 Y 53.7 (48.2 to 59.3)	5 Y 54.7 (48.7 to 60.7)	pre 37.4 ± 15.1	48 weeks 24.7 (20.5 to 28.9)	3 Y 25.4 (19.9 to 31.0)	4 Y 28.6 (22.4 to 34.9)	5 Y 26.9 (20.4 to 33.5)	pre 44.0 ± 12.5	48 weeks 24.2 (17.5 to 31.0)	3 Y 30.9 (23.6 to 38.2)	4 Y 35.7 (29.2 to 42.3)	5 Y 29.1 (22.4 to 35.8)

Y = year, M = month, hUCB-MSC = human umbilical cord blood derived mesenchymal stem cell, BMAC = bone marrow aspiration concentrate, IKDC = International Knee Documentation Committee score, WOMAC = Western Ontario and McMaster Universities Osteoarthritis Index, VAS = visual analogue scale, pre = preoperative, final = final follow-up.

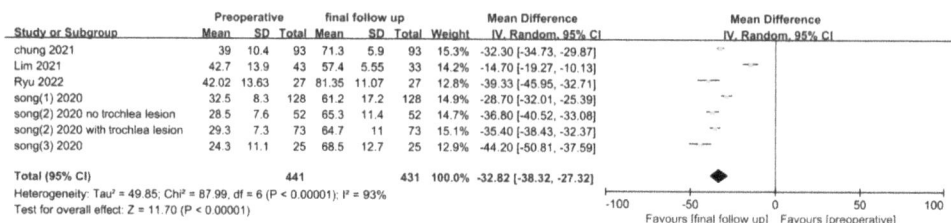

Figure 2. Forest plot of mean differences in IKDC subjective scores between pre-operation and at final follow-up.

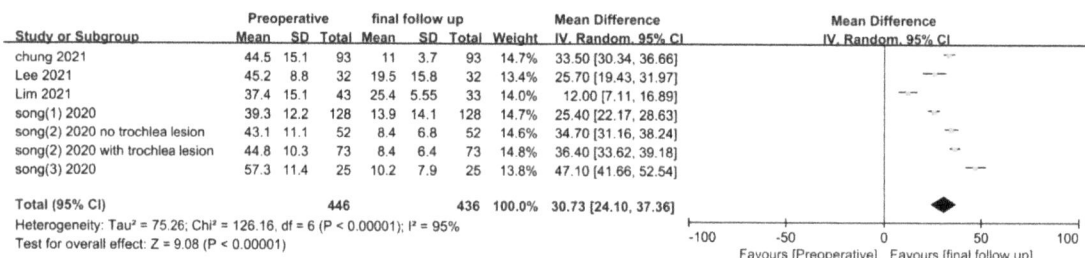

Figure 3. Forest plot of mean differences in WOMAC scores pre-operation and at final follow-up.

3.4.3. VAS Score

The preoperative and final follow-up VAS scores were extracted from five studies and analyzed. Here, 348 patients with preoperative scores and 338 patients with final follow-up scores were included. The final follow-up period ranged from a minimum of 2 years to a maximum of 36.1 months (Table 2). The data of the studies [17,21] in which VAS scores were evaluated based on a total of 100 points were divided by 10, and the standard was unified into a total of 10 points for analysis. As before, 3-year follow-up data were used from the study by Lim et al. [17], and the data of Song et al. [18] were divided into two groups and analyzed. In pooled analysis, the VAS final follow-up scores were significantly decreased (MD, 4.81; 95% CI, 3.17–6.46; $p < 0.00001$) compared to preoperative scores, with significant heterogeneity ($I^2 = 98\%$, $p < 0.00001$) (Figure 4).

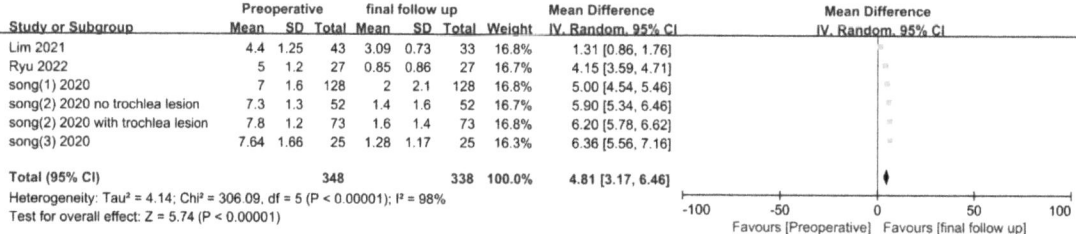

Figure 4. Forest plot of mean difference in VAS scores between pre-operation and final follow-up.

3.4.4. M-MOCART Score

The M-MOCART score was measured in two of the seven studies included in the analysis (Supplementary Materials File S3). In the study by Song et al. [19], 34 patients received M-MOCART scores, and the mean score at 3–6 months after surgery was 30.58 points. According to MRI scans performed $\geq$ 1 year after surgery (mean, 21.2 months), the mean score increased to 55.44 points. Ryu et al. [20] measured the M-MOCART score using MRI scans at 1 year and 2 years after surgery in 27 patients, recording mean respective scores of 69.63 and 73.7 points. In both studies, the M-MOCART score after ≥1 year was sufficient compared to the general results of other cartilage repair surgeries [24,25]. However, evidence confirming whether the M-MOCART score correlates with clinical outcome is insufficient, and the M-MOCART score should be considered an auxiliary indicator of repaired cartilage quality [25]. In the study by Ryu et al. [20], the M-MOCART scores of 25 patients in the BMAC group were measured and compared with those of the hUCB-MSC group. Ultimately, the results of the BMAC group at 1 year and 2 years were 65.4 and 70.2 points, with the hUCB-MSC group showing better results, although there was no significant difference.

3.4.5. Comparison with BMAC and Microfracture Procedures

Comparisons with a control group were performed in three studies. In one study, the group only treated with microfracture surgery was set as a control group [17]; in two studies, the group treated with BMAC procedures was set as a control group [20,22]. The clinical outcome data of the control group are included in Table 4. In the study by Lim et al. [17], compared to the microfracture group, IKDC scores at 48 weeks did not show a significant difference in the hUCB-MSC group, with a mean of 53.4 points versus a mean of 53.5 points. However, at 3 years of follow-up, the hUCB-MSC group had a mean score of 57.4 points and the microfracture group had a mean score of 49.0 points, confirming that better results were obtained in the hUCB-MSC group. Moreover, this trend continues in the 4- and 5-year follow-up comparisons. WOMAC scores also showed no significant difference between the groups, with a mean of 24.7 points for the hUCB-MSC group and a mean of 26.2 points for the microfracture group at 48 weeks; in contrast, at 3 years of follow-up, the hUCB-MSC group had a mean score of 25.4 points versus the microfracture group mean score of 34.5 points, indicating better results in the hUCB-MSC group. Again, this trend persists in the 4- and 5-year follow-up comparisons. In addition, considering the VAS scores, the results of the hUCB-MSC group appear better in 3-, 4-, and 5-year follow-up comparisons with the microfracture group. Regardless of the scoring system, a divergence between groups seems to appear from the third year onward; although the microfracture group had good results until 48 weeks, this good result was not maintained thereafter. In the study by Ryu et al. [20], the outcome of hUCB-MSC therapy at 2 years of follow-up was compared with that of BMAC, and the hUCB-MSC group had a mean IKDC score of 81.35 points compared to the 80.287 points of the BMAC group, showing no significant difference. There was also no significant difference in VAS scores, with means of 0.85 and 0.92 points, respectively. In the study by Lee et al. [22], the outcome of the hUCB-MSC group was evaluated at a mean of 15.6 months, while that of the BMAC group was evaluated at a mean of 20.7 months. WOMAC scores were slightly better in the hUCB-MSC group, with a mean of 19.5 points, compared to the BMAC group with a mean of 23.4 points, but there was no significant difference. In addition to the WOMAC score, the Hospital for Special Surgery score and the pain and function Knee Society scores were also calculated but did not show significant differences between groups, although the results of the hUCB-MSC group were slightly better.

4. Discussion

In the past, arthroplasty was the most common treatment for osteoarthritis; recently, joint-preserving surgery has been developed. In particular, in Korea, the cartilage regeneration procedure performed together with correction of varus or valgus alignment through corrective osteotomy is gradually increasing in popularity [26]. In line with this, stem cell therapy for cartilage defects and osteoarthritis has developed through many studies. Previously, stem cell therapy mainly used BMAC, AD-MSCs, and ADSVF, but research on hUCB-MSCs has been active since Cartistem® was approved by Korea's Food and Drug Administration. As there is a large number of MSCs in umbilical cord blood, its use has been expanded in various fields [27]. To date, a disadvantage to using stem cells has been that the procedure is invasive, and the cells are difficult to obtain in sufficient number from bone marrow and adipose tissue. On the other hand, sourcing hUCB-MSCs can result in collection of a constant and sufficient number of stem cells in a non-invasive manner. In addition, these cells are hypoimmunogenic and do not cause immune-related problems. In addition, unlike with embryonic stem cells, there are no ethical problems [5,28]. Finally, hUCB-MSCs boast higher proliferation, karyotype stability after prolonged expansion, and easier chondrogenic differentiation compared to MSCs extracted from bone marrow and adipose tissue [29]. Therefore, cartilage regeneration therapy using hUCB-MSCs is considered more effective than conventional treatment and is being used in clinical trials. Many retrospective studies have been announced and usually report satisfactory results. Several case reports have also been published, one of which reported satisfactory results using hUCB-MSCs as a treatment for juvenile osteochondritis dissecans [30].

Therefore, we summarized the published therapeutic effects of hUCB-MSCs and present our opinions. First, hUCB-MSC therapy is a new clinical treatment, and its safety must be confirmed. There appear to be no severe adverse effects (AEs) among the studies published to date; however, there were reports of general AEs in three studies. In the study by Park et al. [28], there were no serious AEs, and one patient experienced an elevation of antithyroglobulin antibody level, which was reported as a treatment-emergent AE, but it spontaneously normalized without any special treatment. Ryu et al. [20] reported three cases of adhesions, but this is a minor complication of arthroscopic surgery, and the frequency in this study was not particularly high. Chung et al. [23] reported that temporary knee swelling was observed up to 1 month after surgery in some patients, but it was self-limiting, and there were no other serious AEs. In the study by Lim et al. [17], there were no other surgical-related serious AEs other than surgical site pain, the final reported serious AEs were also not related to the use of hUCB-MSCs, and there were no immunological reactions. Therefore, the safety of hUCB-MSCs is supported by the available research results.

In several studies included in this review, subgroup analyses were conducted. In four studies with subgroup analyses according to age [17–20], excluding one other study [21], age did not affect the results. In three studies [17–19], lesion size did not affect the results. Considering the process of obtaining stem cells from bone marrow or adipose tissue, there may only be a small number of stem cells extracted from a patient of old age, and there may be an overall decrease in their quality with a low differentiation potential. However, as mentioned earlier, hUCB-MSC therapy involves using a product of a certain quality and number of stem cells, and the results can be seen above. However, implanted MSCs are known to promote the regeneration of host cells with a paracrine effect rather than turning them into cartilage, so it may not be described only by stem cell quality [31,32]. In addition, some studies have reported good pain level and functional outcome when using high-dose MSCs [33], indicating the need for additional research.

In pooled data analysis of seven studies included in this systematic review, IKDC, WOMAC, and VAS scores all showed statistically significant improvements at final follow-up compared to the preoperative evaluation. This means that clinical outcomes can be effectively improved through cartilage regeneration surgery using hUCB-MSCs. The final follow-up duration of the included studies varied, but the mean is ≥ 15.6 months, and considering that most of the studies included a follow-up period of about 2 years, this means that the clinical outcome of the hUCB-MSC therapy was sufficiently improved and maintained during the short-term follow-up. It is known that the clinical symptoms recur before two years if there is a failure in cartilage regeneration. Therefore, a favorable short-term outcome is implied when the improvement of clinical outcome is maintained during the 2-year follow-up [34]. In addition, three studies [17–19] showed good results in clinical outcomes measured after a mean period of ≥ 3 years. Several studies reported good quality of regenerated cartilage for up to 2 years after microfracture surgery and then gradually deteriorated [35,36]. In the study by Lim et al. [17], the microfracture group had a worse outcome from the third year onward, while the hUCB-MSC group maintained an improved outcome until 5 years of follow-up. With hUCB-MSC therapy, it can be inferred that the quality of regenerated cartilage is good, and regenerated cartilage is more hyaline-like than microfracture alone. In addition, Suh et al. [37] compared radiological changes after surgery between a group that received hUCB-MSC therapy and a group that received microfracture surgery, with both groups receiving HTO as concomitant surgery, and found that the hUCB-MSC group had a significant increase in joint space width increment ($p < 0.05$) of 0.6 mm compared to that of just 0.1 mm in the microfracture group.

Among the studies included in this systematic review, two [20,22] considered BMAC, and no significant differences were seen in the IKDC, WOMAC, VAS, and M-MOCART scores. However, Lee et al. performed second-look arthroscopy in all patients, and the hUCB-MSC group had better ICRS grade results in the medial femoral condyle and medial tibial condyle, so it seems that hUCB-MSC therapy facilitates better cartilage regeneration. Ryu et al. also performed second-look arthroscopy in some patients and measured the ICRS grade, and they reported no significant difference. However, the study by Ryu et al. includes a difference in the mean age of the hUCB-MSC group and BMAC group (53.93 vs. 39.64 years). In other words, the BMAC group may have experienced better results because younger people have better healing potential. Considering these points, more data must be accumulated to compare the clinical outcomes of cartilage regeneration. In the study by Yang et al. [38], which was excluded from this analysis because there was a risk of overlapping patient groups, the results of hUCB-MSC and BMAC treatments were compared by performing propensity score matching for sex, age, body mass index, and lesion size. No significant differences between the two groups in the measurement of IKDC score, Knee Injury and Osteoarthritis Outcome Score, Short-Form 36 score, or Tegner Activity Score were found. However, following ICRS Cartilage Repair Assessment grading, which was carried out through second-look arthroscopy, the score of the hUCB-MSC group (n = 44) was 9.2 ± 2.2 points, and that of the BMAC group was (n = 37) 7.2 ± 3.0 points. In other words, the hUCB-MSC group experienced significantly better cartilage regeneration. Based on these results, hUCB-MSC therapy can be considered to lead to slightly better-quality cartilage regeneration than BMAC. However, there is still little comparative research with BMAC, and more is needed, with long-term results ≥ 3 years considered crucial.

Our study has some limitations. First, among the studies included in our analysis, six were retrospective studies, and one was an extended follow-up data analysis after RCT. Meta-analysis based on RCT studies could not be performed due to the small number of studies. In order to form a more scientific basis for the effect of hUCB-MSCs, studies analyzing multiple RCTs will be needed. Second, in the studies included in our investigation, several patient characteristics such as age, sex, defect size, and follow-up duration varied, and it is believed that this may have affected the heterogeneity of the results. Lastly, three of the studies included in this meta-analysis were published by a single center, and two of the remaining studies were also published by another single center. We checked the inclusion criteria with the study authors to confirm that there were no overlapping patients and proceeded with our analysis; however, this is a potential cause of bias. All of these limitations are considered to be caused by the insufficient number of studies published so far.

5. Conclusions

Cartilage regeneration surgery using hUCB-MSCs is expected to lead to better results than conventional stem cell therapy or other cartilage repair procedures. Through this review, the safety, efficacy, and quality of repaired cartilage associated with this procedure were demonstrated. In the future, a number of comparative studies considering other stem cell therapies or cartilage repair procedures will be published, and we expect that the relatively superior effect of hUCB-MSC therapy will be demonstrated. Based on this, we hope that the treatment of cartilage defects and osteoarthritis will be improved.

Supplementary Materials: The following supporting information can be downloaded at: https://www.mdpi.com/article/10.3390/medicina58121801/s1, Supplementary File S1: Keywords and search results. Supplementary File S2: Funnel plot of IKDC, WOMAC, and VAS scores. Supplementary File S3: M-MOCART score and second-look arthroscopic findings of included studies.

Author Contributions: Conceptualization, D.H.L. and S.J.K.; methodology, D.H.L., S.A.K. and J.-S.S.; data curation, D.H.L., S.A.K. and J.-S.S.; writing—original draft preparation, D.H.L. and B.-H.K.; writing—review and editing, D.H.L. and S.J.K.; visualization, D.H.L.; supervision, S.J.K. and A.A.S.; project administration, D.H.L. and S.J.K. All authors have read and agreed to the published version of the manuscript.

Funding: This research received no external funding.

Institutional Review Board Statement: Not applicable.

Informed Consent Statement: Not applicable.

Data Availability Statement: The data presented in this study are available in the main article and Supplementary Materials Files.

Acknowledgments: We thank Seung Jae Lee, librarian of the Medical Library of The Catholic University of Korea, Seoul, Republic of Korea, for helping with the data search.

Conflicts of Interest: The authors declare no conflict of interest.

References

1. Angadi, D.S.; Macdonald, H.; Atwal, N. Autologous cell-free serum preparations in the management of knee osteoarthritis: What is the current clinical evidence? *Knee Surg. Relat. Res.* **2020**, *32*, 16. [CrossRef]
2. Hodler, J.; Resnick, D. Current status of imaging of articular cartilage. *Skelet. Radiol.* **1996**, *25*, 703–709. [CrossRef]
3. Williams, R.J., III; Harnly, H.W. Microfracture: Indications, technique, and results. *Instr. Course Lect.* **2007**, *56*, 419–428.
4. Orth, P.; Gao, L.; Madry, H. Microfracture for cartilage repair in the knee: A systematic review of the contemporary literature. *Knee Surg. Sport. Traumatol. Arthrosc.* **2020**, *28*, 670–706. [CrossRef]
5. Lee, D.H.; Kim, S.J.; Kim, S.A.; Ju, G.I. Past, present, and future of cartilage restoration: From localized defect to arthritis. *Knee Surg. Relat. Res.* **2022**, *34*, 1. [CrossRef]
6. Zamborsky, R.; Danisovic, L. Surgical techniques for knee cartilage repair: An updated large-scale systematic review and network meta-analysis of randomized controlled trials. *Arthrosc. J. Arthrosc. Relat. Surg.* **2020**, *36*, 845–858. [CrossRef] [PubMed]
7. Letsiou, S.; Felix, R.C.; Cardoso, J.C.R.; Anjos, L.; Mestre, A.L.; Gomes, H.L.; Power, D.M. Cartilage acidic protein 1 promotes increased cell viability, cell proliferation and energy metabolism in primary human dermal fibroblasts. *Biochimie* **2020**, *171–172*, 72–78. [CrossRef] [PubMed]
8. Na, H.S.; Lee, S.-Y.; Lee, D.H.; Woo, J.S.; Choi, S.-Y.; Cho, K.-H.; Kim, S.; Go, E.J.; Lee, A.R.; Choi, J.-W. Soluble CCR2 gene therapy controls joint inflammation, cartilage damage, and the progression of osteoarthritis by targeting MCP-1 in a monosodium iodoacetate (MIA)-induced OA rat model. *J. Transl. Med.* **2022**, *20*, 482. [CrossRef] [PubMed]
9. Park, Y.-B.; Ha, C.-W.; Rhim, J.H.; Lee, H.-J. Stem cell therapy for articular cartilage repair: Review of the entity of cell populations used and the result of the clinical application of each entity. *Am. J. Sport. Med.* **2018**, *46*, 2540–2552. [CrossRef]
10. Jeyaraman, M.; Muthu, S.; Ganie, P.A. Does the source of mesenchymal stem cell have an effect in the management of osteoarthritis of the knee? Meta-analysis of randomized controlled trials. *Cartilage* **2021**, *13*, 1532S–1547S. [CrossRef]
11. Moon, S.W.; Park, S.; Oh, M.; Wang, J.H. Outcomes of human umbilical cord blood-derived mesenchymal stem cells in enhancing tendon-graft healing in anterior cruciate ligament reconstruction: An exploratory study. *Knee Surg. Relat. Res.* **2021**, *33*, 32. [CrossRef] [PubMed]
12. Harris, D.T. Cord blood stem cells: A review of potential neurological applications. *Stem Cell Rev.* **2008**, *4*, 269–274. [CrossRef] [PubMed]
13. Harris, D.T. Non-haematological uses of cord blood stem cells. *Br. J. Haematol.* **2009**, *147*, 177–184. [CrossRef] [PubMed]
14. Klontzas, M.E.; Kenanidis, E.I.; Heliotis, M.; Tsiridis, E.; Mantalaris, A. Bone and cartilage regeneration with the use of umbilical cord mesenchymal stem cells. *Expert. Opin. Biol. Ther.* **2015**, *15*, 1541–1552. [CrossRef]
15. Page, M.J.; McKenzie, J.E.; Bossuyt, P.M.; Boutron, I.; Hoffmann, T.C.; Mulrow, C.D.; Shamseer, L.; Tetzlaff, J.M.; Akl, E.A.; Brennan, S.E. The PRISMA 2020 statement: An updated guideline for reporting systematic reviews. *Syst. Rev.* **2021**, *10*, 89. [CrossRef]
16. Wells, G.; Shea, B.; O'connell, D.; Peterson, J.; Welch, V.; Losos, M.; Tugwell, P. The Newcastle-Ottawa Scale (NOS) for Assessing the Quality of Nonrandomised Studies in Meta-Analyses. Available online: http://www3.med.unipmn.it/dispense_ebm/2009-2010/Corso%20Perfezionamento%20EBM_Faggiano/NOS_oxford.pdf (accessed on 13 May 2020).

17. Lim, H.C.; Park, Y.B.; Ha, C.W.; Cole, B.J.; Lee, B.K.; Jeong, H.J.; Kim, M.K.; Bin, S.I.; Choi, C.H.; Choi, C.H.; et al. Allogeneic Umbilical Cord Blood-Derived Mesenchymal Stem Cell Implantation Versus Microfracture for Large, Full-Thickness Cartilage Defects in Older Patients: A Multicenter Randomized Clinical Trial and Extended 5-Year Clinical Follow-up. *Orthop. J. Sport. Med.* **2021**, *9*, 2325967120973052. [CrossRef]
18. Song, J.S.; Hong, K.T.; Kong, C.G.; Kim, N.M.; Jung, J.Y.; Park, H.S.; Kim, Y.J.; Chang, K.B.; Kim, S.J. High tibial osteotomy with human umbilical cord blood-derived mesenchymal stem cells implantation for knee cartilage regeneration. *World J. Stem Cells* **2020**, *12*, 514–526. [CrossRef]
19. Song, J.S.; Hong, K.T.; Kim, N.M.; Jung, J.Y.; Park, H.S.; Lee, S.H.; Cho, Y.J.; Kim, S.J. Implantation of allogenic umbilical cord blood-derived mesenchymal stem cells improves knee osteoarthritis outcomes: Two-year follow-up. *Regen. Ther.* **2020**, *14*, 32–39. [CrossRef] [PubMed]
20. Ryu, D.J.; Jeon, Y.S.; Park, J.S.; Bae, G.C.; Kim, J.S.; Kim, M.K. Comparison of Bone Marrow Aspirate Concentrate and Allogenic Human Umbilical Cord Blood Derived Mesenchymal Stem Cell Implantation on Chondral Defect of Knee: Assessment of Clinical and Magnetic Resonance Imaging Outcomes at 2-Year Follow-Up. *Cell Transpl.* **2020**, *29*, 963689720943581. [CrossRef] [PubMed]
21. Song, J.S.; Hong, K.T.; Kim, N.M.; Park, H.S.; Choi, N.H. Human umbilical cord blood-derived mesenchymal stem cell implantation for osteoarthritis of the knee. *Arch. Orthop. Trauma Surg.* **2020**, *140*, 503–509. [CrossRef]
22. Lee, N.H.; Na, S.M.; Ahn, H.W.; Kang, J.K.; Seon, J.K.; Song, E.K. Allogenic Human Umbilical Cord Blood-Derived Mesenchymal Stem Cells Are More Effective Than Bone Marrow Aspiration Concentrate for Cartilage Regeneration After High Tibial Osteotomy in Medial Unicompartmental Osteoarthritis of Knee. *Arthroscopy* **2021**, *37*, 2521–2530. [CrossRef]
23. Chung, Y.W.; Yang, H.Y.; Kang, S.J.; Song, E.K.; Seon, J.K. Allogeneic umbilical cord-blood-derived mesenchymal stem cells combined with high tibial osteotomy: A retrospective study on safety and early results. *Int. Orthop.* **2021**, *45*, 481–488. [CrossRef]
24. Anderson, D.E.; Williams III, R.J.; DeBerardino, T.M.; Taylor, D.C.; Ma, C.B.; Kane, M.S.; Crawford, D.C. Magnetic resonance imaging characterization and clinical outcomes after NeoCart surgical therapy as a primary reparative treatment for knee cartilage injuries. *Am. J. Sport. Med.* **2017**, *45*, 875–883. [CrossRef]
25. De Windt, T.S.; Welsch, G.H.; Brittberg, M.; Vonk, L.A.; Marlovits, S.; Trattnig, S.; Saris, D.B. Is magnetic resonance imaging reliable in predicting clinical outcome after articular cartilage repair of the knee? A systematic review and meta-analysis. *Am. J. Sport. Med.* **2013**, *41*, 1695–1702. [CrossRef] [PubMed]
26. Koh, I.J.; Kim, M.W.; Kim, J.H.; Han, S.Y.; In, Y. Trends in high tibial osteotomy and knee arthroplasty utilizations and demographics in Korea from 2009 to 2013. *J. Arthroplast.* **2015**, *30*, 939–944. [CrossRef]
27. Taghizadeh, R.; Cetrulo, K.; Cetrulo, C. Wharton's Jelly stem cells: Future clinical applications. *Placenta* **2011**, *32*, S311–S315. [CrossRef] [PubMed]
28. Park, Y.B.; Ha, C.W.; Lee, C.H.; Yoon, Y.C.; Park, Y.G. Cartilage Regeneration in Osteoarthritic Patients by a Composite of Allogeneic Umbilical Cord Blood-Derived Mesenchymal Stem Cells and Hyaluronate Hydrogel: Results from a Clinical Trial for Safety and Proof-of-Concept with 7 Years of Extended Follow-Up. *Stem Cells Transl. Med.* **2017**, *6*, 613–621. [CrossRef] [PubMed]
29. Zhang, X.; Hirai, M.; Cantero, S.; Ciubotariu, R.; Dobrila, L.; Hirsh, A.; Igura, K.; Satoh, H.; Yokomi, I.; Nishimura, T. Isolation and characterization of mesenchymal stem cells from human umbilical cord blood: Reevaluation of critical factors for successful isolation and high ability to proliferate and differentiate to chondrocytes as compared to mesenchymal stem cells from bone marrow and adipose tissue. *J. Cell. Biochem.* **2011**, *112*, 1206–1218. [PubMed]
30. Song, J.S.; Hong, K.T.; Kim, N.M.; Jung, J.Y.; Park, H.S.; Kim, Y.C.; Shetty, A.A.; Kim, S.J. Allogenic umbilical cord blood-derived mesenchymal stem cells implantation for the treatment of juvenile osteochondritis dissecans of the knee. *J. Clin. Orthop. Trauma* **2019**, *10*, S20–S25. [CrossRef]
31. Liang, X.; Ding, Y.; Zhang, Y.; Tse, H.-F.; Lian, Q. Paracrine mechanisms of mesenchymal stem cell-based therapy: Current status and perspectives. *Cell Transplant.* **2014**, *23*, 1045–1059. [CrossRef]
32. Gnecchi, M.; Danieli, P.; Malpasso, G.; Ciuffreda, M.C. Paracrine mechanisms of mesenchymal stem cells in tissue repair. *Mesenchymal Stem Cells* **2016**, *1416*, 123–146.
33. Jo, C.H.; Chai, J.W.; Jeong, E.C.; Oh, S.; Shin, J.S.; Shim, H.; Yoon, K.S. Intra-articular injection of mesenchymal stem cells for the treatment of osteoarthritis of the knee: A 2-year follow-up study. *Am. J. Sport. Med.* **2017**, *45*, 2774–2783. [CrossRef] [PubMed]
34. Mithoefer, K.; McAdams, T.; Williams, R.J.; Kreuz, P.C.; Mandelbaum, B.R. Clinical efficacy of the microfracture technique for articular cartilage repair in the knee: An evidence-based systematic analysis. *Am. J. Sport. Med.* **2009**, *37*, 2053–2063. [CrossRef]
35. Goyal, D.; Keyhani, S.; Lee, E.H.; Hui, J.H.P. Evidence-based status of microfracture technique: A systematic review of level I and II studies. *Arthrosc. J. Arthrosc. Relat. Surg.* **2013**, *29*, 1579–1588. [CrossRef] [PubMed]
36. Bert, J.M. Abandoning microfracture of the knee: Has the time come? *Arthrosc. J. Arthrosc. Relat. Surg.* **2015**, *31*, 501–505. [CrossRef] [PubMed]
37. Suh, D.W.; Han, S.B.; Yeo, W.J.; Cheong, K.; So, S.Y.; Kyung, B.S. Human umbilical cord-blood-derived mesenchymal stem cell can improve the clinical outcome and Joint space width after high tibial osteotomy. *Knee* **2021**, *33*, 31–37. [CrossRef]
38. Yang, H.Y.; Song, E.K.; Kang, S.J.; Kwak, W.K.; Kang, J.K.; Seon, J.K. Allogenic umbilical cord blood-derived mesenchymal stromal cell implantation was superior to bone marrow aspirate concentrate augmentation for cartilage regeneration despite similar clinical outcomes. *Knee Surg. Sport. Traumatol Arthrosc.* **2022**, *30*, 208–218. [CrossRef]

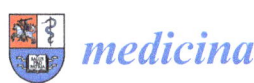

Review

Autologous Collagen-Induced Chondrogenesis: From Bench to Clinical Development

You Seung Chun [1], Seon Ae Kim [1], Yun Hwan Kim [1], Joong Hoon Lee [1], Asode Ananthram Shetty [2] and Seok Jung Kim [1,*]

1. Department of Orthopedic Surgery, College of Medicine, The Catholic University of Korea, Seoul 06591, Republic of Korea
2. Institute of Medical Sciences, Faculty of Health and Wellbeing, Canterbury Christ Church University, Chatham Maritime, Kent ME4 4UF, UK
* Correspondence: peter@catholic.ac.kr; Tel.: +82-31-820-3654; Fax: +82-31-847-3671

Abstract: Microfracture is a common technique that uses bone marrow components to stimulate cartilage regeneration. However, the clinical results of microfracture range from poor to good. To enhance cartilage healing, several reinforcing techniques have been developed, including porcine-derived collagen scaffold, hyaluronic acid, and chitosan. Autologous collagen-induced chondrogenesis (ACIC) is a single-step surgical technique for cartilage regeneration that combines gel-type atelocollagen scaffolding with microfracture. Even though ACIC is a relatively new technique, literature show excellent clinical results. In addition, all procedures of ACIC are performed arthroscopically, which is increasing in preference among surgeons and patients. The ACIC technique also is called the Shetty–Kim technique because it was developed from the works of A.A. Shetty and S.J. Kim. This is an up-to-date review of the history of ACIC.

Keywords: atelocollagen; microfracture; cartilage repair; knee; ACIC

1. Introduction

The articular cartilage is a thin layer of viscoelastic connective tissue that complicates repair of the cartilage. Studies have emphasized the importance of repairing articular cartilage to delay arthroplasty. Multiple drilling techniques have been used to treat articular cartilage defects. In 1959, Pridie [1] said, "If these sclerotic areas were drilled and the holes were not too far apart, smooth fibro-cartilage would spread over the surface." He introduced the drilling of the subchondral bone to heal cartilage defects.

Steadman et al. [2] modified this method to avoid thermal necrosis from drilling, using bone marrow from the subchondral bone to form a clot on the defect holes (Figure 1). The clot contained mesenchymal stem cells (MSCs) and abundant growth factors, inducing repair by fibrous and hyaline-like cartilage [3] (Figure 2).

Multiple drilling techniques produce predominantly fibrocartilage [4]; therefore, several methods have been introduced to produce hyaline-like cartilage. Autologous chondrocyte implantation is considered an ideal procedure to induce hyaline-like cartilage. However, it requires a two-stage procedure, damages the donor site cartilage, and has a high cost.

The limitation of the marrow stimulation technique is that bone marrow stem cells and growth factors are released into the joint rather than remaining at an articular surface. Collagen gel or scaffold has been used to overcome this limitation by providing mechanical stability to form clots [5]. Cell-free type I collagen gels or scaffolds combined with marrow stimulation, such as multiple drilling, have shown good outcomes regarding the induction of hyaline-like cartilage [6–8]. Autologous matrix-induced chondrogenesis (AMIC) uses a porcine collagen matrix to provide a biological scaffold.

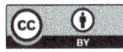

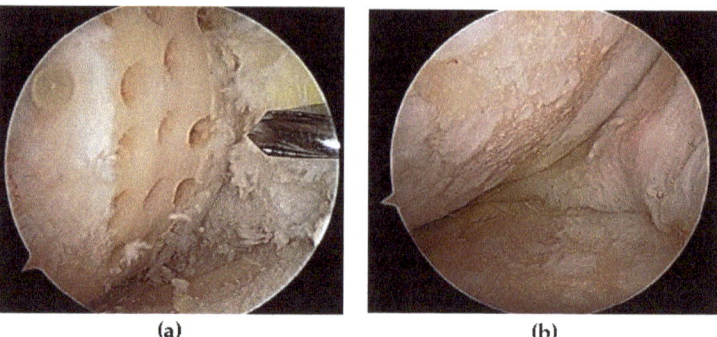

Figure 1. (**a**) Multiple holes drilled into a cartilage defect; (**b**) second-look arthroscopy 2 years later.

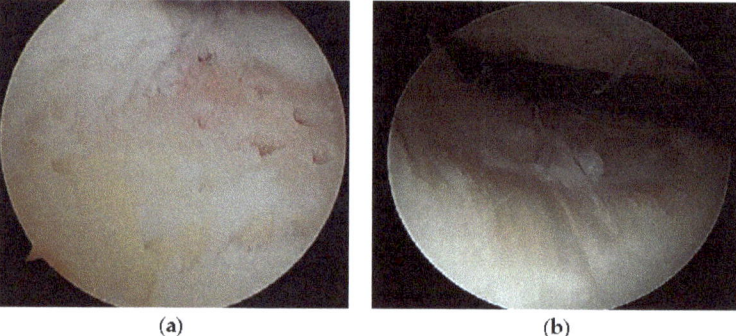

Figure 2. (**a**) Microfracture of a cartilage defect of the trochlea; (**b**) second-look arthroscopy 2 years later.

Despite its popularity since 2000, the AMIC technique requires an open surgical incision for the preparation of the defect and the application of the collagen membrane. To overcome this weakness, autologous collagen-induced chondrogenesis (ACIC) was developed, for which the procedures are performed arthroscopically. For ACIC, atelocollagen gel is used as a scaffold instead of the membrane used in AMIC. Atelocollagen is a highly purified type I collagen obtained following the treatment of skin dermis with pepsin and telopeptide removal, which reduces immunogenicity.

This article reviews the developmental history with a basic scientific rationale and the various techniques and results of ACIC for the repairing of knee cartilage.

2. Basic Science and Methods for Chondrogenesis

2.1. Basic Science of Cartilage Injury

Articular cartilage is a thin, viscoelastic layer of connective tissue 2–3 mm thick [9] (Figure 3). It is of mesodermal origin and is characterized by a cellular component immersed within an extracellular matrix composed of polysaccharides, fibrous protein, and interstitial fluid [10]. The cartilage has no direct supply of blood, nerve signals, or nutrition and relies on diffusion through the surrounding tissues.

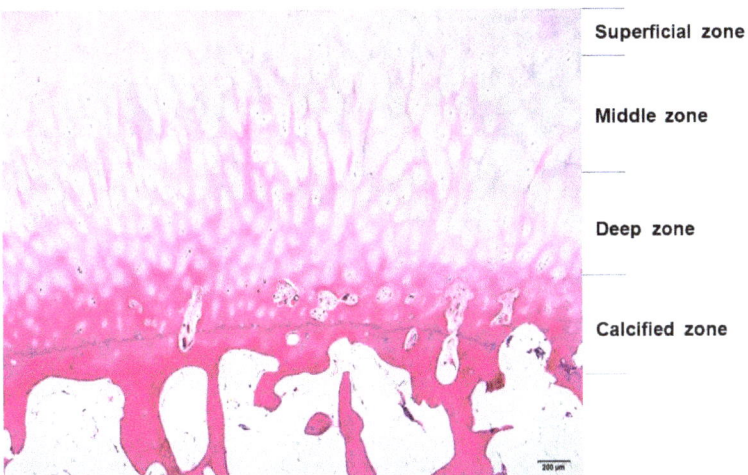

Figure 3. The structure of articular cartilage, comprised of four zones: superficial, middle, deep, and calcified. Among zones, there are differences in collagen fibers, arrangement of chondrocytes, and distribution of proteoglycans and glycosaminoglycans (GAGs). Hematoxylin and eosin staining. Scale bar, 200 µm.

Cartilage can be damaged easily by acute trauma or repetitive microtrauma and is exposed to mechanical stress during active daily living. Such stress can be increased to 10 or 20 times the body weight during sports activities [9]. Acute cartilage injury initiates a repair process that starts with the formation of a blood clot containing bone marrow cells that form fibrocartilaginous tissue. However, repeated microtraumas damage chondrocytes, decrease production of proteoglycan, and damage collagen meshwork. As this meshwork limits water penetration, damage leads to swelling and stiffness of the tissue. Responses to cartilage injury involve both anabolic and catabolic reactions. Aggrecan-degrading enzyme disintegrin, metalloproteinase with thrombospondin motif 5 (ADAMTS-5), and collagenase matrix metalloproteinase 13 (MMP-13), which degrades type II collagen, all contribute to the breakdown of cartilage. However, the induction of chondroprotective genes leads to anabolic effects on the cartilage [11] (Figure 4).

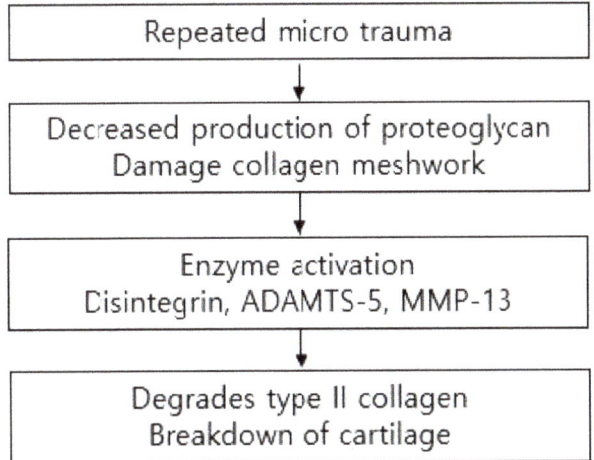

Figure 4. Mechanism leading to the breakdown of cartilage.

2.2. Microfracture and Enhanced Microfracture

Microfracture is a minimally invasive technique that uses an arthroscope to drill small, equidistant holes in subchondral bone, at least 3–4 mm apart and 4 mm in depth, with 3–4 holes per a 1 cm area [12]. This procedure induces the migration of MSCs from the bone marrow to the cartilage defect to allow the formation of fibrocartilage [13]. Kruez et al. reported that microfracture showed good short-term results in small cartilage defects but poorer results at 18 months after surgery, as reflected by Cincinnati Knee Rating System and International Cartilage Repair Society (ICRS) scores. This effect is clearer in large defects and in defects of the patellofemoral joint [14], where subchondral osteophytes develop in 20–50% of cases [15].

AMIC adds a collagen scaffold to multiple drilled holes in a cartilage defect. The scaffold of the collagen binds MSCs and growth factors to the cartilage defect, enhancing regeneration [16,17]. MSCs from microfracture have the same phenotypic plasticity as chondrogenic cells in the cartilage basal zone. With AMIC, MSCs are distributed on the membrane, which acts as the roof of a "biological chamber" [18]. A systematic review conducted in 2022 by Migliorini et al. reported that AMIC showed better clinical scores and a lower rate of revision, compared to microfracture [19].

AMIC requires an open procedure to attach the collagen matrix to the cartilage defect (Figure 5). Even a small defect in articular cartilage needs a large incision for the AMIC procedure, which can delay patient recovery.

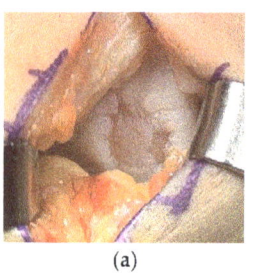 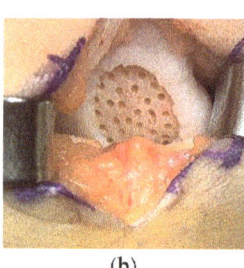 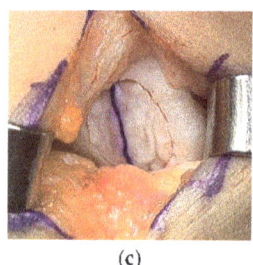 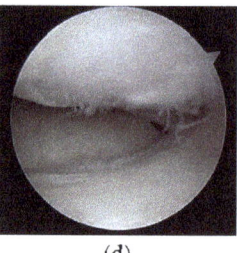

(a) (b) (c) (d)

Figure 5. (a) Cartilage defect, (b) after defect preparation, (c) membrane-covered defect, and (d) second-look arthroscopy 2 years later. Image courtesy of Prof. Sung-Hwan Kim.

To overcome this, ACIC was introduced as an alternative in 2009. Together, Shetty and Kim developed the ACIC technique to be performed with arthroscopy, leaving wounds only for the arthroscopic portal incisions [20]. In this procedure, atelocollagen gel is mixed with fibrin and thrombin and used as a scaffold. The mixture is applied on the cartilage defect after microdrilling the defect under CO_2 gas insufflation to maintain the collagen clot in the chondral defect area.

2.3. Autologous Collagen-Induced Chondrogenesis (ACIC)
2.3.1. Basic Science of ACIC

Atelocollagen is a porcine type I collagen that has been treated to detach the telomeres (Figure 6). This process suppresses immunologic reactions, increasing the effects of the surrounding environment on the collagen.

Atelocollagen induces MSCs to differentiate into chondrocytes (Figure 7). The process is examined by the expression of genes such as Sox9, type II collagen, and aggrecan. Jeong et al. conducted an animal study with rabbits involving a circular, articular cartilage defect 4 mm in diameter in the trochlear region. The 10 rabbits in the control group were not treated, and the 10 rabbits in the experimental group underwent injections of atelocollagen mixed with fibrin. After 12 weeks, the cartilage was examined. The experimental group had regenerated smooth, hyaline-like cartilage, whereas the control group showed incomplete and irregular cartilage [21] (Figure 8).

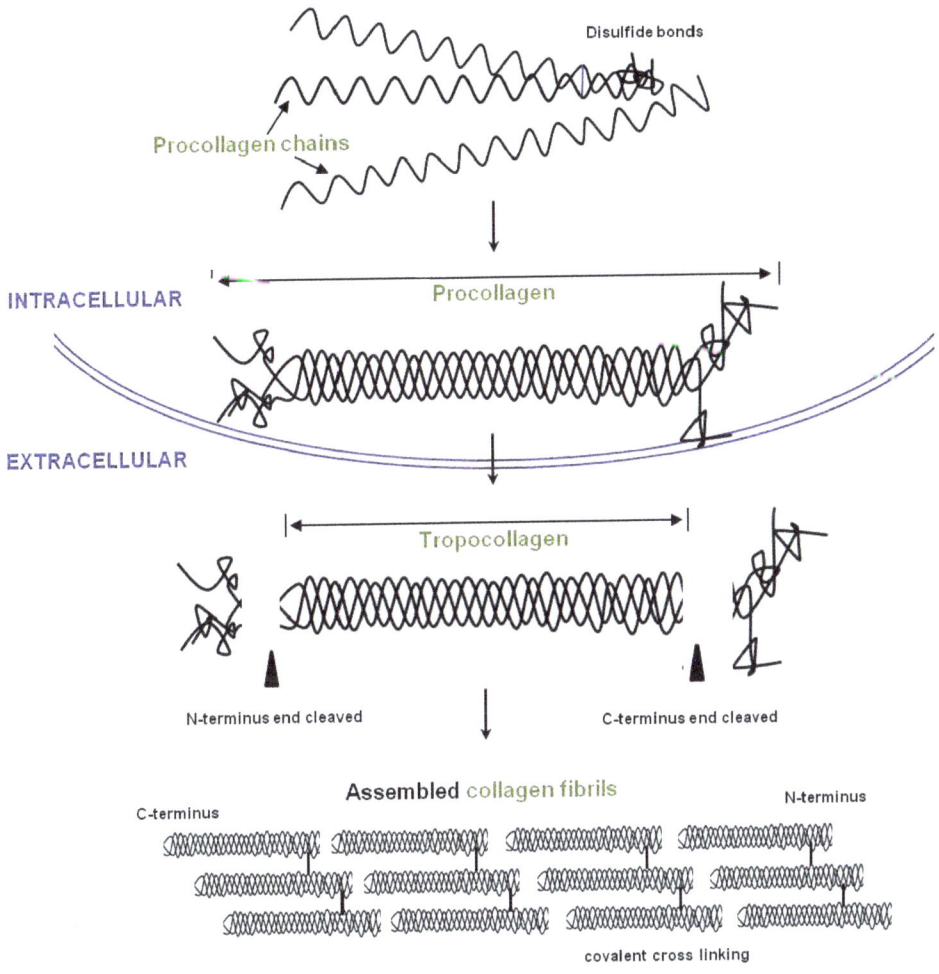

Figure 6. Overview of collagen production. Procollagen chains are synthesized and form a helix in the endoplasmic reticulum (ER). Propeptides are removed by proteinases, and the fibrils are assembled into collagen fibers in the extracellular space (EC).

Many clinical trials have used atelocollagen as an enhancing material for microfractures in a cartilage defect [20–22]. A recent study showed that atelocollagen promotes the chondrogenic differentiation of human adipose-derived MSCs. Chondrogenic genes and proteins were evaluated by RT-qPCR and ELISA, showing differentiation on day 21 [23]. MRI follow-up was conducted at 1 year and showed good cartilage defect filling [20].

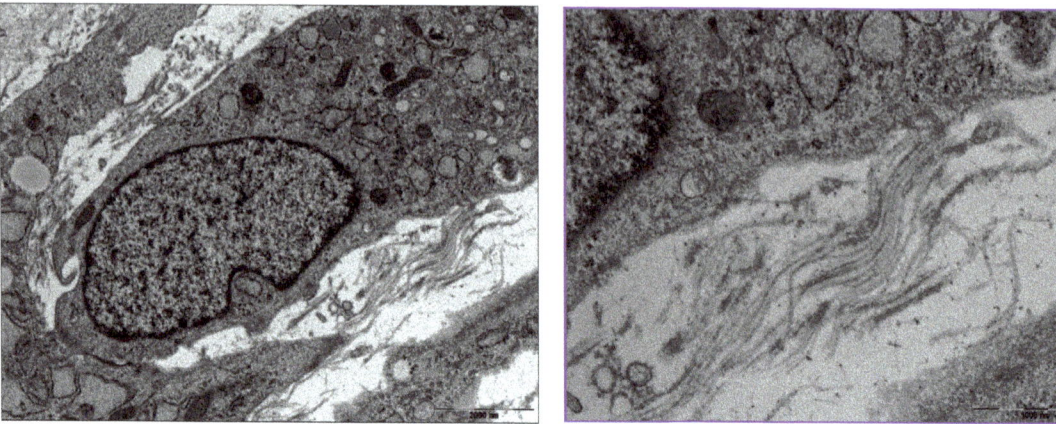

Figure 7. Transmission electron microscopy of differentiated mesenchymal stem cells (MSCs) into chondrocytes and extracellular collagen fibrils (box). (**Left**) Scale bar, 2000 nm; (**Right**) scale bar, 1000 nm.

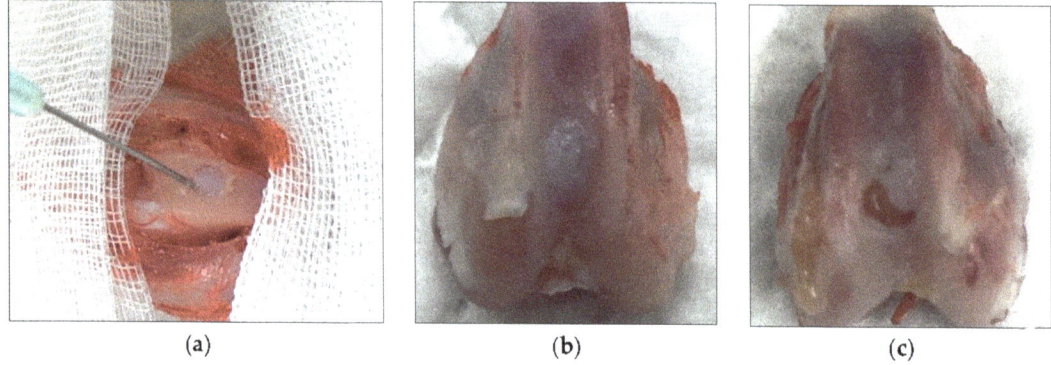

Figure 8. (**a**) Injection of atelocollagen mixed with fibrin into the trochlear defect of a rabbit knee. (**b**) Atelocollagen injection group after 12 weeks. (**c**) Control group without injection after 12 weeks.

2.3.2. Surgical Technique

ACIC is performed in the same manner as routine knee arthroscopy (Figure 9). The articular cartilage is evaluated and mapped according to ICRS guidelines. The lesion is debrided until the margins show stable vertical cartilage. The surface is lightly abraded with a curette or burr to debride sclerotic subchondral bone. Microdrilling is performed, and the subchondral bone is drilled with a 3.5 mm diameter bit up to a depth of 6–10 mm, with a 3 mm interval. After that, the arthroscopic water of the knee joint is drained, and the joint is insufflated with CO_2 (Figure 9). The surface of the subchondral bone is dried with cotton to promote adhesion by the collagen mixture. Atelocollagen gel mixed with fibrinogen and thrombin (ratio—fibrin 1: thrombin 0.2 and atelocollagen 0.8) is prepared and applied under arthroscopy. The applied mixture is assessed for stability in the cartilage defect by observing the range of motion of the knee after 2 min [20,24] (Figure 10).

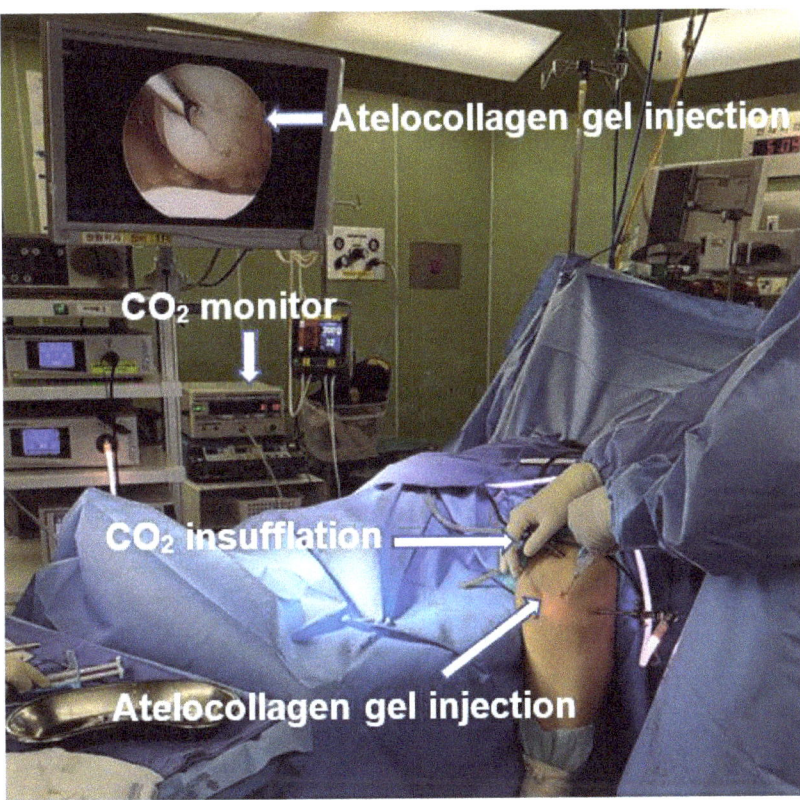

Figure 9. Arthroscopic settings for ACIC.

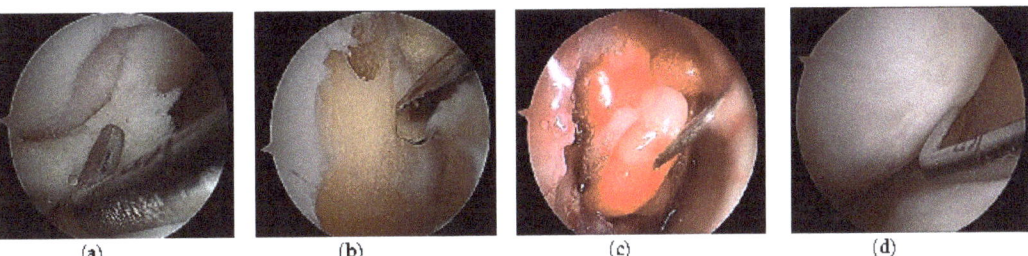

Figure 10. (**a**) Cartilage defect, (**b**) defect preparation and multiple drilling, (**c**) collagen gel injection into the defect under CO_2 gas insufflation, and (**d**) second-look arthroscopy at 2 years later.

2.3.3. Post-Operative Protocol

Patients are recommended to undergo continuous passive motion (CPM) rehabilitation for 4 h/day post-operatively for 4–6 weeks. Patients with a femoral condyle lesion are allowed partial weight-bearing at 6 weeks, and progression to full weight-bearing is encouraged at 3 months. Cartilage being repaired in patellar and trochlear lesions is protected with a knee brace locked at 0–20% movement, which is gradually increased to 90% over 6 weeks. Full weight-bearing is encouraged with protected knee motion right after the surgery [24].

2.3.4. Clinical Results

Clinical studies of ACIC were collected through PubMed, the Cochrane library, and ScienceDirect, with keywords "autologous collagen-induced chondrogenesis" and "porcine, collagen, chondrogenesis"; there have been several studies using ACIC on the knee or the talus. Excluding studies about the talus, five studies were analyzed. Two studies were randomized, controlled trials (RCTs), one study was a matched, comparative study, and two were noncomparative studies. (Table 1)

Table 1. Summary of clinical studies on ACIC for knee chondral defects.

Authors	No. of Patients	Study Design	Cohort Group	Clinical Scores	MRI Evaluation
Kim, M.S. [25]	100	Multicenter RCT	Microfracture	KOOS pain, VAS; significant difference	MOCART
Silva [26]	11	Comparative study	Microfracture	SF-36, IKDC; significant difference	none
Kim, S.J. [24]	30	Longitudinal study		Lysholm, KOOS, IKDC	MOCART
Shetty [20]	10	Longitudinal study		Lysholm	MOCART

KOOS: Knee Injury and Osteoarthritis Outcome Score, MOCART: Magnetic Resonance Observation of Cartilage Repair Tissue, IKDC: International Knee Documentation Committee.

Kim M.S. et al. compared porcine-derived collagen-augmented chondrogenesis to microfracture in 2020 in a multicenter, randomized control study. One hundred patients were randomly assigned to a microfracture or an investigational group. Clinical and MRI outcomes were assessed at 12 and 24 months post-operatively. Magnetic resonance observation of cartilage repair tissue (MOCART) assessment was used to analyze cartilage tissue repair. MOCART score, VAS score, and KOOS pain score were significantly improved in the test group. In addition, the investigational group showed better filling of the cartilage defect in the knee joint [25].

Silva et al. compared ACIC to microfracture in 2020 based on clinical scores at 6 months and 24 months. Eleven patients who underwent ACIC were compared with 11 age- and sex-matched patients who underwent a microfracture-only procedure. The ACIC group showed a significantly better SF36 mental function, International Knee Documentation Committee (IKDC) score, and VAS score at 24 months [26].

Kim S.J. et al. evaluated 30 patients with ICRS grade III/IVa symptomatic knees who were treated with ACIC. Patients were followed for 6 years, and the Lysholm score, Knee Injury and Osteoarthritis Outcome Score (KOOS), and IKDC score were significantly improved. Radiological evaluation was performed using MRI at 6 months, 1 year, and 3 years using the MOCART scoring system. The mean MOCART score was 78, similar to those of other successful cartilage repair techniques [24].

Shetty et al. evaluated 10 patients with symptomatic chondral defects who were treated with ACIC. Morphological and biochemical MRIs were performed at the 1-year follow-up, and the Lysholm score was assessed at the 2-year follow-up. MRIs showed good cartilage defect filling and suggested hyaline-like repair tissue, and the Lysholm score was significantly improved [20].

3. Discussion

Mithoefer et al. conducted a systematic review about microfracture in 2009. Microfracture was a good first-line treatment for cartilage defect but did have a few disadvantages. The short-term outcome was good, but the long-term outcome was inconclusive, due to insufficient data. Shortcomings of microfracture included limited regeneration of hyaline-like cartilage, variable volume of cartilage repair, and functional deterioration [15]. As a consequence, many cartilage regeneration techniques were designed to overcome these limitations of microfracture. ACIC not only improved short-term clinical outcomes, it also significantly improved long-term clinical outcomes at 6 years [24].

ACIC is one of the methods for enhancing cartilage repair; it has no donor site comorbidity and is performed using arthroscopy in a single stage. An animal study and an in vitro study showed that atelocollagen promotes hyaline-like cartilage regeneration [21,23]. These encouraging outcomes and the concept of a single-stage cartilage resurfacing technique are attractive for many surgeons.

Though ACIC is performed mostly under arthroscopy, one study involved a mini open procedure. A multicenter study by Kim M.S. et al. involved an open procedure applying atelocollagen at the chondral defect, whereas S Kim S.J. used CO_2 gas to inflate the joint space while applying atelocollagen. CO_2 gas allows the gravity-independent application of the gel mixture without opening the joint. Thus, all procedures can be conducted under arthroscopy, minimizing soft tissue damage. The method of microfracture may influence the outcomes of cartilage regeneration. Kim S.J. used a 3.5 mm diameter drill up to a depth of 10 mm, with a 3 mm interval. On the other hand, the multicenter study of Kim M.S. did not specify the technique of microfracture. A fibrin and thrombin mixture is used to stabilize the collagen scaffold; however, the mixture ratio varies among studies. Since the collagen scaffold plays a major role in the good outcome of the microfracture technique, the durability of the collagen scaffold may influence the outcomes of cartilage regeneration.

Clinical trials about ACIC are limited. Silva et al. compared ACIC with microfracture in an RCT, another of which was performed by Kim M.S. et al. In addition, Kim S.J. et al. and Shetty et al. found better clinical results and superior MRI findings to microfracture.

This review showed the need to standardize reporting of the AMIC technique to enable future comparisons of efficacy and determine the effects of various technical variations [5]. Some of the technical factors that should be reported are as follows:

(1) Arthroscopic or open surgery
(2) Method of subchondral drilling or microfracture
(3) Type of gel used
(4) Fixation of the matrix or scaffold
(5) Postoperative rehabilitation

In addition, we suggest that the measures for outcomes be standardized. The most common outcome instruments are KOOS, Lysholm, and IKDC scoring. We suggest that these three instruments be used in studies with follow-ups of at least 1–2 years for adequate comparison. MRI protocols for cartilage assessment, such as the modified MOCART score suggested by Marlovits et al., [27], should be routine to allow the comparison of follow-up radiographic studies.

An advantage of ACIC is its cost-effectiveness, compared to ACI. In the UK, the cost of ACI is three times that of ACIC [28]. In addition, ACIC has no donor site morbidity and is performed in one stage.

There are some limitations of ACIC. The few prospective studies of ACIC each had a small sample size. While the results were positive and showed the usefulness of ACIC, comparison studies to other enhanced microfracture techniques are needed.

4. Conclusions

Our review of the ACIC technique suggests it is a promising cartilage repair technique. The outcome scores and MRI results are promising, but there are few comparative studies with other cell-based cartilage methods. Ideal conditions for chondrogenesis should be studied.

Author Contributions: Conceptualization, S.J.K. and A.A.S.; investigation, Y.H.K. and J.H.L.; writing—draft preparation, Y.S.C.; description of surgical methods, S.J.K.; description of basic science, S.A.K.; administration, Y.S.C.; supervision, S.J.K. All authors have read and agreed to the published version of the manuscript.

Funding: This research received no external funding.

Data Availability Statement: Previous studies included in this study can be found on PubMed.

Conflicts of Interest: The authors declare no conflict of interest.

References

1. Martin, R.; Jakob, R.P. Review of K.H. Pridie (1959) on "A method of resurfacing osteoarthritic knee joints". *J. ISAKOS* **2022**, *7*, 39–46. [CrossRef] [PubMed]
2. Steadman, J.R.; Briggs, K.K.; Rodrigo, J.J.; Kocher, M.S.; Gill, T.J.; Rodkey, W.G. Outcomes of microfracture for traumatic chondral defects of the knee: Average 11-year follow-up. *Arthroscopy* **2003**, *19*, 477–484. [CrossRef] [PubMed]
3. Hunziker, E.B. Articular cartilage repair: Basic science and clinical progress. A review of the current status and prospects. *Osteoarthr. Cartil.* **2002**, *10*, 432–463. [CrossRef] [PubMed]
4. Redler, L.H.; Caldwell, J.M.; Schulz, B.M.; Levine, W.N. Management of articular cartilage defects of the knee. *Phys. Sportsmed.* **2012**, *40*, 20–35. [CrossRef]
5. Lee, Y.H.; Suzer, F.; Thermann, H. Autologous Matrix-Induced Chondrogenesis in the Knee: A Review. *Cartilage* **2014**, *5*, 145–153. [CrossRef]
6. Efe, T.; Theisen, C.; Fuchs-Winkelmann, S.; Stein, T.; Getgood, A.; Rominger, M.B.; Paletta, J.R.; Schofer, M.D. Cell-free collagen type I matrix for repair of cartilage defects-clinical and magnetic resonance imaging results. *Knee Surg. Sports Traumatol. Arthrosc.* **2012**, *20*, 1915–1922. [CrossRef]
7. Benthien, J.P.; Behrens, P. The treatment of chondral and osteochondral defects of the knee with autologous matrix-induced chondrogenesis (AMIC): Method description and recent developments. *Knee Surg. Sports Traumatol. Arthrosc.* **2011**, *19*, 1316–1319. [CrossRef]
8. Dhollander, A.A.; De Neve, F.; Almqvist, K.F.; Verdonk, R.; Lambrecht, S.; Elewaut, D.; Verbruggen, G.; Verdonk, P.C. Autologous matrix-induced chondrogenesis combined with platelet-rich plasma gel: Technical description and a five pilot patients report. *Knee Surg. Sports Traumatol. Arthrosc.* **2011**, *19*, 536–542. [CrossRef]
9. Solanki, K.; Shanmugasundaram, S.; Shetty, N.; Kim, S.J. Articular cartilage repair & joint preservation: A review of the current status of biological approach. *J. Clin. Orthop. Trauma* **2021**, *22*, 101602.
10. Armiento, A.R.; Alini, M.; Stoddart, M.J. Articular fibrocartilage—Why does hyaline cartilage fail to repair? *Adv. Drug Deliv. Rev.* **2019**, *146*, 289–305. [CrossRef]
11. Burleigh, A.; Chanalaris, A.; Gardiner, M.D.; Driscoll, C.; Boruc, O.; Saklatvala, J.; Vincent, T.L. Joint immobilization prevents murine osteoarthritis and reveals the highly mechanosensitive nature of protease expression in vivo. *Arthritis Rheum.* **2012**, *64*, 2278–2288. [CrossRef] [PubMed]
12. Steadman, J.R.; Rodkey, W.G.; Rodrigo, J.J. Microfracture: Surgical technique and rehabilitation to treat chondral defects. *Clin. Orthop. Relat. Res.* **2001**, S362–S369. [CrossRef] [PubMed]
13. Gao, L.; Goebel, L.K.H.; Orth, P.; Cucchiarini, M.; Madry, H. Subchondral drilling for articular cartilage repair: A systematic review of translational research. *Dis. Model. Mech.* **2018**, *11*, dmm034280. [CrossRef]
14. Kreuz, P.C.; Steinwachs, M.R.; Erggelet, C.; Krause, S.J.; Konrad, G.; Uhl, M.; Sudkamp, N. Results after microfracture of full-thickness chondral defects in different compartments in the knee. *Osteoarthr. Cartil.* **2006**, *14*, 1119–1125. [CrossRef]
15. Mithoefer, K.; McAdams, T.; Williams, R.J.; Kreuz, P.C.; Mandelbaum, B.R. Clinical efficacy of the microfracture technique for articular cartilage repair in the knee: An evidence-based systematic analysis. *Am. J. Sports Med.* **2009**, *37*, 2053–2063. [CrossRef]
16. Benthien, J.P.; Behrens, P. Autologous matrix-induced chondrogenesis (AMIC). A one-step procedure for retropatellar articular resurfacing. *Acta Orthop. Belg.* **2010**, *76*, 260–263.
17. Kramer, J.; Böhrnsen, F.; Lindner, U.; Behrens, P.; Schlenke, P.; Rohwedel, J. In vivo matrix-guided human mesenchymal stem cells. *Cell. Mol. Life Sci.* **2006**, *63*, 616–626. [CrossRef]
18. Tallheden, T.; Dennis, J.E.; Lennon, D.P.; Sjögren-Jansson, E.; Caplan, A.I.; Lindahl, A. Phenotypic plasticity of human articular chondrocytes. *JBJS* **2003**, *85* (Suppl. 2), 93–100. [CrossRef]
19. Migliorini, F.; Maffulli, N.; Baroncini, A.; Bell, A.; Hildebrand, F.; Schenker, H. Autologous matrix-induced chondrogenesis is effective for focal chondral defects of the knee. *Sci. Rep.* **2022**, *12*, 9328. [CrossRef]
20. Shetty, A.A.; Kim, S.J.; Bilagi, P.; Stelzeneder, D. Autologous collagen-induced chondrogenesis: Single-stage arthroscopic cartilage repair technique. *Orthopedics* **2013**, *36*, e648–e652. [CrossRef]
21. Jeong, I.H.; Shetty, A.A.; Kim, S.J.; Jang, J.D.; Kim, Y.J.; Chung, Y.G.; Choi, N.Y.; Liu, C.H. Autologous collagen-induced chondrogenesis using fibrin and atelocollagen mixture. *Cells Tissues Organs* **2013**, *198*, 278–288. [CrossRef] [PubMed]
22. Shetty, A.A.; Kim, S.J.; Shetty, V.; Jang, J.D.; Huh, S.W.; Lee, D.H. Autologous collagen induced chondrogenesis (ACIC: Shetty-Kim technique)—A matrix based acellular single stage arthroscopic cartilage repair technique. *J. Clin. Orthop. Trauma* **2016**, *7*, 164–169. [CrossRef] [PubMed]
23. Kim, S.A.; Sur, Y.J.; Cho, M.L.; Go, E.J.; Kim, Y.H.; Shetty, A.A.; Kim, S.J. Atelocollagen promotes chondrogenic differentiation of human adipose-derived mesenchymal stem cells. *Sci. Rep.* **2020**, *10*, 10678. [CrossRef]
24. Kim, S.J.; Shetty, A.A.; Kurian, N.M.; Ahmed, S.; Shetty, N.; Stelzeneder, D.; Shin, Y.W.; Cho, Y.J.; Lee, S.H. Articular cartilage repair using autologous collagen-induced chondrogenesis (ACIC): A pragmatic and cost-effective enhancement of a traditional technique. *Knee Surg. Sports Traumatol. Arthrosc.* **2020**, *28*, 2598–2603. [CrossRef]

25. Kim, M.S.; Chun, C.H.; Wang, J.H.; Kim, J.G.; Kang, S.B.; Yoo, J.D.; Chon, J.G.; Kim, M.K.; Moon, C.W.; Chang, C.B.; et al. Microfractures Versus a Porcine-Derived Collagen-Augmented Chondrogenesis Technique for Treating Knee Cartilage Defects: A Multicenter Randomized Controlled Trial. *Arthroscopy* **2020**, *36*, 1612–1624. [CrossRef]
26. Silva, A.N.; Lim, W.J.; Cheok, J.W.G.; Gatot, C.; Tan, H.C.A. Autologous collagen-induced chondrogenesis versus microfracture for chondral defects of the knee: Surgical technique and 2-year comparison outcome study. *J. Orthop.* **2020**, *22*, 294–299. [CrossRef]
27. Marlovits, S.; Singer, P.; Zeller, P.; Mandl, I.; Haller, J.; Trattnig, S. Magnetic resonance observation of cartilage repair tissue (MOCART) for the evaluation of autologous chondrocyte transplantation: Determination of interobserver variability and correlation to clinical outcome after 2 years. *Eur. J. Radiol.* **2006**, *57*, 16–23. [CrossRef] [PubMed]
28. Mistry, H.; Connock, M.; Pink, J.; Shyangdan, D.; Clar, C.; Royle, P.; Court, R.; Biant, L.C.; Metcalfe, A.; Waugh, N. Autologous chondrocyte implantation in the knee: Systematic review and economic evaluation. *Health Technol. Assess.* **2017**, *21*, 1–294. [CrossRef]

Disclaimer/Publisher's Note: The statements, opinions and data contained in all publications are solely those of the individual author(s) and contributor(s) and not of MDPI and/or the editor(s). MDPI and/or the editor(s) disclaim responsibility for any injury to people or property resulting from any ideas, methods, instructions or products referred to in the content.

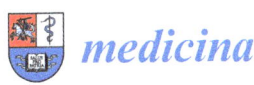

Article

Allogeneic Umbilical Cord-Blood-Derived Mesenchymal Stem Cells and Hyaluronate Composite Combined with High Tibial Osteotomy for Medial Knee Osteoarthritis with Full-Thickness Cartilage Defects

Yong-Beom Park [1,*], Han-Jun Lee [2], Hyun-Cheul Nam [2] and Jung-Gwan Park [3]

1. Department of Orthopedic Surgery, Chung-Ang University Gwangmyeong Hospital, Chung-Ang University College of Medicine, Seoul 06911, Republic of Korea
2. Department of Orthopedic Surgery, Chung-Ang University Hospital, Chung-Ang University College of Medicine, Seoul 06973, Republic of Korea
3. Department of Orthopedic Surgery, Madisesang Hospital, Seoul 02038, Republic of Korea
* Correspondence: whybe78@cau.ac.kr

Abstract: *Background and Objectives*: Although the effects of cartilage repair in patients who are undergoing high tibial osteotomy (HTO) remains controversial, cartilage repair may be required for the full-thickness cartilage defect because of a concern of lower clinical outcome. The purpose of this study was to investigate clinical outcome and cartilage repair following implantation of allogeneic umbilical cord-blood-derived MSCs (UCB-MSCs)–hyaluronate composite in patients who received HTO for medial knee osteoarthritis (OA) with full-thickness cartilage defect. *Materials and Methods*: Inclusion criteria were patients with a medial knee OA, a full-thickness cartilage defect (International Cartilage Repair Society (ICRS) grade IV) ≥ 3 cm^2 of the medial femoral condyle, and a varus deformity $\geq 5°$. The full-thickness cartilage defect was treated with implantation of an allogeneic UCB-MSCs–hyaluronate composite following medial open-wedge HTO. Visual analogue scale for pain and Western Ontario and McMaster Universities Osteoarthritis Index (WOMAC) score were assessed at each follow-up. Cartilage repair was assessed by the ICRS cartilage repair assessment system at second-look arthroscopy when the plate was removed. *Results*: Twelve patients (mean age 56.1 years; mean defect size: 4.5 cm^2) were included, and 10 patients underwent second-look arthroscopy during plate removal after a minimum of 1 year after the HTO. At the final follow-up of mean 2.9 years (range; 1–6 years), all clinical outcomes had improved. At second-look arthroscopy, repaired tissue was observed in all cases. One case (10%) showed grade I, seven (70%) cases showed grade II, and two (20%) cases showed grade III according to ICRS cartilage repair assessment system, which meant that 80% showed an overall repair assessment of "normal" or "nearly normal". *Conclusion*: Allogeneic UCB-MSCs-HA composite implantation combined with HTO resulted in favorable clinical outcome and cartilage repair in all cases. These findings suggest that UCB-MSCs-HA composite implantation combined with HTO would be a good therapeutic option for patients with knee OA and full-thickness cartilage defects.

Keywords: osteoarthritis; cartilage; high tibial osteotomy; stem cells; umbilical cord blood

1. Introduction

High tibial osteotomy (HTO) is a well-established treatment option in knee osteoarthritis (OA) with varus deformity [1–3]. Shifting the mechanical axis of the lower extremity to the lateral side decreases the contact pressure on the medial compartment, which can provide the biological environment to prevent further degenerative changes [4,5]. Although several studies reported favorable short-term and mid-term outcomes after HTO, favorable long-term outcomes may be associate with adequate cartilage repair [6,7].

Although several therapeutic approaches to restore the cartilage have been investigated, the currently available options are not optimal for cartilage repair in knee OA. For the treatment of osteoarthritic cartilage defects, however, microfracture has been used [8,9], but it showed the deterioration of clinical outcomes over time [10].

Recently, mesenchymal stem cells (MSCs) have been gaining attention as a potential cell source for cartilage repair in older patients because of their unique properties, including immunomodulatory and anti-inflammatory capacities, and paracrine activity [11–16]. Allogeneic umbilical cord-blood-derived MSCs (UCB-MSCs) have advantages of non-invasive cell collection, high expansion capacity, hypo-immunogenicity, and immunomodulatory capacity [17–19]. Allogeneic UCB-MSCs implantation showed the safety and efficacy of cartilage repair in older patients with knee OA [20–24]. However, clinical outcomes and cartilage repair after allogeneic UCB-MSCs implantation combined with HTO have been reported rarely [25–27].

The purpose of this study was to investigate clinical outcome and cartilage repair following implantation of allogeneic UCB-MSCs–hyaluronate (UCB-MSCs-HA) composite combined with HTO for older patients who had medial knee OA with large full-thickness cartilage defect. It was hypothesized that an implantation of UCB-MSCs-HA composite would result in good cartilage remodeling and favorable clinical outcomes.

2. Materials and Methods

A total of 62 patients who underwent HTO between 2016 and 2021 were retrospectively reviewed for study inclusion. HTO was indicated for patients who had isolated medial compartmental OA and varus malalignment of the lower extremity (varus deformity $\geq 5°$) without ligament instability. Patients who underwent HTO and concomitant implantation of a UCB-MSCs-HA composite (Cartistem®) for medial compartmental OA and a full-thickness cartilage defect (International Cartilage Repair Society (ICRS) grade IV) ≥ 3 cm^2 of the medial femoral condyle were included. Patients with a history of previous knee surgery, other cartilage repair procedure such as microfracture, and follow-up loss were excluded. Finally, 12 patients were included for this study (Figure 1). This study was approved by the institutional review board of our hospital (IRB No. 2109-025-19385).

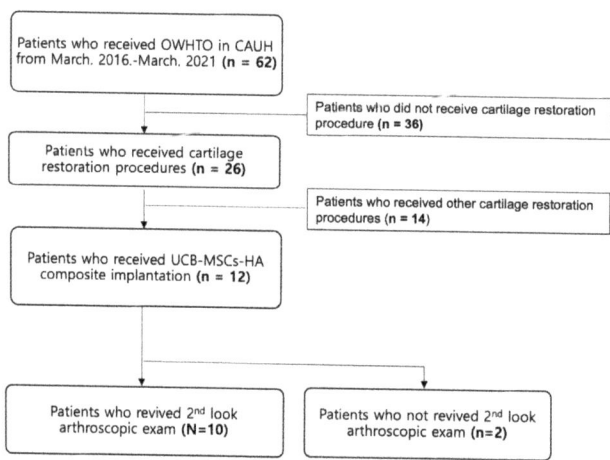

Figure 1. Flow diagram of the included patients.

3. UCB-MSCs-HA Composite

The medicinal product (UCB-MSCs-HA composite, Cartistem®) of this study was approved by the Korea Food and Drug Administration in 2012. Allogeneic UCB-MSCs were taken from donor UCB stored at a cord blood bank and were produced according to good manufacturing practice guidelines by Medipost (Seoul, South Korea). This product comprises 1.5 mL of UCB-MSCs (7.5×10^6) and 4% HA.

4. Surgical Technique

A standard arthroscopy was performed to assess cartilage defects, and arthroscopic procedures including debridement of the cartilage flaps, meniscectomy, or meniscal repair were performed if necessary. Biplanar open-wedge HTO was then performed according to preoperative planning to achieve a valgus alignment of 3–5°.

After HTO, the UCB-MSCs-HA composite was implanted following the previously reported technique [20,21]. A small arthrotomy was made to expose the cartilage defect on the femoral condyle. Cartilage defects was prepared for healthy underlying bone and peripheral margin. Multiple drill holes (4 mm × 4 mm (diameter × depth)) in the subchondral bone were made to place the UCB-MSCs-HA composite. In addition, multiple drill holes with small diameter of 1.4 mm were made between the larger drill holes for better integration. The UCB-MSCs-HA composite was implanted into the drill holes carefully (Figure 2).

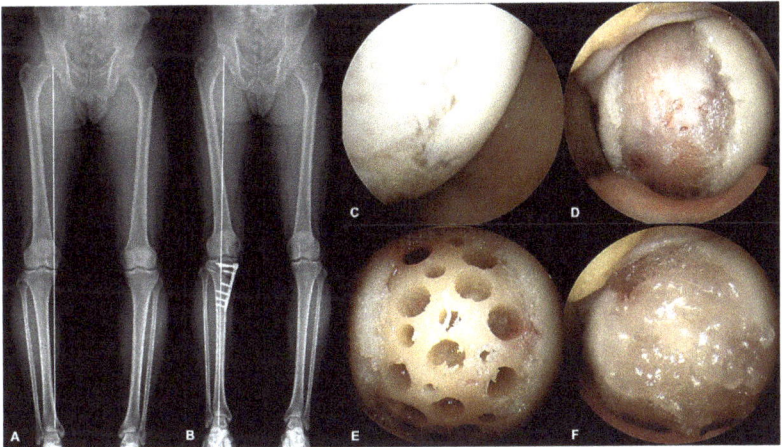

Figure 2. Surgical procedure of implantation for the allogeneic UCB-MSCs-HA composite and combined HTO. (**A**) Preoperative whole-lower-extremity radiograph showed varus limb alignment. (**B**) Postoperative whole-lower-extremity radiograph showed valgus limb alignment after HTO. (**C**) Arthroscopic inspection and confirmation of ICRS 3 and 4 cartilage defect. (**D**) Cartilage defect preparation for underlying healthy subchondral bone and peripheral margin. (**E**) Multiple drill holes in the cartilage defect site. (**F**) Implantation of the UCB-MSCs-HA composite into drill holes and cartilage defect surface (Cartistem®).

5. Postoperative Rehabilitation

Venous impulse pumps were prescribed to prevent deep vein thrombosis. Quadriceps-strengthening and straight-leg-raising exercises were performed immediately after surgery. Additionally, a range-of-motion (ROM) exercise was allowed from postoperative day 1 and progressed as tolerated. Partial-weight bearing with crutch ambulation was allowed during 6 weeks, and full-weight bearing was allowed after 12 weeks. The second arthroscopy was performed during plate removal after the union of the osteotomy site.

6. Outcome Measures

Clinical and radiological evaluation were performed preoperatively at 1, 3, and 6 months; postoperatively at 1 year; and annually thereafter. A 100 mm visual analogue scale (VAS) for pain and Western Ontario and McMaster Universities Osteoarthritis Index (WOMAC) [28] were evaluated. Anteroposterior, lateral, and merchant views and whole-lower-extremity radiographs were obtained for radiological evaluation, including lower-limb alignment and Kellgren–Lawrence grade. The cartilage repair of the medial femoral condyle was assessed visually during second-look arthroscopy using ICRS Macroscopic Assessment of Cartilage Repair [29]. ICRS Macroscopic Assessment of Cartilage Repair consists of three items: degree of defect repair, integration to border zone, and macroscopic appearance, which is graded as the following: normal as grade I, nearly normal as grade II, abnormal as grade III, and severely abnormal as grade IV.

7. Statistical Analysis

VAS and WOMAC score for pain and Wilcoxon signed-rank test were used. All statistical analyses were executed using IBM SPSS statistics version 23.0 (IBM Corp., Armonk, NY, USA); a p-value < 0.05 was considered significant.

8. Results

Twelve patients (9 women and 3 men) were included in this study. A mean age was 54.3 ± 7.8 years (range, 42–66 years). Seven patients had meniscal problems, which was treated by meniscectomy. The mean follow-up was 2.9 years (range, 1 to 6 years). The mean cartilage defect size of the medial femoral condyle was 4.5 cm^2 (range, 4 to 6.9 cm^2) (Table 1).

Table 1. Demographics and Baseline Characteristics of patients of this study.

	UCB-MSCs-HA Composite
Age years (mean ± SD)	54.3 ± 7.8
Sex n (%)	
Male	3 (25.0)
Female	9 (75.0)
BMI (body mass index) kg/m^2 (mean ± SD)	25.9 ± 2.8
HKA angle	173.3 ± 2.8
Osteoarthritis n (%)	
K-L grade I	0
K-L grade II	2 (16.7)
K-L grade III	9 (75.0)
K-L grade IV	1 (8.3)
Pain on 100 mm VAS * (mean ± SD)	61.6 ± 7.9
WOMAC score † (mean ± SD)	46.6 ± 5.3
Cartilage Defect Characteristics	
Size cm^2 (mean ± SD)	4.5 ± 1.0
Location n (%)	
MFC	9 (75.0)
MFC and MTP	3 (25.0)

Kellgren–Lawrence (K-L) grade II or III, sustaining typical bipolar lesions with varying degrees of severity. * Pain on the 100 mm visual analogue scale (VAS) ranges from 0 to 100, with higher score indicating worse results. † Western Ontario and McMaster Universities Osteoarthritis Index (WOMAC) ranges from 0 to 92, with higher score indicating worse results.

At final follow-up, the VAS pain score was significantly improved from 61.6 to 11.4 and the WOMAC score from 46.6 to 12.3 (p < 0.05, Figure 3). The lower-limb alignment was changed from varus 6.7 to valgus 2.2.

At an average of 18 months after a UCB-MSCs-HA composite implantation combined with HTO, 10 patients underwent second-look arthroscopy during plate removal. At second-look arthroscopy, repaired tissue was observed in all cases. The mean total score of ICRS Macroscopic Assessment of Cartilage Repair was 8.4 (range, 5 to 12 points) (Table 2). One case (10%) showed grade I, seven (70%) cases showed grade II, and two (20%) cases showed grade III (Figure 4), which meant that 80% of the repaired cartilage was classified as "normal" or "nearly normal".

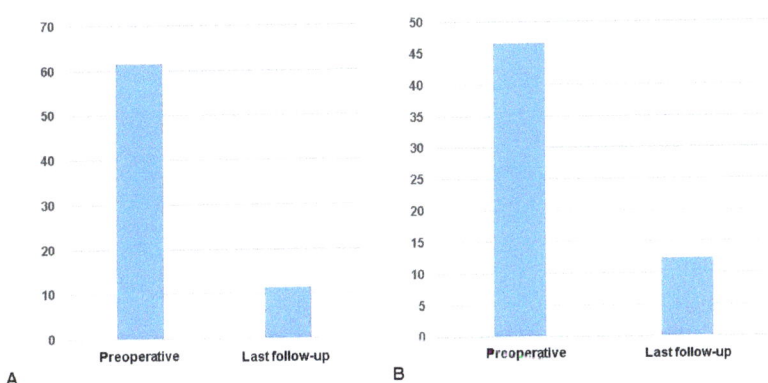

Figure 3. Clinical outcomes after the UCB-MSCs-HA composite implantation combined with HTO. (**A**) Pain on the 100 mm visual analogue scale (VAS) score; (**B**) Western Ontario and McMaster Universities Osteoarthritis Index (WOMAC) score.

Table 2. Cartilage repair assessment of second arthroscopic findings.

	Score	Mean ± SD
Degree of defect repair		
Level with surrounding cartilage	4	
75% repair of defect depth	3	
50% repair of defect depth	2	3.5 ± 0.5
25% repair of defect depth	1	
0% repair of defect depth	0	
Integration to the border zone		
Complete integration with surrounding cartilage	4	
Demarcating border < 1 mm	3	
2/4 of graft integrated, 1/4 with a notable border >1 mm width	2	2.5 ± 1.1
1/2 of graft integrated with surrounding cartilage, 1/2 with a notable border >1 mm	1	
From no contact to 1/4 of graft integrated with surrounding cartilage	0	
Macroscopic appearance		
Intact smooth surface	4	
Fibrillated surface	3	
Small, scattered fissures or cracks	2	2.4 ± 1.0
Several small or few but large fissures	1	
Total degeneration of the grafted area	0	
Total score (mean ± SD)	0–12	8.4 ± 2.3
Grading system *		n (%)
Grade 1: Normal	12	1 (10)
Grade 2: Nearly normal	8–11	7 (70)
Grade 3: Abnormal	5–7	2 (20)
Grade 4: Severely abnormal	0–4	0 (0)

* Grade was classified according to the total score.

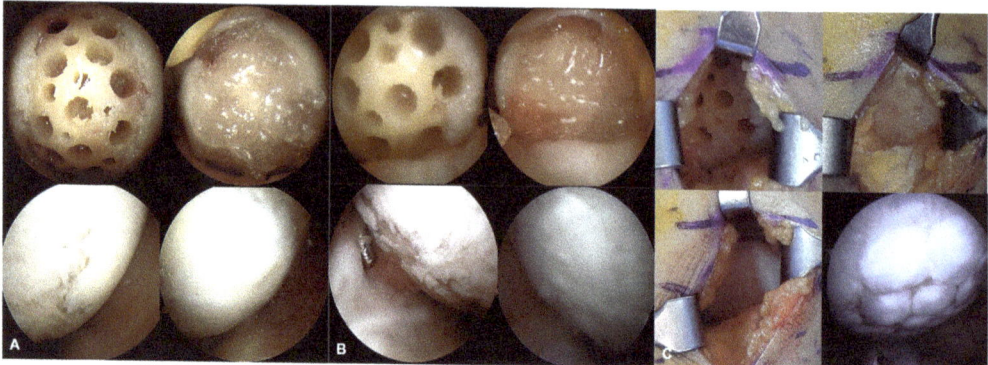

Figure 4. Evaluation of the repaired cartilage according to the ICRS Macroscopic Assessment of Cartilage Repair during second look arthroscopy. (**A**) A case of ICRS cartilage repair assessment score of 12, which was grade I in overall repair assessment, i.e., "normal". (**B**) A case of ICRS cartilage repair assessment score of 9, which was grade II in overall repair assessment, i.e., "nearly normal". (**C**) A case of ICRS cartilage repair assessment score of 5, which was grade II in overall repair assessment, i.e., "abnormal".

9. Discussion

This study demonstrated that implantation of an allogeneic UCB-MSCs-HA composite combined with HTO provides favorable clinical outcome and cartilage restoration for full-thickness cartilage defects in knee OA with varus deformity. The consistent regenerative response was observed in all cases despite large full-thickness cartilage defects in knee OA, which may suggest that UCB-MSCs-HA implantation is required for better outcomes in patients who planned to undergo HTO for medial compartmental OA with large full-thickness cartilage defects and varus deformity.

The repaired cartilage was observed in all cases during second-look arthroscopy after UCB-MSCs-HA composite implantation with concomitant HTO. A limited number of studies has reported that only HTO without cartilage repair procedure could provide cartilage repair potentially in some cases due to the change of the biomechanical environment [4,5]. However, the quality and quantity of the repaired cartilage were still insufficient. In addition, a randomized controlled trial regarding MSCs implantation combined with HTO reported a higher proportion of cartilage repair compared to HTO only [30]. A recent meta-analysis including four comparative studies reported that intra-articular MSCs administration combined with HTO showed better cartilage repair compared with the HTO alone [31]. In line with previous a meta-analysis, intra-articular UCB-MSCs-HA composite implantation combined with HTO in this study showed cartilage repair in all patients with medial compartmental OA with large full-thickness cartilage defects and varus deformity. Taken together with the results of this study and those of the meta-analysis, intra-articular MSCs administration could enhance cartilage repair in patients who underwent HTO for the treatment of knee OA and varus deformity.

Interestingly, regardless of the status of cartilage repair, pain and function at final follow-up was significantly improved compared to preoperative evaluation. Several studies have demonstrated that HTO could provide satisfactory pain and functional improvements [5,32,33], which may be induced by the decrease of contact pressure on the medial compartment by shifting the load from the medial to lateral compartment [4,5]. A recent meta-analysis study reported that intra-articular MSCs administration combined with HTO may improve clinical outcomes as compared to HTO alone [31]. In line with a previous meta-analysis, intra-articular UCB-MSCs-HA composite implantation combined with HTO in this study showed significant improvement in pain and function in all patients with knee OA with large full-thickness cartilage defects and varus deformity. Taken together, cartilage repair with MSCs administration in patients who underwent HTO could be a viable option for improved clinical outcomes at long-term follow-up.

To date, there has been no reliable cartilage repair procedure for favorable outcomes in osteoarthritic cartilage defects [34]. Microfracture, the most common of a small cartilage defects, generally leads to fibrous repair tissue with unsatisfactory durability [8,9]. Autologous chondrocyte implantation (ACI) is usually recommended for younger patients with large focal chondral defects [35]. Both procedures are generally limited to restoring cartilage in large defects of older patients, with outcomes tending to deteriorate over time [10]. Some recent studies have demonstrated that surgical implantation of UCB-MSCs-HA composite could result in reliable cartilage repair in osteoarthritic cartilage defects. In this regard, surgical implantation of the UCB-MSCs-HA composite was selected for the cartilage repair procedure in this study. In accordance with previous studies with UCB-MSCs-HA composite, cartilage repair was observed in all cases despite full-thickness large cartilage defects more than 4 cm^2. Therefore, surgical implantation of UCB-MSCs-HA composite could be a reliable option for cartilage repair in osteoarthritic knees.

Some limitations of this study need to be addressed. First, this study was retrospective and did not include a control group. However, clinical outcome including cartilage repair after allogeneic UCB-MSCs implantation combined with HTO has rarely been reported [25–27]. Second, a small number of patients were included in this study. However, the regenerated cartilage was evaluated via second-look arthroscopy. In addition, only patients with a large full-thickness osteoarthritic cartilage defects were included in this study. Finally, magnetic resonance or biopsy for histological evaluation was not performed in this study, which would be a more reliable means for determining the properties of repaired cartilage. However, a direct visual evaluation of the repaired cartilage is one of the most reliable validated assessment tools for cartilage repair.

In conclusion, this study showed that allogeneic UCB-MSCs-HA composite implantation combined with HTO resulted in favorable clinical outcome and cartilage repair in all cases. These findings suggest that UCB-MSCs-HA composite implantation combined with HTO would be a good therapeutic option for patients with knee OA and full-thickness large cartilage defects.

Author Contributions: Y.-B.P., study concepts/design and manuscript drafting/revision; H.-J.L., data acquisition/analysis and manuscript revision; H.-C.N., data acquisition/analysis and manuscript revision; J.-G.P. and H.-C.N., data acquisition/analysis and manuscript revision. All authors have read and agreed to the published version of the manuscript.

Funding: This research received no external funding.

Institutional Review Board Statement: This study was approved by the institutional ethical review board.

Informed Consent Statement: Patient consent was waived because this study is a retrospective record review.

Data Availability Statement: Not applicable.

Acknowledgments: Authors would like to acknowledge support from Yoo-Sun Won at our institution for obtaining clinical data acquisition.

Conflicts of Interest: The authors declare no conflict of interest.

References

1. Bode, G.; von Heyden, J.; Pestka, J.; Schmal, H.; Salzmann, G.; Südkamp, N.; Niemeyer, P. Prospective 5-year survival rate data following open-wedge valgus high tibial osteotomy. *Knee Surg. Sports Traumatol. Arthrosc.* **2015**, *23*, 1949–1955. [CrossRef] [PubMed]
2. Rupp, M.C.; Muench, L.N.; Ehmann, Y.J.; Themessl, A.; Winkler, P.W.; Mehl, J.; Imhoff, A.B.; Feucht, M.J. Improved Clinical Outcome and High Rate of Return to Low-Impact Sport and Work after Knee Double Level Osteotomy for Bifocal Varus Malalignment. *Arthroscopy* **2022**, *38*, 1944–1953. [CrossRef] [PubMed]

3. Takahara, Y.; Nakashima, H.; Itani, S.; Katayama, H.; Miyazato, K.; Iwasaki, Y.; Kato, H.; Uchida, Y. Mid-term results of medial open-wedge high tibial osteotomy based on radiological grading of osteoarthritis. *Arch. Orthop. Trauma Surg.* **2021**. [CrossRef]
4. Jung, W.H.; Takeuchi, R.; Chun, C.W.; Lee, J.S.; Ha, J.H.; Kim, J.H.; Jeong, J.H. Second-look arthroscopic assessment of cartilage regeneration after medial opening-wedge high tibial osteotomy. *Arthroscopy* **2014**, *30*, 72–79. [CrossRef] [PubMed]
5. Kim, K.I.; Seo, M.C.; Song, S.J.; Bae, D.K.; Kim, D.H.; Lee, S.H. Change of Chondral Lesions and Predictive Factors After Medial Open-Wedge High Tibial Osteotomy with a Locked Plate System. *Am. J. Sports Med.* **2017**, *45*, 1615–1621. [CrossRef]
6. Bode, L.; Eberbach, H.; Brenner, A.S.; Kloos, F.; Niemeyer, P.; Schmal, H.; Suedkamp, N.P.; Bode, G. 10-Year Survival Rates after High Tibial Osteotomy Using Angular Stable Internal Plate Fixation: Case Series with Subgroup Analysis of Outcomes after Combined Autologous Chondrocyte Implantation and High Tibial Osteotomy. *Orthop. J. Sports Med.* **2022**, *10*, 23259671221078003. [CrossRef]
7. Schuster, P.; Geßlein, M.; Schlumberger, M.; Mayer, P.; Mayr, R.; Oremek, D.; Frank, S.; Schulz-Jahrsdörfer, M.; Richter, J. Ten-Year Results of Medial Open-Wedge High Tibial Osteotomy and Chondral Resurfacing in Severe Medial Osteoarthritis and Varus Malalignment. *Am. J. Sports Med.* **2018**, *46*, 1362–1370. [CrossRef]
8. Bae, D.K.; Yoon, K.H.; Song, S.J. Cartilage healing after microfracture in osteoarthritic knees. *Arthroscopy* **2006**, *22*, 367–374. [CrossRef]
9. Yen, Y.M.; Cascio, B.; O'Brien, L.; Stalzer, S.; Millett, P.J.; Steadman, J.R. Treatment of osteoarthritis of the knee with microfracture and rehabilitation. *Med. Sci. Sports Exerc.* **2008**, *40*, 200–205. [CrossRef]
10. Mithoefer, K.; McAdams, T.; Williams, R.J.; Kreuz, P.C.; Mandelbaum, B.R. Clinical efficacy of the microfracture technique for articular cartilage repair in the knee: An evidence-based systematic analysis. *Am. J. Sports Med.* **2009**, *37*, 2053–2063. [CrossRef]
11. Nauta, A.J.; Fibbe, W.E. Immunomodulatory properties of mesenchymal stromal cells. *Blood* **2007**, *110*, 3499–3506. [CrossRef]
12. Caplan, A.I.; Dennis, J.E. Mesenchymal stem cells as trophic mediators. *J. Cell. Biochem.* **2006**, *98*, 1076–1084. [CrossRef]
13. Ha, C.W.; Park, Y.B.; Kim, S.H.; Lee, H.J. Intra-articular Mesenchymal Stem Cells in Osteoarthritis of the Knee: A Systematic Review of Clinical Outcomes and Evidence of Cartilage Repair. *Arthroscopy* **2019**, *35*, 277–288.e272. [CrossRef]
14. Kim, S.H.; Djaja, Y.P.; Park, Y.B.; Park, J.G.; Ko, Y.B.; Ha, C.W. Intra-articular Injection of Culture-Expanded Mesenchymal Stem Cells Without Adjuvant Surgery in Knee Osteoarthritis: A Systematic Review and Meta-analysis. *Am. J. Sports Med.* **2020**, *48*, 2839–2849. [CrossRef]
15. Kim, S.H.; Ha, C.W.; Park, Y.B.; Nam, E.; Lee, J.E.; Lee, H.J. Intra-articular injection of mesenchymal stem cells for clinical outcomes and cartilage repair in osteoarthritis of the knee: A meta-analysis of randomized controlled trials. *Arch. Orthop. Trauma Surg.* **2019**, *139*, 971–980. [CrossRef]
16. Park, Y.B.; Ha, C.W.; Rhim, J.H.; Lee, H.J. Stem Cell Therapy for Articular Cartilage Repair: Review of the Entity of Cell Populations Used and the Result of the Clinical Application of Each Entity. *Am. J. Sports Med.* **2018**, *46*, 2540–2552. [CrossRef]
17. Flynn, A.; Barry, F.; O'Brien, T. UC blood-derived mesenchymal stromal cells: An overview. *Cytotherapy* **2007**, *9*, 717–726. [CrossRef]
18. Kern, S.; Eichler, H.; Stoeve, J.; Kluter, H.; Bieback, K. Comparative analysis of mesenchymal stem cells from bone marrow, umbilical cord blood, or adipose tissue. *Stem Cells* **2006**, *24*, 1294–1301. [CrossRef]
19. Park, Y.B.; Ha, C.W.; Kim, J.A.; Kim, S.; Park, Y.G. Comparison of Undifferentiated Versus Chondrogenic Predifferentiated Mesenchymal Stem Cells Derived from Human Umbilical Cord Blood for Cartilage Repair in a Rat Model. *Am. J. Sports Med.* **2019**, *47*, 451–461. [CrossRef]
20. Lim, H.C.; Park, Y.B.; Ha, C.W.; Cole, B.J.; Lee, B.K.; Jeong, H.J.; Kim, M.K.; Bin, S.I.; Choi, C.H.; Choi, C.H.; et al. Allogeneic Umbilical Cord Blood-Derived Mesenchymal Stem Cell Implantation Versus Microfracture for Large, Full-Thickness Cartilage Defects in Older Patients: A Multicenter Randomized Clinical Trial and Extended 5-Year Clinical Follow-up. *Orthop. J. Sports Med.* **2021**, *9*, 2325967120973052. [CrossRef]
21. Park, Y.B.; Ha, C.W.; Lee, C.H.; Yoon, Y.C.; Park, Y.G. Cartilage regeneration in osteoarthritic patients by a composite of allogeneic umbilical cord blood-derived mesenchymal stem cells and hyaluronate hydrogel: Results from a clinical trial for safety and proof-of-concept with 7 years of extended follow-up. *Stem Cells Transl. Med.* **2017**, *6*, 613–621. [CrossRef] [PubMed]
22. Song, J.S.; Hong, K.T.; Kim, N.M.; Jung, J.Y.; Park, H.S.; Lee, S.H.; Cho, Y.J.; Kim, S.J. Implantation of allogenic umbilical cord blood-derived mesenchymal stem cells improves knee osteoarthritis outcomes: Two-year follow-up. *Regen. Ther.* **2020**, *14*, 32–39. [CrossRef] [PubMed]
23. Song, J.S.; Hong, K.T.; Kim, N.M.; Park, H.S.; Choi, N.H. Human umbilical cord blood-derived mesenchymal stem cell implantation for osteoarthritis of the knee. *Arch. Orthop. Trauma Surg.* **2020**, *140*, 503–509. [CrossRef] [PubMed]
24. Yang, H.Y.; Song, E.K.; Kang, S.J.; Kwak, W.K.; Kang, J.K.; Seon, J.K. Allogenic umbilical cord blood-derived mesenchymal stromal cell implantation was superior to bone marrow aspirate concentrate augmentation for cartilage regeneration despite similar clinical outcomes. *Knee Surg. Sports Traumatol. Arthrosc.* **2022**, *30*, 208–218. [CrossRef]
25. Chung, Y.W.; Yang, H.Y.; Kang, S.J.; Song, E.K.; Seon, J.K. Allogeneic umbilical cord blood-derived mesenchymal stem cells combined with high tibial osteotomy: A retrospective study on safety and early results. *Int. Orthop.* **2021**, *45*, 481–488. [CrossRef]
26. Lee, N.H.; Na, S.M.; Ahn, H.W.; Kang, J.K.; Seon, J.K.; Song, E.K. Allogenic Human Umbilical Cord Blood-Derived Mesenchymal Stem Cells Are More Effective Than Bone Marrow Aspiration Concentrate for Cartilage Regeneration After High Tibial Osteotomy in Medial Unicompartmental Osteoarthritis of Knee. *Arthroscopy* **2021**, *37*, 2521–2530. [CrossRef]

27. Song, J.S.; Hong, K.T.; Kong, C.G.; Kim, N.M.; Jung, J.Y.; Park, H.S.; Kim, Y.J.; Chang, K.B.; Kim, S.J. High tibial osteotomy with human umbilical cord blood-derived mesenchymal stem cells implantation for knee cartilage regeneration. *World J. Stem Cells* **2020**, *12*, 514–526. [CrossRef]
28. Bellamy, N.; Buchanan, W.W.; Goldsmith, C.H.; Campbell, J.; Stitt, L.W. Validation study of WOMAC: A health status instrument for measuring clinically important patient relevant outcomes to antirheumatic drug therapy in patients with osteoarthritis of the hip or knee. *J. Rheumatol.* **1988**, *15*, 1833–1840.
29. Van den Borne, M.P.; Raijmakers, N.J.; Vanlauwe, J.; Victor, J.; de Jong, S.N.; Bellemans, J.; Saris, D.B. International Cartilage Repair Society (ICRS) and Oswestry macroscopic cartilage evaluation scores validated for use in autologous chondrocyte implantation (ACI) and microfracture. *Osteoarthr. Cartil.* **2007**, *15*, 1397–1402. [CrossRef]
30. Wong, K.L.; Lee, K.B.; Tai, B.C.; Law, P.; Lee, E.H.; Hui, J.H. Injectable cultured bone marrow-derived mesenchymal stem cells in varus knees with cartilage defects undergoing high tibial osteotomy: A prospective, randomized controlled clinical trial with 2 years' follow-up. *Arthroscopy* **2013**, *29*, 2020–2028. [CrossRef]
31. Tan, S.H.S.; Kwan, Y.T.; Neo, W.J.; Chong, J.Y.; Kuek, T.Y.J.; See, J.Z.F.; Hui, J.H. Outcomes of High Tibial Osteotomy with Versus without Mesenchymal Stem Cell Augmentation: A Systematic Review and Meta-Analysis. *Orthop. J. Sports Med.* **2021**, *9*, 23259671211014840. [CrossRef]
32. Na, B.R.; Yang, H.Y.; Seo, J.W.; Lee, C.H.; Seon, J.K. Effect of medial open wedge high tibial osteotomy on progression of patellofemoral osteoarthritis. *Knee Surg. Relat. Res.* **2022**, *34*, 42. [CrossRef]
33. Kim, J.H.; Kim, H.J.; Lee, D.H. Survival of opening versus closing wedge high tibial osteotomy: A meta-analysis. *Sci. Rep.* **2017**, *7*, 7296. [CrossRef]
34. Filardo, G.; Vannini, F.; Marcacci, M.; Andriolo, L.; Ferruzzi, A.; Giannini, S.; Kon, E. Matrix-assisted autologous chondrocyte transplantation for cartilage regeneration in osteoarthritic knees: Results and failures at midterm follow-up. *Am. J. Sports Med.* **2013**, *41*, 95–100. [CrossRef]
35. Harris, J.D.; Siston, R.A.; Pan, X.; Flanigan, D.C. Autologous chondrocyte implantation: A systematic review. *J. Bone Joint Surg. Am.* **2010**, *92*, 2220–2233. [CrossRef]

Disclaimer/Publisher's Note: The statements, opinions and data contained in all publications are solely those of the individual author(s) and contributor(s) and not of MDPI and/or the editor(s). MDPI and/or the editor(s) disclaim responsibility for any injury to people or property resulting from any ideas, methods, instructions or products referred to in the content.

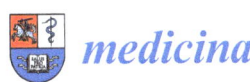

Article

Relationship between Outerbridge Scale and Chondropathy Femorotibial Joint in Relation to Gender and Age—The Use of 1.5T and 3.0T MRI Scanners

Dominik Sieroń [1,*], Izabella Jabłońska [2], Paweł Niemiec [3], Dawid Lukoszek [4], Karol Szyluk [5,6], Ivan Platzek [7], Hugo Meusburger [1], Georgios Delimpasis [1] and Andreas Christe [1]

1. Department of Radiology SLS, Inselgroup, Bern University Hospital, University of Bern, Freiburgstrasse 10, 3010 Bern, Switzerland
2. Recreation and Treatment Center "Glinik" 1, Wysowa-Zdrój 101 str, 38-316 Wysowa-Zdrój, Poland
3. Department of Biochemistry and Medical Genetics, School of Health Sciences in Katowice, Medical University of Silesia in Katowice, Medyków 18 str, 40-752 Katowice, Poland
4. Dawid Lukoszek Physiotherapy Osteopathy, 42-690 Hanusek, Poland
5. Department of Physiotherapy, Faculty of Health Sciences in Katowice, Medical University of Silesia in Katowice, 40-752 Katowice, Poland
6. Department of Orthopaedic and Trauma Surgery, District Hospital of Orthopaedics and Trauma Surgery, Bytomska 62 str, 41-940 Piekary Śląskie, Poland
7. Department of Radiology, Dresden University Hospital, Fetscherstr. 74, 01307 Dresden, Germany
* Correspondence: dominik.sieron.ch@gmail.com

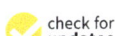

Abstract: *Background and Objective*: Magnetic resonance imaging (MRI) enables the effective evaluation of chondromalacia of the knee joint. Cartilage disease is affected by many factors, including gender, age, and body mass index (BMI). The aim of this study was to check the relationship between the severity of chondromalacia of the femoro-tibial joint and age, gender, and BMI assessed with 1.5T and 3.0T MRI scanners. *Materials and Methods*: The cross-observational study included 324 patients—159 (49%) females and 165 (51%) males aged 8–87 (45.1 ± 20.9). The BMI of study group was between 14.3 and 47.3 (27.7 ± 5.02). 1.5T and 3.0T MRI scanners were used in the study. The articular cartilage of the knee joint was assessed using the Outerbridge scale. *Results*: The age of the patients showed a significant correlation with Outerbrige for each compartment of the femorotibial joint (Spearman's rank correlation rho: 0.69–0.74, $p < 0.0001$). A higher correlation between BMI and Outerbridge was noted in the femur medial (rho = 0.45, $p < 0.001$) and the tibia medial (rho = 0.43, $p < 0.001$) than in the femur lateral (rho = 0.29, $p < 0.001$) and the tibia lateral compartment (rho = 0.34, $p < 0.001$). *Conclusions*: The severity of chondromalacia significantly depends on age and BMI level, regardless of gender.

Keywords: femorotibial joint; chondromalacia; aging; body mass index; magnetic resonance imaging

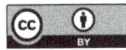

1. Introduction

Chondromalacia is a disease affecting the hyaline cartilage that covers the articular surfaces of bones. It causes the cartilage to soften and often leads to tearing and erosion of the cartilage. The environment and physical stress both have an effect on this cartilage. Degeneration of the cartilage also occurs in response to microtraumatic wear. Repeated activities that cause compressive stress on the joint or increased loads on the joint can lead to chondromalacia [1–3]. Aging also affects the hyaline cartilage. As we age the number of chondrocytes in cartilage decreases, which correlates with a decrease in the number of proteoglycans produced. This reduction leads to a decrease in the water content of cartilage. A loss of elastic properties develops in the cartilage due to the gradual loss of collagen fibril cross-linking, which also occurs with age. With age, the superficial zone is the first to be damaged [4].

The Outerbridge scale is most commonly used to assess chondromalacia. This classification allows us to categorize cartilage degeneration into four degrees of advancement. It is common to find several degenerative processes at varying levels of severity in the same knee joint [5,6]. MRI is an effective and non-invasive method for evaluating the articular cartilage of the knee joint. This method can be used to detect and monitor degenerative changes that may lead to osteoarthritis [7]. Typical MRI scans (PD and fat-suppressed T2-weighted) can assess the characteristics of cartilage pathology [8]. Together with existing grading scales that assess articular cartilage, MRI can be considered a highly accurate and non-invasive cartilage diagnostic tool [9], with an accuracy of up to 91% [10].

Obesity has a direct correlation with the degeneration of the osteo-articular system. Being overweight causes increased pressure on the articular surfaces of small and large joints, which results in faster wear of the articular surfaces, including cartilage, and its accelerated degeneration [11].

Osteoarthritis (OA) is the most common form of arthritis, affecting approximately 90 million adults (36.8% of the adult population) in the United States alone [12] and hundreds of millions of people worldwide. The disease primarily affects the articular hyaline cartilage in stressed joints, such as the knee joint. Other tissues such as the synovial membrane of the joint capsule and subchondral bone are also affected and contribute to disease progression. As the disease advances, severe cartilage degeneration, joint space narrowing, subchondral bone thickening, osteophyte [13] or bone spur formation, and joint inflammation with associated swelling and pain occur [14]. Increased risk factors for OA are numerous and include obesity, being of the female gender, age, congenital structural defects of the joint, and acute joint trauma [15]. Scientific evidence from systematic reviews show that the progression of knee degenerative changes increases with age and excess weight. In addition, studies indicate that BMI is a significant indicator of the degeneration of articular cartilage in individual compartments of the same knee [16–18]. Furthermore, we were interested in the normal range of chondromalacia depending on age, gender and BMI using the Outerbridge classification as quantification of cartilage degeneration. Age and BMI could be used as a direct replacement for the Outerbridge score without the need to perform an MRI.

Due to the large amount of research on patellofemoral chondromalacia, we wanted to improve our understanding of femorotibial cartilage degeneration and check its characteristics. The aim of the study was to investigate the correlation between the severity of chondromalacia of the femorotibial joints and BMI, broken down into categories based on age and gender. Additionally, the differences between using a 1.5T and a 3.0T MRI scanner in the assessment of the knee cartilage were checked.

2. Materials and Methods

2.1. Study Design

The IRB (Institutional Review Board) states that the presented retrospective studies containing irreversibly anonymized data in our institution do not require the approval of the bioethics committee. In the current observational cross-sectional study, we analyzed the effect of BMI and demographic variables (including age and gender of patients) on the severity of femorotibial joint chondromalacia in consecutive incoming patients undergoing evaluations of knee joint lesions from 2018 to 2019. Patients were recruited from community and clinical hospitals as well as private facilities in Zamość Elblag, Jelenia Góra, and Bielsko Biala (Poland). The medial (femur and tibia separately) and lateral (femur and tibia separately) compartments of the knee joint were evaluated.

The following work is the most recent in a series of scientific publications on chondromalacia of the knee joint. Earlier work included radiological measurements to assess chondromalacia of the knee joint [19]. A paper on chondromalacia of the patellofemoral joint in correlation with BMI depending on age and gender is currently being published. All work was performed based on the same study group and their respective MRI scans.

2.2. Description of the Participants

The study group included 324 patients, 159 (47.1%) women and 165 (52.9%) men. A total of 155 (47.8%) patients, including 70 (45.2%) women and 85 (54.8%) men, were examined on the 1.5T scanner, while 169 (52.2%) patients, including 89 (52.7%) women and 80 (47.3%) men, were examined on the 3.0T scanner. Four age classes were defined for the study: <30 years (94 participants); 30–45 years (61 participants); 46–60 years (78 participants); >60 years (91 participants).

2.3. Inclusion and Exclusion Criteria

Inclusion criteria: patients with pain or suspected osteoarthritis or post-traumatic lesions who on the order of an orthopedist, surgeon, or physiotherapist submitted for an MRI. Several patients also submitted for a private scan at their own request due to complaints of joint pain.

Exclusion criteria: previous knee surgery or chronic post-traumatic changes of the knee.

2.4. Evaluation of Cartilage Chondromalacia

To assess cartilage chondromalacia, we used the 5-level Outerbridge classification (Table 1) using fat-saturated proton density sequences—a modified classification for arthroscopic cartilage assessment [16–19]. Three board-certified radiologists with 12, 25 and 32 years of experience in musculoskeletal imaging classified the MR images according to the Outerbridge score. Cases were randomly and equally distributed among the radiologists. The MRI scans reported by the radiologists did not overlap. For this reason, consistency between radiologists was not assessed.

Table 1. Outerbridge classification [19–23].

Grade	Macroscopy	MRI
Grade 0	Normal cartilage	Normal cartilage
Grade 1	Rough surface; chondral softening; focal thickening	Inhomogeneous; high signal; surface intact; cartilage swelling
Grade 2	Irregular surface defects; <50% of cartilage thickness	Superficial ulceration, fissuring, fibrillation; <50% of cartilage thickness
Grade 3	Loss of >50% cartilage thickness	Ulceration fissuring, fibrillation; >50% of depth of cartilage
Grade 4	Cartilage loss	Full thickness chondral wear with exposure of subchondral bone

2.5. Image Acquisition

The study was evaluated on an iMac pro (Apple, Cupertino, CA, USA) using the FDA approved OsiriX MD software (version 11.0, Pixmeo SARL, Bernex, Switzerland). MRIs were performed on 3.0T scanners (Ingenia 3.0T, Philips, Amsterdam, The Netherlands) and on 1.5T GE scanners (SIGNA, GE, Milwaukee, WI, USA) GE at different facilities located in clinical hospitals and private facilities in Zamość, Elbląg, Jelenia Góra, and Bielsko-Biala. All MRI studies were irreversibly anonymized [16].

The following diagnostic sequence protocol was used in the study: axial, sagittal and coronal PD FS, sagittal and coronal T1 (all with a slice thickness of 3 mm), 3D high-resolution PD FS with a slice thickness from 0.8 to 1 mm. The same protocol we used in the earlier publication [19].

2.6. Statistical Analysis

A Chi-square (χ^2) test of independence was used to analyze the difference of chondromalacia in the various age, sex and MRI-unit groups. The correlation between the age subgroups and Outerbridge scale chondromalacia lesion scores, the C contingency co-efficient, was calculated, and the R-Spearman rank correlation was checked. The comparison of correlation coefficients was performed using the z statistic.

Subsequently, the correlation between BMI level and Outerbridge chondromalacia lesion scores was tested using the Kruskal–Wallis test, ANOVA, post-hoc analysis (Conover test), the trend for mean values (Me) of BMI level in each Outerbridge scale grade, the Jockheere–Terpstra trend test, and the R-Spearman (rho). The analysis was performed for the whole group, 1.5T and 3.0T, for females and males—separately for 1.5T and 3.0T—and a pooled analysis of Outerbridge score 0/1/2 vs. 3/4 was performed. The continuity coefficient was used as a measure of the relationship between the age subgroup and Outerbridge scale grade. The use of the χ^2 test provided the basis for the calculation of the C coefficient. Our table had dimensions of 4 × 4; in this case Cmax = 0.866. To compare the impact of the different variables (age, BMI, sex and MRI scanner type) on the Outerbridge score, a logistic regression model was used with the dependent dichotomous variable being no or slight degeneration (Outerbridge score 0/1/2) and severe degeneration (Outerbridge score 3/4).

3. Results

3.1. Age

Age demonstrated significant correlation coefficients (Spearman rank correlation, $p < 0.001$) with Outerbridge for the femur lateral (rho = 0.69), tibia lateral (rho = 0.71), femur medial (0.72), tibia medial (rho = 0.74) (Table 2, Figure 1).

Table 2. Relationship between the Outerbridge scale and age for particular compartments of the femorotibial joint.

Correlated Variables	N	R_s Spearman	T (N-2)	p
Femur Lateral & Age	324	0.69	16.9308	<0.001
Femur Medial & Age	324	0.72	18.8962	<0.001
Tibia Lateral & Age	324	0.71	18.3634	<0.001
Tibia Medial & Age	324	0.74	20.0209	<0.001

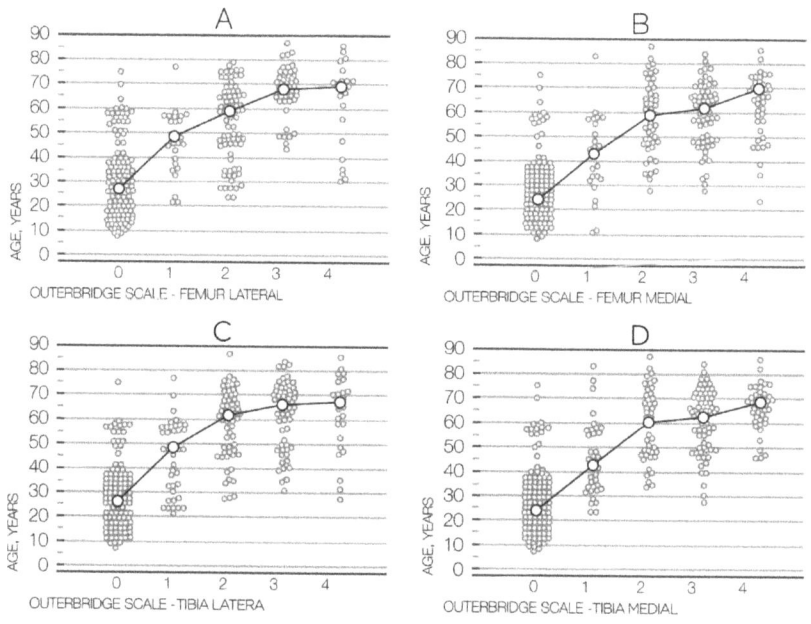

Figure 1. Relationship between the Outerbridge scale and age for femur lateral (**A**), femur medial (**B**), tibia lateral (**C**), and tibia medial (**D**).

3.2. BMI

The mean BMI for the entire study group was 27.7; SD: 5.02. The highest values of BMI were noted in the patients diagnosed with Outerbridge Scale 2 for the tibia lateral and

Outerbridge Scale 4 for the femur medial and tibia medial. For the individual parameters of the Outerbridge scale, the mean BMI is presented in Table 3.

Table 3. BMI for Outerbridge scale.

Outerbridge	BMI (Mean ± SD)			
	Femur Lateral	Tibia Lateral	Femur Medial	Tibia Medial
Grade 0	26.0 ± 4.88	25.7 ± 4.92	25.3 ± 4.47	25.4 ± 4.55
Grade 1	29.1 ± 5.31	28.8 ± 4.97	26.4 ± 4.17	28.2 ± 4.71
Grade 2	29.4 ± 4.49	29.6 ± 4.54	29.4 ± 3.85	28.3 ± 3.97
Grade 3	29.6 ± 5.00	28.8 ± 4.06	29.9 ± 4.90	28.3 ± 3.97
Grade 4	27.0 ± 3.54	29.4 ± 5.33	30.3 ± 5.01	29.6 ± 4.78

3.2.1. Femur Lateral

A statistically significant positive correlation was found between BMI level and Outerbridge parameter score (rho = 0.29, $p < 0.001$) (Figure 2A).

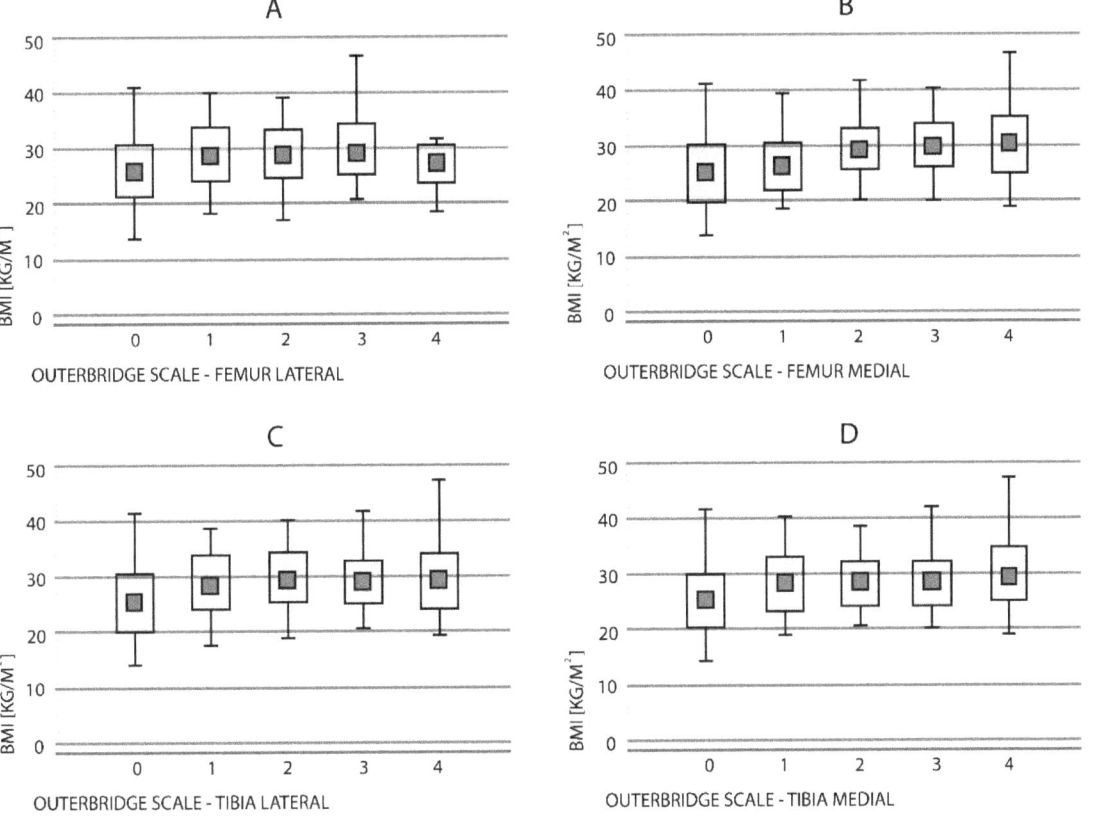

Figure 2. Relationship between BMI and Outerbridge scores using both scanners (1.5T and 3.0T) in the entire study group for femur lateral (**A**), femur medial (**B**), tibia lateral (**C**), and tibia medial (**D**).

There was a statistically significant difference in BMI level according to the Outerbridge parameter score (KW, $p < 0.001$) in the entire study group of patients (scanner 1.5T and 3.0T).

For the femur lateral, there were no significant statistical differences between the Outerbridge subgroups (1 and 2 vs. 3 and 4) in terms of the BMI level (U-test, $p = 0.39$).

The grade 0 Outerbridge parameter score showed a statistically significant lower mean BMI level compared to grades 1, 2 and 3 ($p < 0.05$).

3.2.2. Femur Medial

There was a statistically significant positive correlation between the BMI level and Outerbridge parameter score (rho = 0.45, $p < 0.001$) for both scanners (Figure 2B).

There was a statistically significant difference in BMI level between the Outerbridge scores ($p < 0.001$) in the entire study group.

For the femur medial, there were significant statistical differences between the Outerbridge subgroups (1 and 2 vs. 3 and 4) in terms of the BMI level ($p = 0.01$).

The grade 0 Outerbridge parameter score showed a statistically significant lower mean BMI level compared to grades 2, 3 and 4 ($p < 0.05$).

3.2.3. Tibia Lateral

A significant correlation was found between the BMI level and Outerbridge parameter score (rho = 0.34, $p < 0.001$) for both scanners (Figure 2C).

The parameters' Outerbridge scores significantly differed statistically in terms of the BMI ($p = 0.0001$) for both scanners.

For the tibia lateral, no significant differences were found between the Outerbridge subgroups (1 and 2 vs. 3 and 4) in terms of the BMI level ($p = 0.72$)

The grade 0 Outerbridge parameter score showed a statistically significant lower mean BMI level compared to the level of the rest of the parameters ($p < 0.05$).

3.2.4. Tibia Medial

There was a statistically significant relationship between the BMI level and Outerbridge parameter score (rho = 0.42, $p < 0.001$) at this location (Figure 2D).

The Outerbridge score parameters were significantly statistically different in terms of the BMI level ($p < 0.001$) at this location.

The Outerbridge subgroups (1 and 2 vs. 3 and 4) differed significantly in terms of the BMI level for the tibia medial ($p = 0.017$).

The grade 0 Outerbridge parameter score showed a statistically significant lower mean BMI level compared to the level of the rest of the parameters ($p < 0.05$).

3.3. Gender

There were no significant differences between women and men in the Outerbridge assessment for each knee joint compartment in each age subgroup (test χ^2, $p > 0.05$).

3.3.1. Women

For women, age demonstrated the following correlation coefficients (Spearman rank correlation, $p < 0.001$) with Outerbridge: for the femur lateral (rho = 0.72), the tibia lateral (rho = 0.71), the femur medial (rho = 0.70), and the tibia medial (rho = 0.70).

3.3.2. Men

For men, age demonstrated the following correlation coefficients (Spearman rank correlation, $p < 0.001$) with Outerbridge: for the femur lateral (rho = 0.66), the tibia lateral (rho = 0.71), the femur medial (rho = 0.74), and the tibia medial (rho = 0.77).

3.4. Type of Scanners (1.5T vs. 3.0T)

The demographics of the two groups were as follows: A total of 70 (45.2%) females and 85 (54.8%) males were examined on the 1.5T scanner, while 89 (52.7%) females and 80 (47.3%) males were examined on the 3.0T scanner. The average age of the 1.5T and 3.0T group was 43.8 ± 18.7 and 46.9 ± 23.5 years, while the mean BMI of the 1.5T and 3.0T group added up to 28.2 ± 5.0 and 27.1 ± 5.2.

Significant differences were found between the scanner type (1.5T vs. 3.0T) in the Outerbridge assessment for the femur lateral ($\chi2$, $p = 0.002$), tibia lateral ($\chi2$, $p = 0.006$), femur medial ($\chi2$, $p = 0.034$), and tibia medial ($\chi2$, $p = 0.007$) in the entire study group:

For the 1.5T scanner, the Outerbridge scale scores were in general higher than for the 3.0T scanner (Table 4).

Table 4. Outerbridge Scale for each compartment of femorotibial joint.

	Outerbridge Scale	
	1.5T MRI scanner	3.0T MRI Scanner
Femur Lateral	1.387 ± 1.306	1.225 ± 1.400
Tibia Lateral	1.581 ± 1.391	1.207 ± 1.379
Femur Medial	1.794 ± 1.528	1.367 ± 1.503
Tibia Medial	1.709 ± 1.503	1.260 ± 1.485

When all joint compartments were evaluated together, the correlation coefficient of the Outerbridge and BMI at 1.5T/3.0T was 0.3997/0.3303 ($p = 0.1314$) and the correlation of the Outerbridge and age at 1.5T/3.0T was 0.687/0.777 ($p < 0.001$).

3.5. Logistic Regression of Age, BMI, Sex and MRI Scanner Type on Outerbridge Score

Age, BMI and MRI scanner type played a significant role in predicting the severity of knee degeneration (Outerbridge 3 and 4) with the following logistic regression formula:

$$\text{Logit (Outerbridge 3/4)} = 0.0888 \times A + 0.0864 \times B + 0.0604 \times M - 0.717 \times T - 6.58 \quad (1)$$

A (age), B (BMI), M (male patient) and T (1.5 Tesla MRI) demonstrated odd ratios of 1.093 (95% CI: 1.073 to 1.113), 1.090 (95% CI: 1.026 to 1.159), 1.062 (95% CI: 0.578 to 1.953) and 0.488 (95% CI: 0.265 to 0.901), respectively. According to the p-value, the influence was strongest for the age ($p < 0.001$), followed by BMI ($p = 0.005$) and MRI type ($p = 0.022$); sex did not have a significant impact on degeneration prediction ($p = 0.85$).

4. Discussion

The results showed a significant correlation between the Outerbridge chondromalacia score and BMI and age. A similar correlation was noted in a study by Matada, who additionally noted that a significant increase in larger knee cartilage lesions occurs in individuals > 50 years and BMI > 25 [24]. Chondromalacia changes are noted when assessing structural changes in osteoarthritis [21]. Risk factors for symptomatic knee joint changes due to osteoarthritis include obesity and age [25]. The relationship between BMI and knee OA is mainly linear [26].

4.1. Gender

Previous studies have noted differences in the extent of cartilage loss of the femorotibial joint between men and women, with greater degeneration observed in women than in men [27–29]. Despite these reports lacking clarity, the hypothesized mechanism for the significant progression of knee cartilage disorders involves biomechanical and hormonal factors that distinguish women from men [28]. In women, the progression of degenerative changes of the knee joint significantly increases after the age of 50 in the postmenopausal period [27]. A cross-sectional study found that women taking hormone therapy in the postmenopausal period exhibit greater cartilage volume [30]. Possible biomechanical differences in gait and the knee joint in women may also accelerate the development of OA [31,32]. Our study showed no significant difference in the Outerbridge scores between women and men. Additionally, the correlation of Outerbridge and age/BMI was the same between both genders.

4.2. Aging

The development of knee osteoarthritis is closely related to aging [33,34]. The catabolic–anabolic imbalance of cartilage causes matrix destruction through excessive oxidation of antioxidant systems in chondrocytes, including glutathione and peroxiredoxins [35]. Joint components that undergo changes due to aging also contribute to the degeneration of hyaline cartilage. Osteoporosis or the weakening of the quadriceps muscle of the thigh leads to the dysfunction of the femorotibial joint, increasing the maximum stresses on the cartilage [36–38]. In the analysis of this study, a significant relationship was found between the presence of greater chondromolytic changes and increasing age for this group.

4.3. BMI

For the entire group, a positive correlation was found between BMI and Outerbridge scores. A higher correlation between BMI and Outerbridge was found in the medial compartments, femur medial (rho = 0.45) and tibia medial (rho = 0.42), than the lateral compartments, femur lateral (rho = 0.29) and tibia lateral (rho = 0.34). It should be noted that obesity is not only associated with osteoarthritic changes of the knee joint in the mechanical but also in the metabolic background [39–41]. Through research, adipokines, leptin, and resistin, which have endocrine functions in adipose tissue, have been identified [38]. In vivo, findings have indicated that there is a detrimental effect on chondrocyte proliferation as well as the initiation of extracellular matrix metalloproteinase expression, resulting in reduced cartilage volume [42].

4.4. MRI and the Assessment of Cartilage Chondromalacia

A comparison of knee joint images from the same patients on the 1.5T and 3.0T apparatus in Wang's study, followed by arthroscopy, concluded that the visualization of anatomical structures and the confidence in making diagnoses of cartilage lesions are both improved when using 3.0T scanners. The reliability (88.2% vs. 86.4%) and sensitivity (51.3% vs. 42.9%) of the 3.0T device was improved compared with the 1.5T. The correct assessment of cartilage damage differed in favor of the 3.0T apparatus (51.3 vs. 42.9%) [43]. A study by Mandell, who used a similar methodology to Wang in examining a larger group, inferred no significant differences between the 1.5T and 3.0T [44]. In contrast, a systematic review and meta-analysis concluded that the 3.0T scanners were significantly more reliable for imaging articular cartilage [10] with age-related degeneration. In our study, the 1.5T scanner scored higher Outerbridge levels in all compartments compared to the 3.0T unit, but the correlation coefficients of Outerbridge and BMI did not differ, and the correlation coefficient of Outerbridge and age was even significantly higher than with the 3.0T unit. Therefore, one explanation for the higher Outerbridge scores of the 1.5T scanner could be a possible geographical inclusion inhomogeneity. From our results, it seems that both the 1.5T and the 3.0T apparatuses are effective methods of evaluating Outerbridge cartilage according to the BMI level. On the other hand, the 3.0T apparatus may have an advantage in terms of age correlation.

4.5. Limitations

One major drawback of our study is the lack of a comparison of the same group of subjects using the 1.5T and 3.0T apparatus. The lack of a characterization of the group in terms of additional injuries such as ACL, meniscus, fat pad, and other factors such as physical activity or quadriceps thigh muscle strength made it impossible to test for differences in Outerbridge scores. The most important limitation of the study is the BMI used, which shows low sensitivity in obesity research and non-specificity in chondromalacia studies [45].

5. Conclusions

Assessing the degree of cartilage degenerative changes with 1.5T and 3.0T MRI is an effective form of lesion classification using the Outerbridge scale.

A positive correlation was observed between the degree of chondromalacia in both compartments of the femorotibial joint and the body mass index and age of the subject.

No differences were noted between men and women in the assessment of articular cartilage.

Our suggestion for further research is a longitudinal follow-up to evaluate the effect of the duration of obesity during life on cartilage changes and to see which apparatus, the 1.5T or 3.0T, is more effective in monitoring patients with OA. In order to provide a complete answer to the question of whether age and BMI can be used as a variable in the Outerbridge scale without the use of MRI, a predictive model study with multivariable analysis should be performed, taking into account many factors causing a predisposition to chondropathy of the femorotibial joint.

Author Contributions: Conceptualization, D.S.; I.J.; methodology, D.S.; A.C.; software, D.L.; K.S.; P.N.; I.P.; H.M.; G.D.; validation, D.S.; A.C.; P.N.; I.P.; H.M.; G.D.; formal analysis, D.L.; K.S.; D.S.; A.C.; I.P.; P.N.; H.M.; G.D.; investigation, D.S.; I.J.; I.P.; H.M.; G.D.; resources, D.S.; data curation, D.S.; I.J.; writing—original draft preparation, D.S.; I.J.; writing—review and editing, D.L.; K.S.; I.J.; A.C.; P.N.; I.P.; H.M.; G.D.; visualization, D.L.; K.S.; supervision, A.C.; K.S. All authors have read and agreed to the published version of the manuscript.

Funding: This research received no external funding.

Institutional Review Board Statement: The IRB approval could be waived due to the retrospective and irreversibly anonymized patent data.

Informed Consent Statement: Not applicable.

Data Availability Statement: Data are available upon special request.

Conflicts of Interest: The authors declare no conflict of interest.

References

1. Carballo, C.; Nakagawa, Y.; Sekiya, I.; Rodeo, S. Basic Science of Articular Cartilage. *Clin. Sport. Med.* **2017**, *36*, 413–425. [CrossRef] [PubMed]
2. Ekman, S.; Carlson, C. The Pathophysiology of Osteochondrosis. Veterinary Clinics of North America. *Small Anim. Pract.* **1998**, *28*, 17–32. [CrossRef]
3. Wong, B.; Bae, W.; Chun, J.; Gratz, K.; Lotz, M.; Robert, L. Sah Biomechanics of cartilage articulation: Effects of lubrication and degeneration on shear deformation. *Arthritis Rheum.* **2008**, *58*, 2065–2074. [CrossRef]
4. Sacitharan, P.; Vincent, T. Cellular ageing mechanisms in osteoarthritis. *Mamm. Genome* **2016**, *27*, 421–429. [CrossRef] [PubMed]
5. Slattery, C.; Kweon, C. Classifications in Brief: Outerbridge Classification of Chondral Lesions. *Clin. Orthop. Relat. Res.* **2018**, *476*, 2101–2104. [CrossRef]
6. Reed, M.; Villacis, D.; Hatch, G.; Burke, W.; Colletti, P.; Narvy, S.; Mirzayan, R.; Vangsness, C. 3.0-Tesla MRI and Arthroscopy for Assessment of Knee Articular Cartilage Lesions. *Orthopedics* **2013**, *36*, e1060–e1064. [CrossRef]
7. Burge, A.; Potter, H.; Argentieri, E. Magnetic Resonance Imaging of Articular Cartilage within the Knee. *J. Knee Surg.* **2018**, *31*, 155–165. [CrossRef]
8. Schreiner, A.; Stoker, A.; Bozynski, C.; Kuroki, K.; Stannard, J.; Cook, J. Clinical Application of the Basic Science of Articular Cartilage Pathology and Treatment. *J. Knee Surg.* **2020**, *33*, 1056–1068. [CrossRef]
9. Jungmann, P.; Welsch, G.; Brittberg, M.; Trattnig, S.; Braun, S.; Imhoff, A.; Salzmann, G. Magnetic Resonance Imaging Score and Classification System (AMADEUS) for Assessment of Preoperative Cartilage Defect Severity. *Cartilage* **2016**, *8*, 272–282. [CrossRef]
10. Cheng, Q.; Zhao, F. Comparison of 1.5- and 3.0-T magnetic resonance imaging for evaluating lesions of the knee. *Medicine* **2018**, *97*, e12401. [CrossRef]
11. Wang, L.; Denniston, M.; Lee, S.; Galuska, D.; Lowry, R. Long-term Health and Economic Impact of Preventing and Reducing Overweight and Obesity in Adolescence. *J. Adolesc. Health* **2010**, *46*, 467–473. [CrossRef] [PubMed]
12. Oliveria, S.; Felson, D.; Cirillo, P.; Reed, J.; Walker, A. Body Weight, Body Mass Index, and Incident Symptomatic Osteoarthritis of the Hand, Hip, and Knee. *Epidemiology* **1999**, *10*, 161–166. [CrossRef] [PubMed]
13. Blagojevic, M.; Jinks, C.; Jeffery, A.; Jordan, K. Risk factors for onset of osteoarthritis of the knee in older adults: A systematic review and meta-analysis. *Osteoarthr. Cartil.* **2010**, *18*, 24–33. [CrossRef] [PubMed]
14. Abbate, L.; Stevens, J.; Schwartz, T.; Renner, J.; Helmick, C.; Jordan, J. Anthropometric Measures, Body Composition, Body Fat Distribution, and Knee Osteoarthritis in Women*. *Obesity* **2006**, *14*, 1274–1281. [CrossRef] [PubMed]

15. Lohmander, L.; Gerhardsson de Verdier, M.; Rollof, J.; Nilsson, P.; Engström, G. Incidence of severe knee and hip osteoarthritis in relation to different measures of body mass: A population-based prospective cohort study. *Ann. Rheum. Dis.* **2008**, *68*, 490–496. [CrossRef]
16. Bedson, J.; Croft, P. The discordance between clinical and radiographic knee osteoarthritis: A systematic search and summary of the literature. *BMC Musculoskelet. Disord.* **2008**, *9*, 116. [CrossRef]
17. Zheng, H.; Chen, C. Body mass index and risk of knee osteoarthritis: Systematic review and meta-analysis of prospective studies. *BMJ Open* **2015**, *5*, e007568. [CrossRef]
18. Rai, M.; Sandell, L.; Barrack, T.; Cai, L.; Tycksen, E.; Tang, S.; Silva, M.; Barrack, R. A Microarray Study of Articular Cartilage in Relation to Obesity and Severity of Knee Osteoarthritis. *Cartilage* **2020**, *4*, 458–472. [CrossRef]
19. Sieroń, D.; Jabłońska, I.; Lukoszek, D.; Szyluk, K.; Meusburger, H.; Delimpasis, G.; Kostrzewa, M.; Platzek, I.; Christe, A. Knee Diameter and Cross-Section Area Measurements in MRI as New Promising Methods of Chondromalacia Diagnosis-Pilot Study. *Medicina* **2022**, *58*, 1142. [CrossRef]
20. Park, C.; Song, K.; Kim, J.; Lee, S. Retrospective evaluation of outcomes of bone peg fixation for osteochondral lesion of the talus. *Bone Jt. J.* **2020**, *102-B*, 1349–1353. [CrossRef]
21. Slimi, F.; Zribi, W.; Trigui, M.; Amri, R.; Gouiaa, N.; Abid, C.; Rebai, M.; Boudawara, T.; Jebahi, S.; Keskes, H. The effectiveness of platelet-rich plasma gel on full-thickness cartilage defect repair in a rabbit model. *Bone Jt. Res.* **2021**, *10*, 192–202. [CrossRef] [PubMed]
22. Elder, S.; Clune, J.; Walker, J.; Gloth, P. Suitability of EGCG as a Means of Stabilizing a Porcine Osteochondral Xenograft. *J. Funct. Biomater.* **2017**, *8*, 43. [CrossRef] [PubMed]
23. Eldridge, S.; Barawi, A.; Wang, H.; Roelofs, A.; Kaneva, M.; Guan, Z.; Lydon, H.; Thomas, B.; Thorup, A.; Fernandez, B.; et al. Agrin induces long-term osteochondral regeneration by supporting repair morphogenesis. *Sci. Transl. Med.* **2020**, *12*, eaax9086. [CrossRef] [PubMed]
24. Matada, M.; Holi, M.; Raman, R.; Jayaramu Suvarna, S. Visualization of Cartilage from Knee Joint Magnetic Resonance Images and Quantitative Assessment to Study the Effect of Age, Gender and Body Mass Index (BMI) in Progressive Osteoarthritis (OA). *Curr. Med. Imaging Former. Curr. Med. Imaging Rev.* **2019**, *15*, 565–572. [CrossRef] [PubMed]
25. Murphy, L.; Schwartz, T.; Helmick, C.; Renner, J.; Tudor, G.; Koch, G.; Dragomir, A.; Kalsbeek, W.; Luta, G.; Jordan, J. Lifetime risk of symptomatic knee osteoarthritis. *Arthritis Rheum.* **2008**, *59*, 1207–1213. [CrossRef] [PubMed]
26. Grotle, M.; Hagen, K.; Natvig, B.; Dahl, F.; Kvien, T. Obesity and osteoarthritis in knee, hip and/or hand: An epidemiological study in the general population with 10 years follow-up. *BMC Musculoskelet. Disord.* **2008**, *9*, 132. [CrossRef]
27. Ding, C.; Cicuttini, F.; Blizzard, L.; Scott, F.; Jones, G. A longitudinal study of the effect of sex and age on rate of change in knee cartilage volume in adults. *Rheumatology* **2006**, *46*, 273–279. [CrossRef]
28. Berry, P.; Wluka, A.; Davies-Tuck, M.; Wang, Y.; Strauss, B.; Dixon, J.; Proietto, J.; Jones, G.; Cicuttini, F. The relationship between body composition and structural changes at the knee. *Rheumatology* **2010**, *49*, 2362–2369. [CrossRef]
29. Tsai, C.L.; Liu, T.K. Osteoarthritis in women: Its relationship to estrogen and current trends. *Life Sci.* **1992**, *50*, 1737–1744. [CrossRef]
30. Wluka, A. Users of oestrogen replacement therapy have more knee cartilage than non-users. *Ann. Rheum. Dis.* **2001**, *60*, 332–336. [CrossRef]
31. McKean, K.; Landry, S.; Hubley-Kozey, C.; Dunbar, M.; Stanish, W.; Deluzio, K. Gender differences exist in osteoarthritic gait. *Clin. Biomech.* **2007**, *22*, 400–409. [CrossRef]
32. Hanna, F.; Teichtahl, A.; Wluka, A.; Wang, Y.; Urquhart, D.; English, D.; Giles, G.; Cicuttini, F. Women have increased rates of cartilage loss and progression of cartilage defects at the knee than men. *Menopause* **2009**, *16*, 666–670. [CrossRef] [PubMed]
33. Leong, D.; Sun, H. Events in Articular Chondrocytes with Aging. *Curr. Osteoporos. Rep.* **2011**, *9*, 196–201. [CrossRef] [PubMed]
34. O'Connor, M. Sex differences in osteoarthritis of the hip and knee. *J. Am. Acad. Orthop. Surg.* **2007**, *15*, 22–25. [CrossRef] [PubMed]
35. Loeser, R. The Role of Aging in the Development of Osteoarthritis. *Trans. Am. Clin. Clim. Assoc.* **2017**, *128*, 44–54.
36. Marie, P.; Kassem, M. Extrinsic Mechanisms Involved in Age-Related Defective Bone Formation. *J. Clin. Endocrinol. Metab.* **2011**, *96*, 600–609. [CrossRef]
37. Shirazi, R.; Shirazi-Adl, A. Computational biomechanics of articular cartilage of human knee joint: Effect of osteochondral defects. *J. Biomech.* **2009**, *42*, 2458–2465. [CrossRef] [PubMed]
38. Stevens, J.; Binder-Macleod, S.; Snyder-Mackler, L. Characterization of the human quadriceps muscle in active elders. *Arch. Phys. Med. Rehabil.* **2001**, *82*, 973–978. [CrossRef] [PubMed]
39. Resorlu, M.; Doner, D.; Karatag, O.; Toprak, C. The relationship between chondromalacia patella, medial meniscal tear and medial periarticular bursitis in patients with osteoarthritis. *Radiol. Oncol.* **2017**, *51*, 401–406. [CrossRef]
40. Pereira, D.; Severo, M.; Ramos, E.; Branco, J.; Santos, R.; Costa, L.; Lucas, R.; Barros, H. Potential role of age, sex, body mass index and pain to identify patients with knee osteoarthritis. *Int. J. Rheum. Dis.* **2015**, *20*, 190–198. [CrossRef]
41. Go, D.; Kim, D.; Guermazi, A.; Crema, M.; Hunter, D.; Hwang, H.; Kim, H. Metabolic obesity and the risk of knee osteoarthritis progression in elderly community residents. A 3-year longitudinal cohort study. *Int. J. Rheum. Dis.* **2021**, *25*, 192–200. [CrossRef] [PubMed]
42. Gao, Y.; Zhao, C.; Liu, B.; Dong, N.; Ding, L.; Li, Y.; Liu, J.; Feng, W.; Qi, X.; Jin, X. An update on the association between metabolic syndrome and osteoarthritis and on the potential role of leptin in osteoarthritis. *Cytokine* **2020**, *129*, 155043. [CrossRef] [PubMed]

43. Wong, S.; Steinbach, L.; Zhao, J.; Stehling, C.; Ma, C.; Link, T. Comparative study of imaging at 3.0 T versus 1.5 T of the knee. *Skelet. Radiol.* **2009**, *38*, 761–769. [CrossRef]
44. Mandell, J.; Rhodes, J.; Shah, N.; Gaviola, G.; Gomoll, A.; Smith, S. Routine clinical knee MR reports: Comparison of diagnostic performance at 1.5 T and 3.0 T for assessment of the articular cartilage. *Skelet. Radiol.* **2017**, *46*, 1487–1498. [CrossRef]
45. Vasconcelos, F.; Cordeiro, B.; Rech, C.; Petroski, E. Sensitivity and specificity of the body mass index for the diagnosis of overweight/obesity in elderly. *Cad. Saude Publica* **2010**, *26*, 1519–1527. [CrossRef] [PubMed]

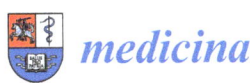

Article

Knee Diameter and Cross-Sectional Area as Biomarkers for Cartilage Knee Degeneration on Magnetic Resonance Images

Elias Primetis [1,†], Dionysios Drakopoulos [1,†], Dominik Sieron [1], Hugo Meusburger [1], Karol Szyluk [2,3], Paweł Niemiec [4], Verena C. Obmann [5], Alan A. Peters [5], Adrian T. Huber [5], Lukas Ebner [5,†], Georgios Delimpasis [1,†] and Andreas Christe [1,5,*,†]

[1] Department of Radiology SLS, Inselgroup, Bern University Hospital, University of Bern, Freiburgstrasse 10, 3010 Bern, Switzerland
[2] Department of Physiotherapy, Faculty of Health Sciences in Katowice, Medical University of Silesia in Katowice, 40-752 Katowice, Poland
[3] District Hospital of Orthopaedics and Trauma Surgery, Bytomska 62 St., 41-940 Piekary Slaskie, Poland
[4] Department of Biochemistry and Medical Genetics, Faculty of Health Sciences in Katowice, Medical University of Silesia in Katowice, 40-752 Katowice, Poland
[5] Department of Diagnostic, Interventional and Pediatric Radiology, Inselspital, Bern University Hospital, University of Bern, 3010 Bern, Switzerland
* Correspondence: andreas.christe@insel.ch
† These authors contributed equally to this work.

Abstract: *Background and Objectives*: Osteoarthritis (OA) of the knee is a degenerative disorder characterized by damage to the joint cartilage, pain, swelling, and walking disability. The purpose of this study was to assess whether demographic and radiologic parameters (knee diameters and knee cross-sectional area from magnetic resonance (MR) images) could be used as surrogate biomarkers for the prediction of OA. *Materials and Methods*: The knee diameters and cross-sectional areas of 481 patients were measured on knee MR images, and the corresponding demographic parameters were extracted from the patients' clinical records. The images were graded based on the modified Outerbridge arthroscopic classification that was used as ground truth. Receiver-operating characteristic (ROC) analysis was performed on the collected data. *Results*: ROC analysis established that age was the most accurate predictor of severe knee cartilage degeneration (corresponding to Outerbridge grades 3 and 4) with an area under the curve (AUC) of the specificity–sensitivity plot of 0.865 ± 0.02. An age over 41 years was associated with a sensitivity and specificity for severe degeneration of 82.8% (CI: 77.5–87.3%), and 76.4% (CI: 70.4–81.6%), respectively. The second-best degeneration predictor was the normalized knee cross-sectional area, with an AUC of 0.767 ± 0.04), followed by BMI (AUC = 0.739 ± 0.02), and normalized knee maximal diameter (AUC = 0.724 ± 0.05), meaning that knee degeneration increases with increasing knee diameter. *Conclusions*: Age is the best predictor of knee damage progression in OA and can be used as surrogate marker for knee degeneration. Knee diameters and cross-sectional area also correlate with the extent of cartilage lesions. Though less-accurate predictors of damage progression than age, they have predictive value and are therefore easily available surrogate markers of OA that can be used also by general practitioners and orthopedic surgeons.

Keywords: Outerbridge; chondromalacia; aging; body mass index; degeneration; magnetic resonance imaging

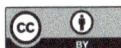

1. Introduction

Osteoarthritis (OA) of the knee is a very common pathology affecting the whole joint but in particular the cartilage [1]. It is classified as primary if its origin is unknown, or secondary if it is subsequent to a specific condition or event like trauma, repetitive micro stress, surgery, or malalignment [2]. OA is a degenerative disease that usually becomes manifest in the elderly [1]. The medial compartment is the most affected, though also the lateral and the patellofemoral compartments are also affected. The cartilage changes characteristic of this condition are accompanied by marginal osteophytes, subchondral bone cyst formation (geodes) and sclerosis, buttressing, and soft tissue changes, namely ganglion cyst formation, and periarticular soft tissue edema. Reactive synovium thickening and intra-articular fluid can also be observed [3,4]. The symptoms, including pain, stiffness and walking disability can increase to the point to deteriorate life quality, leading in some cases to depression [5]. The pathology is prevalent in the obese female population, and correlates with knee diameter [6–9]. Disease frequency and severity increase with increasing age [10,11].

Obesity, previous knee trauma, biomechanical factors, female gender and older age are common known risk factors for the development of osteoarthritis [12–14]. As no drugs are available to treat this condition, the focus is on prevention and management of joint damage progression through interventions on the modifiable risk factors, like the diet and physical exercise [13].

MR imaging (MRI) with 1.5 and 3 Tesla systems has proven to be a suitable technology for both the quantitative and qualitative assessment of joint cartilages [15,16], especially of the knee, and is clearly superior to plain radiography for the evaluation of the hyaline cartilage, as the last methodology provides only indirect signs of chondromalacia, actually not depicting the cartilage itself [17–20]. The Outerbridge scoring system is widely used to evaluate the extent of cartilage degeneration. It is a 5-grade scale: grade 0—normal articular cartilage, grade 1—softening of the cartilage due to biochemical modifications of the cartilage composition, grade 2—extent of cartilage loss <50%, grade 3—extent of cartilage loss >50%, and grade 4—complete cartilage loss accompanied by subchondral bone changes [21].

In spite of the high accuracy of MRI techniques for the assessment of the disease extent, this methodology is expensive and its use is restricted to equipped radiologic facilities and experienced medical staff. Therefore, more easily available tools to detect the disease and monitor its progression are needed.

Starting from the evidence that obese individuals with large knee cross sections often present with extensive cartilage degeneration (chondromalacia) [6], we hypothesized that both knee diameter and cross-sectional area might be employed as easily accessible surrogate biomarkers of chondromalacia. Similarly, given the high prevalence of OA in the obese female population as well as in the elderly [1,7], further parameters like age, gender, and BMI might also be suitable predictors of OA.

2. Materials and Methods

2.1. Ethics

The responsible ethics commission waived the requirement to obtain informed consent from the patients included in this study due to the study's retrospective nature and the irreversible anonymization of patients' identifying information.

2.2. Study Design

Among patients undergoing knee MRI between 2018 and 2019, 481 patients were retrospectively selected from the archives of community and clinical hospitals as well as private clinics in Zamość Elblag, Jelenia Góra and Bielsko-Biala (Poland) based on the inclusion and exclusion criteria listed below. The study was performed according to the STROBE guidelines. A number of 120–121 patients for each of four age groups were selected: <30 years (120); 30–45 years (120); 46–60 years (120); >60 years (121). Demographic data were retrieved from the MRI safety questionnaires of the corresponding clinics (age, sex, height, weight and BMI). The MR images used for this study had been acquired on either 1.5 T (SIGNA, GE, Milwaukee, WI, USA) or 3 T (Ingenia 3.0 T, Philips, Amsterdam, Netherlands) scanners using the following diagnostic sequence protocols: axial, sagittal and coronal PD FS, sagittal and coronal T1 (all with a slice thickness of 3 mm), 3D high-resolution PD FS with a slice thickness from 0.8 to 1 mm. All MRI data were irreversibly anonymized, and evaluated using iMac pro (Apple, Cupertino, CA, USA) with FDA-approved OsiriX MD software (version 11.0, Pixmeo SARL, Bernex, Switzerland). The radiological evaluation of cartilage chondromalacia included the medial, lateral and retropatellar compartments of the knee joint.

2.3. Inclusion and Exclusion Criteria

All patients undergoing an MRI of the knee in the period from 2018 to 2019 at the above-mentioned radiological clinics were eligible for this study. MRI referral was mostly due to knee pain, suspicion of arthrosis or post-traumatic lesions.

Patients with previous surgery, chronic post-traumatic changes, tumorous lesions in the knee joint, and examinations lacking the PD sequences for any reason (abortion of the MRI scan) were not included in the study.

2.4. Image Analysis

Four radiologists with radiology board examination and 10, 12, 17 and 25 years of experience in musculoskeletal radiology analyzed the images. Each radiologist assessed 30 patients from each age group. No double reading was performed, thus inter- and intrareader agreement could not be assessed. To evaluate cartilage chondromalacia, the modified Outerbridge classification (Table 1) for arthroscopic cartilage evaluation was used, and grading scores were attributed based on fat-saturated proton density sequences [22,23]. Besides cartilage assessment using Outerbridge scoring system, the Insall-Salvati index, cross-sectional area of the knee at the level of the upper pole of the patella as well as diameters at the same level were calculated [24].

Table 1. Modified Outerbridge classification.

Grade	Macroscopy	MRI
Grade 0	Normal cartilage	Normal cartilage
Grade 1	Rough surface; chondral softening, focal thickening	Inhomogeneous; high signal; surface intact; cartilage swelling
Grade 2	Irregular surface defects; <50% of cartilage thickness	Superficial ulceration, fissuring, fibrillation; <50% of cartilage thickness
Grade 3	Loss of >50% cartilage thickness	Ulceration fissuring, fibrillation; >50% of depth of cartilage
Grade 4	Cartilage loss	Full thickness chondral wear with exposure of subchondral bone

The following parameters of the knee joint were measured for the subsequent analysis:

(1) On the sagittal PD-weighted images, the patellar ligament and the max. pole to pole distance in the patella were measured to calculate the Insall-Salvati index (Figure 1).
(2) Knee diameters were measured on axial PD-weighted images at the exact level of the patella upper pole (strictly antero-posterior = vertical, and medio-lateral = horizontal, independent of the leg position; Figure 2). The larger of these 2 diameters was taken as "maximal diameter".
(3) The whole knee cross-sectional area at the same level was automatically calculated by the Osirix software (Figure 2),
(4) The largest axial diameter of the distal femur at the level of maximal condyle diameter was measured and used for normalization (Figure 3).

In addition, some individuals tend to use the right more than the left side, or vice versa, and/or may be or may have been active in a sport discipline involving overuse of one side and thus are suffering from repetitive microtrauma. This is potentially related with a differential Outerbridge grading for the two body sides, and therefore the analysis did include specification of the investigated side.

Furthermore, the MRI resolution of images acquired with a 3 T unit is higher than that of images from examinations performed at a 1.5 T unit, suggesting the possibility of earlier detection of (severe) degeneration related with the use of the more powerful 3 T unit [19]. Therefore, the used MRI strength (1.5 T vs. 3 T) Tesla was also included in the evaluation.

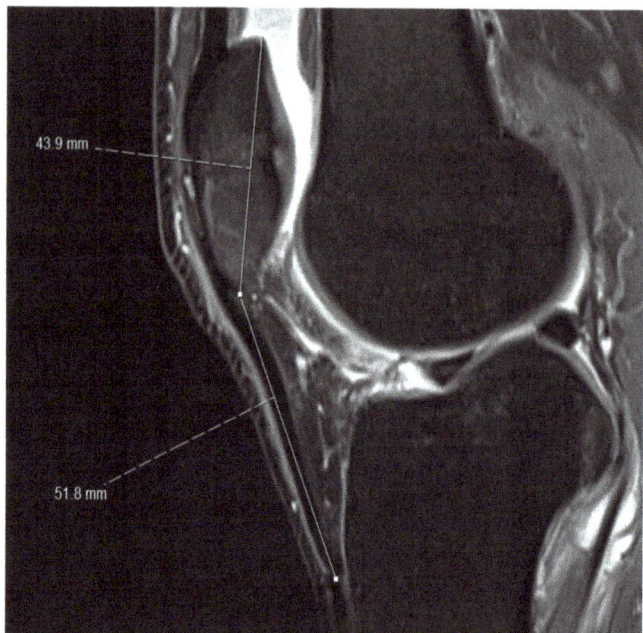

Figure 1. Normal Insall-Salvati index. For the knee in the figure, an Insall Salvati index of 1.18 was obtained by dividing the length of the patellar ligament (51.8 mm) by the patellar pole distance (43.9 mm).

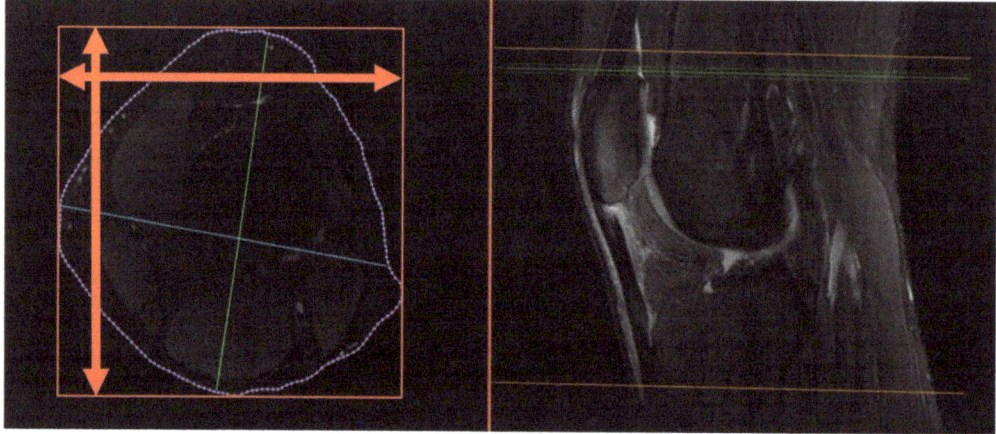

Figure 2. Knee diameters were measured on axial PD-weighted images at the exact level of the patella upper pole, indicated by the green line on the right image. Radiologists measured strictly antero-posterior = vertical and medio-lateral = horizontal (red arrows). The maximal diameter of the knee was not measured (green line on left image).

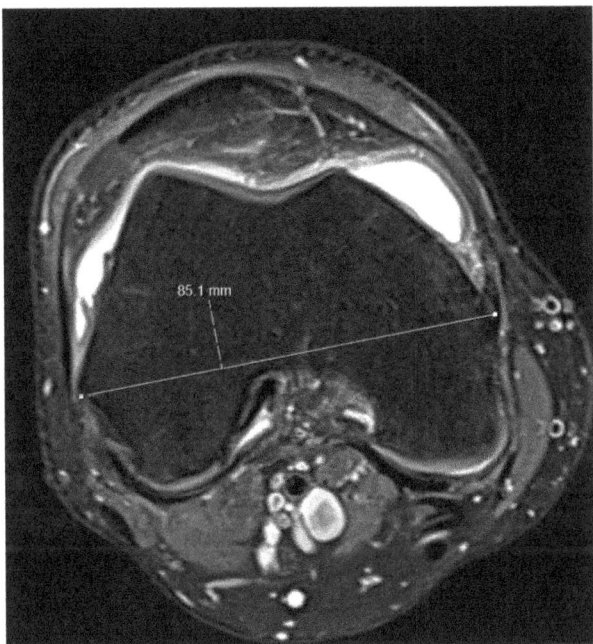

Figure 3. The largest axial femur diameter was measured at the level of the condyles as indicated in the figure.

2.5. Statistical Analysis

The Outerbridge scores were assessed in the lateral, medial and retropatellar compartment. The maximal score of all three compartments was pooled into zero or slight degeneration (Outerbridge 0–2) and severe degeneration (Outerbridge 3 and 4) and was defined as the classifying variable (outcome). A logistic regression was performed with the binary variables (gender (f, m), examination side (right, left), MRI strength (1.5 or 3 T)) to retrieve regression coefficients and odds ratios. Measurements were normalized for 122 patients: the maximal knee diameter and cross-sectional area were normalized by dividing their value by the max femoral diameter to level out the fact that larger patients have larger knees without necessarily suffering from knee degeneration. The non-binary variables (age, height, weight, BMI, Insall-Salvati index, knee cross-sectional area, vertical, horizontal and maximal diameter as well as normalized maximal diameter and cross-sectional area) were analyzed using receiver operating characteristic curves (ROC). The respective areas under the curve (AUC) were used as comparators to establish the most accurate parameter for the prediction of severe cartilage degeneration. AUC comparison was performed based on pairwise comparison of ROC curves. MedCalc® (Version 19.3, Medcalc Software Ltd, Ostend, Belgium) was used for statistical analysis. The significance level was set to $p < 0.05$.

Sample size calculation. The null hypothesis is that an AUC of 0.5 corresponds to random detection probability. The significance level and power of the test were set to 0.05 and 0.8, respectively. The estimated ratio between slight and severe degeneration was 3:1. To reach an AUC of 0.6 and higher (at least 0.1 higher than chance) a sample size of 352 patients was needed.

3. Results

3.1. Demographics and Average Measurements

Gender (f:m) and examination side (right:left) were equally distributed (Table 2). The average age and BMI of the study patients was 45.3 ± 22 years and 27.2 ± 5.4 kg/m^2, respectively. The retropatellar compartment presented the highest level of cartilage degeneration with an average Outerbridge score of 1.9 ± 1.5, followed by the medial and lateral compartment with scores of 1.7 ± 1.5 and 1.5 ± 1.4, respectively. The average maximal knee diameter and cross-sectional area of the knee were 13.8 ± 1.4 cm and 131.6 ± 30.2 cm^2, respectively. The examined parameters and corresponding results are summarized in Table 3.

Table 2. Binary variables distribution.

Gender (f:m)	242:239
Knee (right:left)	241:240
MRI (1.5T:3T)	163:318

Table 3. Summary of non-binary variable statistics.

	N	Mean	Median	SD	25–75 P
age (years)	481	45.33	45	21.66	27 to 62
BMI (kg/m^2)	481	27.21	27	5.39	24 to 30
weight (kg)	481	79.32	80	17.78	69 to 90
height (m)	481	1.70	1.70	0.11	1.63 to 1.78
knee cross-sectional area (cm^2)	481	131.63	128	30.21	111 to 146
horizontal knee diameter (cm)	481	13.42	13.5	1.64	12.4 to 14.4
vertical knee diameter (cm)	481	13.25	13.1	1.46	12.3 to 14.1
maximal knee diameter (cm)	481	13.78	13.7	1.43	12.8 to 14.7
Insall Salvati index	481	1.08	1.08	0.16	0.98 to 1.18
maximal Outerbridge grade per knee	481	2.28	3	1.55	1 to 4
maximal lateral Outerbridge grade	481	1.52	2	1.41	0 to 3
maximal medial Outerbridge grade	481	1.70	2	1.54	0 to 3
maximal retropatellar Outerbridge grade	481	1.89	2	1.46	0 to 3
maximal femur diameter (cm)	122	8.29	8.4	0.71	7.7 to 8.9
normalized knee cross-sectional area	122	15.47	14.36	4.29	13.0 to 16.5
normalized maximal knee diameter	122	0.89	0.894	0.12	0.82 to 0.97

N: number of cases; SD: Standard Deviation; P: Percentile.

3.2. Logistic Regression for Binary Variables

Gender, examined side and MRI scanner strength did not correlate with the evaluated outcome (severe degeneration = Outerbridge grades 3 and 4), proving therefore useless in predicting degeneration, with the following logistic regression formula:

$$\text{Logit (severe degeneration)} = -0.264 * M + 0.068 * R - 0.18 * T + 0.25$$

M: male patient = 1, female patient = 0; R: right knee = 1, left knee = 0; T: 1.5 T scanner = 1, 3 T scanner = 0. These variables demonstrated non-significant odd ratios for degeneration around 1 (Table 4).

Table 4. Logistic regression of dichotomous variables for severe knee degeneration (Outerbridge > 2).

Variable	Odds Ratio	95% CI	Coefficient	Std Error	p-Value
Gender = m	0.768	0.53 to 1.10	−0.26	0.18	0.152
Knee side = right	1.071	0.75 to 1.54	0.07	0.18	0.710
MRI = 1.5 T	0.833	0.57 to 1.22	−0.18	0.19	0.348
Constant			0.25	0.21	0.241

CI: Confidence Interval, m: male; MRI: Magnetic Resonance Imaging; T: Tesla.

3.3. Receiver Operating Characteristic Curves (ROC) for Non-Binary Variables

The parameter that allowed for the most accurate prediction of severe degeneration (Outerbridge grades 3 and 4) was the age, with an AUC of 0.865 ± 0.02 on the specificity-sensitivity plot. For an age over 41 years, sensitivity and specificity for severe degeneration were 82.8% (CI: 77.5–87.3%) and 76.4% (CI: 70.4–81.6%), respectively. The next best predictor for degeneration was the normalized cross section area of the knee (AUC = 0.767 ± 0.04), followed by BMI (AUC = 0.739 ± 0.02) and the normalized maximal diameter of the knee (AUC = 0.724 ± 0.05). The absolute diameters and cross-sectional areas showed AUCs in the range of 0.653–0.685. The Insall-Salvati index proved to be useless for making predictions. The AUC, sensitivity, specificity and relative criteria for all non-binary variables are listed in Table 5 and the ROC curves are depicted in Figure 4.

Table 5. Accuracy (AUC) of demographic and radiologic parameters for the prediction of severe knee degeneration (Outerbridge > 2).

Variable	AUC	Std. Error	p-Value	Criterion	Sensitivity	95% CI	Specificity	95% CI
age	0.865	0.02	<0.0001	>41 years	82.8	77.5–87.3	76.4	70.4–81.6
Height (m)	0.538	0.03	0.1535	≤1.66 m	45.1	38.7–51.6	65.0	58.5–71.0
weight	0.672	0.02	<0.0001	>72 Kg	80.7	75.2–85.5	49.8	43.3–56.3
BMI	0.739	0.02	<0.0001	>24.9	82.8	77.5–87.3	52.7	46.2–59.2
Insall-Salvati index	0.508	0.03	0.7613	>1.25	9.4	6.1–13.8	83.5	78.2–88.0
AREA (cm^2)	0.676	0.02	<0.0001	>117.2 cm^2	80.3	74.8–85.1	49.0	42.4–55.5
vertical diameter (cm)	0.653	0.02	<0.0001	>12.7 cm	74.2	68.2–79.6	52.3	45.8–58.8
horizontal diameter (cm)	0.667	0.02	<0.0001	>13.1 cm	73.0	66.9–78.4	55.7	49.1–62.1
max diameter	0.685	0.02	<0.0001	>13.3	77.1	71.3–82.2	52.3	45.8–58.8
max diameter normalized	0.724	0.05	<0.0001	>1.60	73.3	60.3–83.9	67.7	54.7–79.1
normalized area	0.767	0.04	<0.0001	>14.08	81.7	69.6–90.5	62.9	49.7–74.8

AUC: Area under the curve; CI: Confidence Interval; BMI: Body Mass Index.

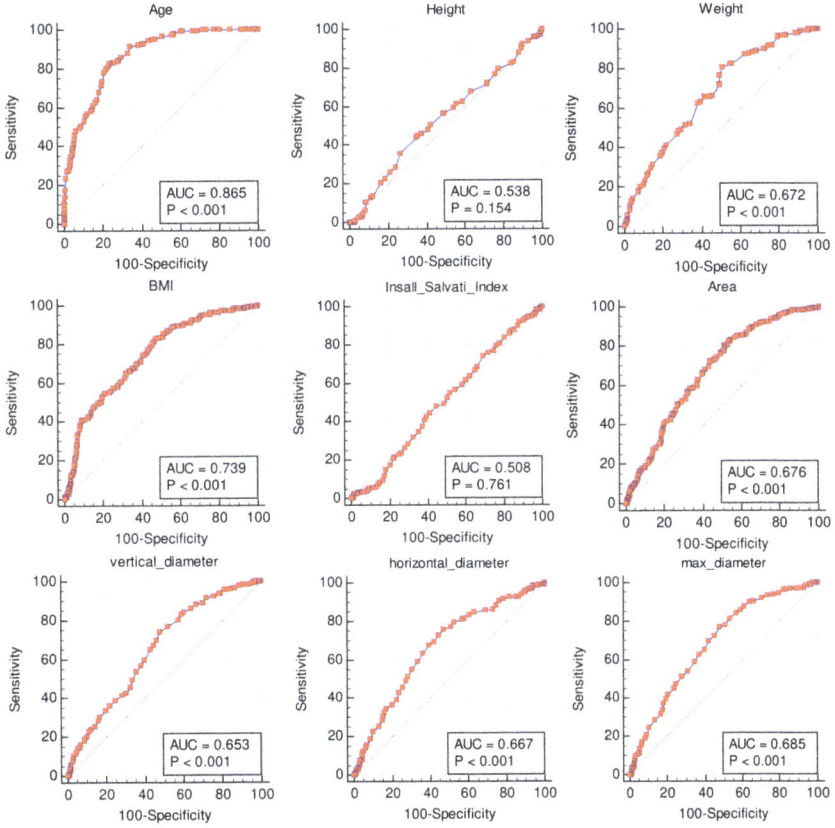

Figure 4. Areas under the curve of the non-binary variables. Top predictors for severe Outerbridge score before normalization are age, BMI and maximal knee diameter.

3.4. Comparisons of ROC Curves

Age has a significantly higher AUC for predicting severe degeneration than BMI ($p < 0.0001$), maximal diameter ($p < 0.0001$) and knee cross-sectional area ($p < 0.0001$). BMI showed a significantly better accuracy for detecting degeneration than maximal diameter ($p = 0.0049$) and knee cross-sectional area ($p = 0.0008$).

For the 122 patients that have been normalized by the maximal femur diameter (Figure 5), age did not demonstrate a significant difference in AUC compared to the normalized maximal diameter ($p = 0.363$) or the normalized knee area ($p = 0.846$). No combination of variables for a multicriteria ROC analysis reached a higher AUC than age alone.

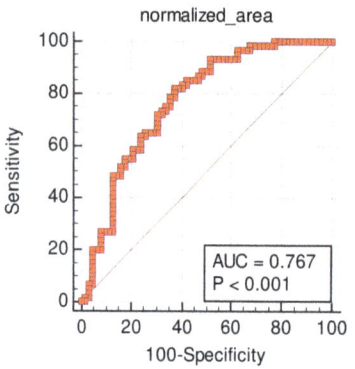 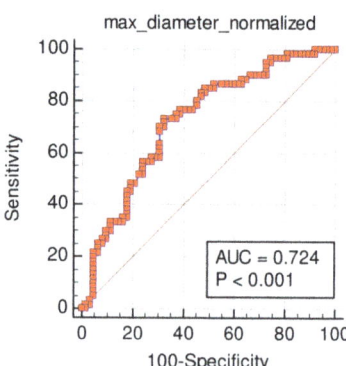

Figure 5. Normalizing the knee cross-sectional area and maximal knee diameter by dividing the measurements by the maximal femur diameter (at the level of the condyles) results in an increase in the respective AUCs.

4. Discussion

The purpose of our study was to assess the areas under the curve of multiple variables (age, height, weight, BMI, Insall-Salvati index, cross section area of the knee, vertical diameter, horizontal diameter, maximal diameter) as well as normalized cross-sectional area and normalized maximal diameter as biomarkers for the prediction of knee cartilage degeneration. The knee images used for this study were acquired using 1.5 T and 3 T MRI scanners. To grade cartilage changes, the modified Outerbridge classification was used. Both 1.5 T and 3.0 T scanners have been proven effective in detecting not only advanced cartilage loss but also mild cartilage changes [25], although previous studies have stressed the superiority of 3.0 T scanners for cartilage assessment [19,26].

Degenerative cartilage changes and subsequent loss in joint cartilage volume are among the first structural changes observed during OA progression, and they are always present in patients with advanced osteoarthritis [21].

Age and obesity are known risk factors for knee pain and osteoarthritis. Previous studies showed that degenerative knee changes increase with increasing obesity measured in terms of BMI and that cartilage loss extent is age-dependent and more pronounced in individuals aged 50+ years [9,19,27–29].

Our study results provide evidence for the fact that knee cartilage changes begin earlier in life with a cut-off for prediction of cartilage degeneration set to 41 years of age, making age the best surrogate biomarker for severe cartilage degeneration.

Many age-dependent factors such as gradual strength loss of quadriceps muscle and increased oxidative stress in the knee joint microenvironment contribute to this process [30–34].

As for obesity, body weight excess promotes knee joint degeneration in a multifactorial way, including both mechanical and metabolic components. On the one side indeed, obesity constitute a chronic overload for the legs' joints, and it also modifies the biomechanics and the axes load of the joints in the lower extremities. On the other side, metabolic factors are affected by obesity, e.g., the proliferation of chondrocytes, which is impaired in overweight individuals, or leptin secretion, a hormone regulating the food intake habits that was shown to also play a role in OA [10,35,36].

Previous attempts have been made to quantify the amount of adipose tissue surrounding the knee, beyond BMI, e.g., by measuring the anteroposterior and sinistro-dexter (medio-lateral) knee diameter as well as by measuring the surface of the knee cross-sectional area, and to evaluate these measurements as possible prognostic indicators for cartilage loss [8]. The rationale behind the evaluation of these parameters with respect to their ability to be prognostic markers was their potential use by clinicians as a simplified way to predict cartilage degeneration, performing the relevant measurements on the x-ray images, where the cartilage is not visible, thus avoiding a more expensive MRI examination, or even by measuring the diameters or the circumference of the knee directly on the patient's body, making imaging unnecessary, at least at the moment a first risk assessment is indicated. Only a weak association was observed between the extent of cartilage loss, as graded by the Outerbridge scale, and the anteroposterior knee diameter, the sinistro-dexter diameter or the knee surface area.

In the present study, we included in our evaluation also the normalized cross-sectional area and the normalized maximal diameter of the knee by dividing the cross-sectional area and the maximal knee diameter by the maximal femoral diameter in a subgroup of 122 patients. The area under the curve was used to evaluate the different parameters as possible predictors. No combination of these parameters proved to be a better predictor of degeneration than age alone. In the 122 patients in which measurements were normalized to the maximal femur diameter, normalized diameter and area measurement showed the same ability to predict severe cartilage degeneration as the age variable did, whereas the absolute measurements of the diameter and area (n = 481) were significantly inferior as surrogate biomarkers than the variable age alone. This signifies that in order for the measurements to be as efficient as age in predicting cartilage degeneration, the measurements need to be normalized.

4.1. Strengths

The large number of patients (481), the inclusion of all knee compartments in the cartilage assessment, the further analysis of knee cross-sectional area and maximal diameter upon normalization and the calculation of the ROC AUC values for all parameters are some of the strengths of our study, making the statistical results of the study more reliable and strengthening the conclusions.

4.2. Limitations

Axial images were not perpendicular to leg axis, which might have caused an overestimation of the diameters, circumference and knee cross-sectional areas. However, we counteracted the above-mentioned bias by simplifying the readout: the strictly vertical and horizontal diameters of the knee were measured and the knee cross-sectional surface was measured automatically by Osirix, allowing greater reproducibility. Furthermore, the Outerbridge classification is a radiological score and not a reliable direct measurement. Although the correlation between the Outerbridge score and arthroscopic or surgical knee findings is high [21], the clinical impact would still be the ground truth. Another limitation is that inter- and intra-reader variability assessments are missing due to the fact that no double reading was performed because of the large size of the dataset under investigation.

5. Conclusions

Our hypothesis that larger knee diameters and cross-sectional area but also gender, obesity (BMI), and the older age are correlated with a larger extent of knee cartilage degeneration proved correct. These parameters can therefore be used as surrogate biomarkers for knee cartilage loss in OA (Outerbridge grades 3 and 4), with age representing the most accurate biomarker, but not the only one. The measurement of the knee diameter directly on the patient's body or on the patient's knee x-ray images can substitute for the use of lengthier and more expensive imaging methodologies and constitute an easily accessible diagnostic tool that not only radiologists but also general practitioners or orthopedic surgeons can use, with a maximal knee diameter over 13 cm being an alarm bell for severe knee cartilage degeneration.

Author Contributions: Conceptualization, A.C., D.S. and H.M.; methodology, A.C., D.S. and H.M.; software, A.C.; Validation, E.P., D.D., G.D., K.S., P.N., A.C. and D.S.; formal analysis, E.P., G.D., K.S., P.N., A.C. and D.S.; investigation, A.C. and D.S.; resources, A.C., L.E., D.S. and H.M.; data curation, D.S., K.S. and P.N.; writing—original draft preparation, E.P., D.D., G.D., D.S. and A.C.; writing—review and editing, E.P., D.D:, H.M., D.S., G.D., K.S., P.N., V.C.O., A.A.P., A.T.H., L.E. and A.C.; visualization, A.C., V.C.O., A.A.P. and A.T.H.; supervision, A.C. and D.S.; project administration, A.C. and L.E. All authors have read and agreed to the published version of the manuscript.

Funding: This research received no external funding.

Institutional Review Board Statement: Ethical review and approval were waived for this study due to the retrospective nature of the study without participation of the patients and the irreversible anonymization of the image data (SIL.KB.1076.2022.MP).

Informed Consent Statement: The responsible ethics commission waived the requirement to obtain informed consent from the patients included in this study due to the study's retrospective nature and the irreversible anonymization of patients' identifying information.

Data Availability Statement: Data are available upon special request.

Acknowledgments: We would like to thank Grazia Maria Cereghetti De Marchi for the distinguished manuscript preparation.

Conflicts of Interest: The authors declare no conflict of interest.

References

1. Sharma, L. Osteoarthritis of the Knee. *N. Engl. J. Med.* **2021**, *384*, 51–59. [CrossRef] [PubMed]
2. Altman, R.; Asch, E.; Bloch, D.; Bole, G.; Borenstein, D.; Brandt, K.; Christy, W.; Cooke, T.D.; Greenwald, R.; Hochberg, M.; et al. Development of criteria for the classification and reporting of osteoarthritis. Classification of osteoarthritis of the knee. Diagnostic and Therapeutic Criteria Committee of the American Rheumatism Association. *Arthritis Rheum.* **1986**, *29*, 1039–1049. [CrossRef] [PubMed]
3. Wong, B.L.; Bae, W.C.; Chun, J.; Gratz, K.R.; Lotz, M.; Sah, R.L. Biomechanics of cartilage articulation: Effects of lubrication and degeneration on shear deformation. *Arthritis Rheum.* **2008**, *58*, 2065–2074. [CrossRef] [PubMed]
4. Carballo, C.B.; Nakagawa, Y.; Sekiya, I.; Rodeo, S.A. Basic Science of Articular Cartilage. *Clin. Sports Med.* **2017**, *36*, 413–425. [CrossRef] [PubMed]
5. Axford, J.; Butt, A.; Heron, C.; Hammond, J.; Morgan, J.; Alavi, A.; Bolton, J.; Bland, M. Prevalence of anxiety and depression in osteoarthritis: Use of the Hospital Anxiety and Depression Scale as a screening tool. *Clin. Rheumatol.* **2010**, *29*, 1277–1283. [CrossRef]
6. Zheng, H.; Chen, C. Body mass index and risk of knee osteoarthritis: Systematic review and meta-analysis of prospective studies. *BMJ Open* **2015**, *5*, e007568. [CrossRef]
7. Hanna, F.S.; Teichtahl, A.J.; Wluka, A.E.; Wang, Y.; Urquhart, D.M.; English, D.R.; Giles, G.G.; Cicuttini, F.M. Women have increased rates of cartilage loss and progression of cartilage defects at the knee than men: A gender study of adults without clinical knee osteoarthritis. *Menopause* **2009**, *16*, 666–670. [CrossRef]
8. Sieron, D.; Jablonska, I.; Lukoszek, D.; Szyluk, K.; Meusburger, H.; Delimpasis, G.; Kostrzewa, M.; Platzek, I.; Christe, A. Knee Diameter and Cross-Section Area Measurements in MRI as New Promising Methods of Chondromalacia Diagnosis-Pilot Study. *Medicina* **2022**, *58*, 1142. [CrossRef]
9. Matada, M.S.; Holi, M.S.; Raman, R.; Jayaramu Suvarna, S.T. Visualization of Cartilage from Knee Joint Magnetic Resonance Images and Quantitative Assessment to Study the Effect of Age, Gender and Body Mass Index (BMI) in Progressive Osteoarthritis (OA). *Curr. Med. Imaging Rev.* **2019**, *15*, 565–572. [CrossRef]
10. Go, D.J.; Kim, D.H.; Guermazi, A.; Crema, M.D.; Hunter, D.J.; Hwang, H.S.; Kim, H.A. Metabolic obesity and the risk of knee osteoarthritis progression in elderly community residents: A 3-year longitudinal cohort study. *Int. J. Rheum. Dis.* **2022**, *25*, 192–200. [CrossRef]
11. Sacitharan, P.K.; Vincent, T.L. Cellular ageing mechanisms in osteoarthritis. *Mamm. Genome* **2016**, *27*, 421–429. [CrossRef]

12. Blagojevic, M.; Jinks, C.; Jeffery, A.; Jordan, K.P. Risk factors for onset of osteoarthritis of the knee in older adults: A systematic review and meta-analysis. *Osteoarthritis Cartilage* **2010**, *18*, 24–33. [CrossRef]
13. Georgiev, T.; Angelov, A.K. Modifiable risk factors in knee osteoarthritis: Treatment implications. *Rheumatol. Int.* **2019**, *39*, 1145–1157. [CrossRef]
14. Martin, K.R.; Kuh, D.; Harris, T.B.; Guralnik, J.M.; Coggon, D.; Wills, A.K. Body mass index, occupational activity, and leisure-time physical activity: An exploration of risk factors and modifiers for knee osteoarthritis in the 1946 British birth cohort. *BMC Musculoskelet. Disord.* **2013**, *14*, 219. [CrossRef]
15. Link, T.M.; Sell, C.A.; Masi, J.N.; Phan, C.; Newitt, D.; Lu, Y.; Steinbach, L.; Majumdar, S. 3.0 vs 1.5 T MRI in the detection of focal cartilage pathology–ROC analysis in an experimental model. *Osteoarthritis Cartilage* **2006**, *14*, 63–70. [CrossRef]
16. Kuo, R.; Panchal, M.; Tanenbaum, L.; Crues, J.V., 3rd. 3.0 Tesla imaging of the musculoskeletal system. *J. Magn. Reson. Imaging* **2007**, *25*, 245–261. [CrossRef]
17. Reed, M.E.; Villacis, D.C.; Hatch, G.F., 3rd; Burke, W.S.; Colletti, P.M.; Narvy, S.J.; Mirzayan, R.; Vangsness, C.T., Jr. 3.0-Tesla MRI and arthroscopy for assessment of knee articular cartilage lesions. *Orthopedics* **2013**, *36*, e1060–e1064. [CrossRef]
18. Argentieri, E.C.; Burge, A.J.; Potter, H.G. Magnetic Resonance Imaging of Articular Cartilage within the Knee. *J. Knee Surg.* **2018**, *31*, 155–165. [CrossRef]
19. Cheng, Q.; Zhao, F.C. Comparison of 1.5- and 3.0-T magnetic resonance imaging for evaluating lesions of the knee: A systematic review and meta-analysis (PRISMA-compliant article). *Medicine* **2018**, *97*, e12401. [CrossRef]
20. Kijowski, R.; Blankenbaker, D.G.; Davis, K.W.; Shinki, K.; Kaplan, L.D.; De Smet, A.A. Comparison of 1.5- and 3.0-T MR imaging for evaluating the articular cartilage of the knee joint. *Radiology* **2009**, *250*, 839–848. [CrossRef]
21. Slattery, C.; Kweon, C.Y. Classifications in Brief: Outerbridge Classification of Chondral Lesions. *Clin. Orthop. Relat. Res.* **2018**, *476*, 2101–2104. [CrossRef] [PubMed]
22. Eldridge, S.E.; Barawi, A.; Wang, H.; Roelofs, A.J.; Kaneva, M.; Guan, Z.; Lydon, H.; Thomas, B.L.; Thorup, A.S.; Fernandez, B.F.; et al. Agrin induces long-term osteochondral regeneration by supporting repair morphogenesis. *Sci. Transl. Med.* **2020**, *12*, aax9086. [CrossRef] [PubMed]
23. Park, C.H.; Song, K.S.; Kim, J.R.; Lee, S.W. Retrospective evaluation of outcomes of bone peg fixation for osteochondral lesion of the talus. *Bone Jt. J.* **2020**, *102*, 1349–1353. [CrossRef] [PubMed]
24. Verhulst, F.V.; van Sambeeck, J.D.P.; Olthuis, G.S.; van der Ree, J.; Koeter, S. Patellar height measurements: Insall-Salvati ratio is most reliable method. *Knee Surg. Sports Traumatol. Arthrosc.* **2020**, *28*, 869–875. [CrossRef] [PubMed]
25. Mandell, J.C.; Rhodes, J.A.; Shah, N.; Gaviola, G.C.; Gomoll, A.H.; Smith, S.E. Routine clinical knee MR reports: Comparison of diagnostic performance at 1.5 T and 3.0 T for assessment of the articular cartilage. *Skeletal. Radiol.* **2017**, *46*, 1487–1498. [CrossRef]
26. Wong, S.; Steinbach, L.; Zhao, J.; Stehling, C.; Ma, C.B.; Link, T.M. Comparative study of imaging at 3.0 T versus 1.5 T of the knee. *Skeletal. Radiol.* **2009**, *38*, 761–769. [CrossRef]
27. O'Connor, M.I. Sex Differences in Osteoarthritis of the Hip and Knee. *J. Am. Acad. Orthop. Surg.* **2007**, *15*, S22–S25. [CrossRef]
28. Grotle, M.; Hagen, K.B.; Natvig, B.; Dahl, F.A.; Kvien, T.K. Obesity and osteoarthritis in knee, hip and/or hand: An epidemiological study in the general population with 10 years follow-up. *BMC Musculoskelet. Disord.* **2008**, *9*, 132. [CrossRef]
29. Murphy, L.; Schwartz, T.A.; Helmick, C.G.; Renner, J.B.; Tudor, G.; Koch, G.; Dragomir, A.; Kalsbeek, W.D.; Luta, G.; Jordan, J.M. Lifetime risk of symptomatic knee osteoarthritis. *Arthritis Rheum.* **2008**, *59*, 1207–1213. [CrossRef]
30. Stevens, J.E.; Binder-Macleod, S.; Snyder-Mackler, L. Characterization of the human quadriceps muscle in active elders. *Arch. Phys. Med. Rehabil.* **2001**, *82*, 973–978. [CrossRef]
31. Loeser, R.F. The Role of Aging in the Development of Osteoarthritis. *Trans. Am. Clin. Climatol. Assoc.* **2017**, *128*, 44–54.
32. Temple-Wong, M.M.; Ren, S.; Quach, P.; Hansen, B.C.; Chen, A.C.; Hasegawa, A.; D'Lima, D.D.; Koziol, J.; Masuda, K.; Lotz, M.K.; et al. Hyaluronan concentration and size distribution in human knee synovial fluid: Variations with age and cartilage degeneration. *Arthritis Res. Ther.* **2016**, *18*, 18. [CrossRef]
33. Kanthawang, T.; Bodden, J.; Joseph, G.B.; Lane, N.E.; Nevitt, M.; McCulloch, C.E.; Link, T.M. Obese and overweight individuals have greater knee synovial inflammation and associated structural and cartilage compositional degeneration: Data from the osteoarthritis initiative. *Skeletal. Radiol.* **2021**, *50*, 217–229. [CrossRef]
34. Hubert, J.; Beil, F.T.; Rolvien, T.; Butscheidt, S.; Hischke, S.; Puschel, K.; Frosch, S.; Mussawy, H.; Ries, C.; Hawellek, T. Cartilage calcification is associated with histological degeneration of the knee joint: A highly prevalent, age-independent systemic process. *Osteoarthritis Cartilage* **2020**, *28*, 1351–1361. [CrossRef]
35. Gao, Y.H.; Zhao, C.W.; Liu, B.; Dong, N.; Ding, L.; Li, Y.R.; Liu, J.G.; Feng, W.; Qi, X.; Jin, X.H. An update on the association between metabolic syndrome and osteoarthritis and on the potential role of leptin in osteoarthritis. *Cytokine* **2020**, *129*, 155043. [CrossRef]
36. Pereira, D.; Severo, M.; Ramos, E.; Branco, J.; Santos, R.A.; Costa, L.; Lucas, R.; Barros, H. Potential role of age, sex, body mass index and pain to identify patients with knee osteoarthritis. *Int. J. Rheum. Dis.* **2017**, *20*, 190–198. [CrossRef]

Disclaimer/Publisher's Note: The statements, opinions and data contained in all publications are solely those of the individual author(s) and contributor(s) and not of MDPI and/or the editor(s). MDPI and/or the editor(s) disclaim responsibility for any injury to people or property resulting from any ideas, methods, instructions or products referred to in the content.

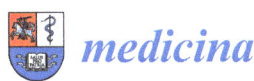

Article

Adjustable-Loop Cortical Suspensory Fixation Results in Greater Tibial Tunnel Widening Compared to Interference Screw Fixation in Primary Anterior Cruciate Ligament Reconstruction

Tae-Jin Lee [1], Ki-Mo Jang [2], Tae-Jin Kim [1], Sang-Min Lee [1] and Ji-Hoon Bae [1,*]

1 Department of Orthopaedic Surgery, Korea University Guro Hospital, Korea University College of Medicine, Seoul 08308, Korea
2 Department of Orthopaedic Surgery, Korea University Anam Hospital, Korea University College of Medicine, Seoul 02841, Korea
* Correspondence: osman@korea.ac.kr; Tel.: +82-2-2626-3296

Abstract: *Background:* Although the use of adjustable-loop suspensory fixation has increased in recent years, the influence of the shortcomings of suspensory fixation, such as the bungee-cord or windshield-wiper effects, on tunnel widening remains to be clarified. *Hypothesis/Purpose:* The purpose of this study was to compare adjustable-loop femoral cortical suspensory fixation and interference screw fixation in terms of tunnel widening and clinical outcomes after anterior cruciate ligament reconstruction (ACLR). We hypothesized that tunnel widening in the adjustable-loop femoral cortical suspensory fixation (AL) group would be comparable to that in the interference screw fixation (IF) group. *Methods:* This study evaluated patients who underwent primary ACLR at our institution between March 2015 and June 2019. The femoral and tibial tunnel diameters were measured using plain radiographs in the immediate postoperative period and 2 years after ACLR. Tunnel widening and clinical outcomes (Lysholm score, 2000 International Knee Documentation Committee subjective score, and Tegner activity level) were compared between the two groups. *Results:* There were 48 patients (mean age, 29.8 ± 12.0 years) in the AL group and 44 patients (mean age, 26.0 ± 9.5 years) in the IF group. Tunnel widening was significantly greater in the AL group than that in the IF group at the tibia anteroposterior (AP) middle (2.03 mm vs. 1.32 mm, $p = 0.017$), tibia AP distal (1.52 mm vs. 0.84 mm, $p = 0.012$), tibia lateral proximal (1.85 mm vs. 1.00 mm, $p = 0.001$), tibia lateral middle (2.36 mm vs. 1.03 mm, $p < 0.001$), and tibia lateral distal (2.34 mm vs. 0.85 mm, $p < 0.001$) levels. There were no significant differences between the two groups with respect to femoral tunnel widening and clinical outcomes. *Conclusions:* Tibial tunnel widening was significantly greater in the AL group than in the IF group at 2 years after primary ACLR. However, the clinical outcomes in the two groups were comparable at 2 years.

Keywords: anterior cruciate ligament; reconstruction; bone tunnel widening; adjustable-loop device; interference screw; hamstring tendon; autograft

Citation: Lee, T.-J.; Jang, K.-M.; Kim, T.-J.; Lee, S.-M.; Bae, J.-H. Adjustable-Loop Cortical Suspensory Fixation Results in Greater Tibial Tunnel Widening Compared to Interference Screw Fixation in Primary Anterior Cruciate Ligament Reconstruction. *Medicina* 2022, 58, 1193. https://doi.org/10.3390/medicina58091193

Academic Editor: Vassilios S. Nikolaou

Received: 8 August 2022
Accepted: 30 August 2022
Published: 1 September 2022

Publisher's Note: MDPI stays neutral with regard to jurisdictional claims in published maps and institutional affiliations.

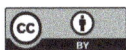

Copyright: © 2022 by the authors. Licensee MDPI, Basel, Switzerland. This article is an open access article distributed under the terms and conditions of the Creative Commons Attribution (CC BY) license (https://creativecommons.org/licenses/by/4.0/).

1. Introduction

Anatomical anterior cruciate ligament (ACL) reconstruction (ACLR) is being performed more frequently than in the past, and the use of adjustable- or fixed-loop devices has increased with the development of suspensory fixation. With suspensory fixation, the graft has full contact within the bone tunnel without any foreign material, which may allow early graft integration. However, femoral cortical suspensory fixation may increase the risk of tunnel widening due to micro-movements at the bone-tendon interface, such as the bungee-cord and windshield-wiper effects along the longitudinal and transverse axes, respectively [1,2].

Micro-movements at the tendon-bone interface, such as the bungee-cord and windshield-wiper effects, have resulted in tunnel widening in experimental animal studies [3]. A recent meta-analysis revealed greater femoral tunnel widening with suspensory fixation using a fixed-loop device for ACLR than that with transfemoral cross-pin fixation [4]. In comparison, interference screw fixation has the advantage of reducing graft movement in the tunnel and synovial fluid influx, although there is a risk of graft and tunnel damage during screw insertion. A recent study also reported that tunnel widening with interference screws was less than that with cortical suspensory fixation [5,6].

The use of adjustable-loop devices has increased to compensate for the micro-movement due to cortical suspensory fixation. Several studies have reported that adjustable-loop devices can reduce micro-movements compared to fixed-loop devices after ACLR [7–10]. However, studies have reported that the adjustable-loop device may cause tunnel widening after surgery [11,12].

Although most previous studies did not report an association between tunnel widening and adverse clinical outcomes, large tunnels may compromise graft fixation during revision surgery or may necessitate two-stage surgery [13–17]. Therefore, the purpose of our study was to compare tunnel widening and clinical outcomes after ACLR with adjustable-loop femoral cortical suspensory fixation to those with interference screw fixation. We hypothesized that tunnel widening in the adjustable-loop femoral cortical suspensory fixation (AL) group would be comparable to that in the interference screw fixation (IF) group.

2. Methods

2.1. Participants

This study retrospectively analyzed data obtained from our prospective longitudinal observational study of primary ACLR between March 2015 and June 2019 at our institutions, namely Korea University Anam Hospital and Korea University Guro Hospital, Seoul, Republic of Korea. All patients were provided written information about the study and informed consent was obtained. Ethical approval was obtained from the institutional review board (IRB) of our hospital (IRB No. 2021GR0105). Patients who underwent primary ACLR were included, and demographic data were collected from electronic medical records.

Patients who met the following inclusion criteria were included: (1) anatomical single-bundle ACLR using hamstring-tendon autograft (outside-in technique); (2) the same tibial fixation technique (interference screw fixation with additional fixation); and (3) a follow-up of at least 2 years. The exclusion criteria were as follows: (1) other ligament injuries requiring surgical treatment, (2) previous knee surgeries, and (3) subsequent injuries (ACL graft failure, meniscus or cartilage injury, or contralateral ACL rupture).

Of the 352 patients who underwent primary ACLR in our institution, 109 met the inclusion and exclusion criteria for the study. The study was conducted on 92 patients who completed serial tests. The AL group included 48 patients and 44 patients were allocated to the IF group. The patient's flow diagram is shown in Figure 1.

2.2. Surgical Technique and Rehabilitation

All patients underwent anatomical single-bundle ACLR. Surgeries were performed by two senior surgeons. One surgeon used an adjustable-loop cortical suspensory device for femoral fixation, and the other surgeon used an interference screw for femoral fixation. Tibial fixation was performed in the same way in both groups. If there was a meniscus tear, concomitant meniscus repair or a meniscectomy was performed, according to meniscal repairability, prior to ACLR.

A two-incision outside-in technique was used for anatomical femoral tunnel placement in all cases. In the AL group, the femoral part of the graft was prepared using adjustable-loop suspensory devices (TightRope [Arthrex, Naples, FL, USA]), and the femoral tunnel was made by retrograde drilling. In the interference screw fixation group (IF group), antegrade drilling and bioabsorbable interference screw (GENESYS Matryx [ConMed, Utica, NY, USA]) were used for femoral fixation. In both groups, a bioabsorbable interference screw was used for tibial fixation after cyclic loading. Additionally, a 6.5-mm cancellous screw and spiked washer (Arthrex, Naples, FL, USA) were used on the tibial side. The femoral and tibial tunnels were of the same size as the graft diameter, and bioabsorbable interference screws of the same size were used. In both group, grafts were inserted up to the distal end of the tibial tunnel. For the femoral tunnel, the suspensory group inserted the grafts into the femoral tunnel 5 mm away from proximal end and the interference group inserted the grafts up to the proximal end of the femoral tunnel (Figure 2).

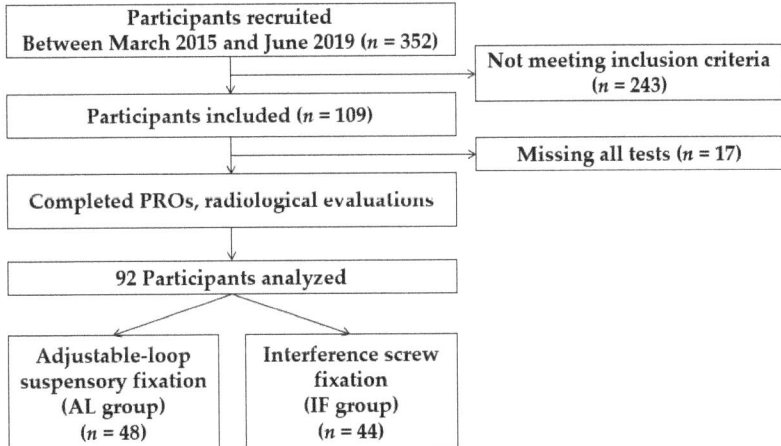

Figure 1. Patient flow diagram. AL, adjustable-loop suspensory fixation; IF, interference screw fixation.

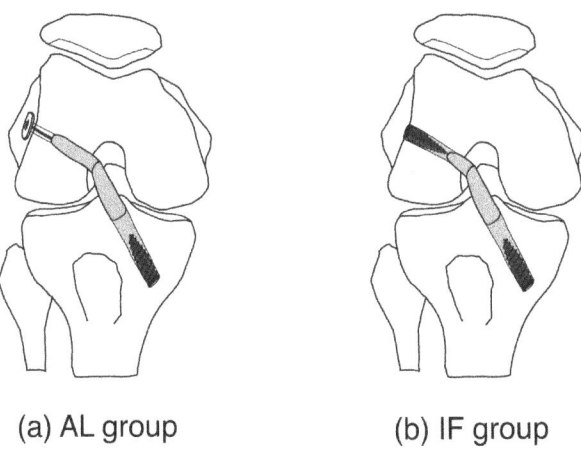

Figure 2. Surgical technique.

After ACLR, all patients underwent the same rehabilitation protocol. A return to previous sports activities was allowed if the patient achieved >80–90% muscle strength compared with that of the contralateral uninjured leg.

2.3. Radiographic Evaluation

Anteroposterior (AP) and lateral radiographs were taken immediately after surgery and at 12 and 24 months after surgery. On the AP and lateral radiographs, the diameters of the femoral and tibial tunnels were measured between the two sclerotic margins perpendicular to the longitudinal axis at the proximal, middle, and distal sites of the tunnel (Figure 3) [11]. Tunnel widening was calculated by subtracting the diameter measured immediately after surgery from that measured 24 months after surgery.

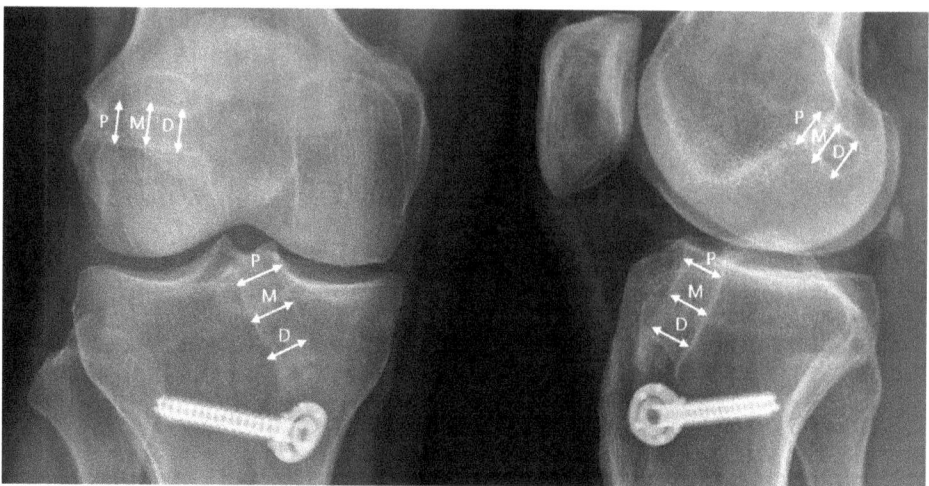

Figure 3. Anteroposterior and lateral radiographs of a right knee showing measurement of each tunnel at proximal (P), middle (M), and distal (D) locations.

All radiographic measurements were performed on the picture archiving and communications system (PACS [INFINITT Healthcare, Seoul, Korea]) using a mouse cursor with automated distance calculation. Two orthopedic surgeons, who were trained in identifying each variable, independently reviewed the radiographs. They performed measurements on two separate occasions, 4 weeks apart.

2.4. Clinical Evaluation

All patients were evaluated during their regular visits to the outpatient clinic at 6, 12, and 24 months after surgery. The independent staff (experienced athletic trainers and physical therapists) from our sports rehabilitation center conducted all the tests and obtained the data. Patients completed three patient-reported outcomes, including the Lysholm Knee Scoring Scale, the 2000 International Knee Documentation Committee (IKDC) subjective scale, and Tegner activity level [18,19].

2.5. Second-Look Arthroscopy and Graft Evaluation Method

Second-look arthroscopy was performed for skin irritation from the tibial fixation screw at least one year after ACLR. During the second-look arthroscopy, newly identified problems that were not present at the time of ACLR were investigated. In addition, a modified graft maturation scoring system (Korea University Medical Center score; KUMC score) was used for graft evaluation based on previous studies [20,21].

Two blinded observers (orthopedic surgeons) scored each parameter, and interobserver and intraobserver reliabilities were evaluated. Total graft maturation scores (KUMC score) and individual parameter scores were compared between the two groups.

2.6. Statistical Analysis

In a pilot study of 10 patients from both groups, tunnel widening was measured, and the mean and standard deviation were calculated. To achieve a power of 80% using a two-group t-test with a two-sided significance level of $p < 0.05$, a sample size of 44 in each treatment group was required when calculated using the value measured at the middle of the lateral tibial view as a variable. Data for the final follow-up were available for 48 patients in the AL group and 44 patients in the IF group. Therefore, a power of 80% was reached.

Demographic variables (including patient sex, age, and body mass index), clinical outcomes, and tunnel widening calculated using radiologic measurements were compared between the two groups. Independent *t*-tests and Mann–Whitney U tests were used for continuous variables. Chi-square tests and Fisher's exact tests were used for categorical variables. Paired-samples *t*-tests and Wilcoxon signed-rank tests were applied to continuous variables within each group.

For each variable, the intraclass and interclass correlation coefficients were calculated to quantify the agreement between the measurements. Correlation coefficients >0.75 and <0.4 represent good and poor agreement, respectively [22]. In addition, all variables were expressed using mean values and standard deviations.

Statistical significance was set at $p < 0.05$. Statistical analysis was performed using SPSS for Windows (version 20.0; IBM Corp., Armonk, NY, USA).

3. Results

Demographic data of the 92 patients are presented in Table 1. No significant differences in age, sex, or body mass index were observed between the two groups.

Table 1. Demographic factors.

	Total ($n = 92$)	AL Group ($n = 48$)	IF Group ($n = 44$)	*p*-Value *
Age (years)	28.0 ± 11.1	29.8 ± 12.0	26.0 ± 9.5	0.081
Sex				0.557
Male, *n* (%)	79 (85.9)	40 (83.3)	39 (88.6)	
Female, *n* (%)	13 (14.1)	8 (16.7)	5 (11.4)	
BMI (kg/m^2)	25.3 ± 3.3	25.7 ± 3.4	24.9 ± 3.3	0.259

Values are given as mean and standard deviation. BMI, body mass index. * Comparisons between the AL and IF groups. AL, adjustable-loop suspensory fixation; IF, interference screw fixation.

3.1. Radiologic Outcomes

Significant tunnel widening was observed at all measured sites between the immediate postoperative period and 2 years after ACLR in both groups (Tables 2 and 3). All correlation coefficients ranged from 0.813 to 0.935, indicating good reliability.

Table 2. Immediate and 2-year postoperative tunnel size in the AL group.

	Immediate Postoperative	2-Year Postoperative	*p*-Value *
Femur AP Proximal (mm)	9.10 ± 1.23	9.86 ± 1.70	**<0.001**
Femur AP Middle (mm)	9.16 ± 1.17	10.30 ± 1.82	**<0.001**
Femur AP Distal (mm)	9.17 ± 1.15	10.45 ± 1.85	**<0.001**
Tibia AP Proximal (mm)	9.33 ± 1.05	10.63 ± 1.42	**<0.001**
Tibia AP Middle (mm)	9.53 ± 1.02	11.56 ± 1.60	**<0.001**
Tibia AP Distal (mm)	9.60 ± 1.07	11.12 ± 1.45	**<0.001**
Femur Lat Proximal (mm)	8.64 ± 1.10	9.62 ± 1.88	**<0.001**
Femur Lat Middle (mm)	8.70 ± 1.12	9.98 ± 1.90	**<0.001**
Femur Lat Distal (mm)	8.70 ± 1.09	9.94 ± 1.85	**<0.001**
Tibia Lat Proximal (mm)	9.09 ± 0.88	10.94 ± 1.42	**<0.001**
Tibia Lat Middle (mm)	9.34 ± 1.02	11.70 ± 1.62	**<0.001**
Tibia Lat Distal (mm)	9.33 ± 1.11	11.67 ± 1.61	**<0.001**

Bold indicates statistical significance ($p < 0.05$). Values are given as mean and standard deviation. * Comparisons between the immediate and 2-year postoperative values. Lat, lateral. AP, anterior posterior; Lat, lateral.

The tunnel widening in the AL group was significantly greater than that in the IF group at the tibia AP middle, tibia AP distal, tibia lateral proximal, tibia lateral middle, and tibia lateral distal (Table 4).

Table 3. Immediate and 2-year postoperative tunnel size in the IF group.

	Immediate Postoperative	2-Year Postoperative	p-Value *
Femur AP Proximal (mm)	9.61 ± 1.42	10.54 ± 1.51	<0.001
Femur AP Middle (mm)	9.43 ± 1.44	10.79 ± 1.53	<0.001
Femur AP Distal (mm)	9.20 ± 1.18	10.76 ± 1.37	<0.001
Tibia AP Proximal (mm)	9.48 ± 0.85	10.81 ± 1.39	<0.001
Tibia AP Middle (mm)	9.58 ± 0.89	10.89 ± 1.06	<0.001
Tibia AP Distal (mm)	9.53 ± 0.84	10.37 ± 1.05	<0.001
Femur Lat Proximal (mm)	9.19 ± 1.30	9.74 ± 1.13	<0.001
Femur Lat Middle (mm)	8.95 ± 1.09	9.86 ± 1.10	<0.001
Femur Lat Distal (mm)	8.79 ± 0.89	9.99 ± 1.02	<0.001
Tibia Lat Proximal (mm)	9.38 ± 0.87	10.38 ± 1.17	<0.001
Tibia Lat Middle (mm)	9.47 ± 0.82	10.50 ± 0.99	<0.001
Tibia Lat Distal (mm)	9.45 ± 0.87	10.30 ± 1.08	<0.001

Bold indicates statistical significance ($p < 0.05$). Values are given as mean and standard deviation. * Comparisons between the immediate and 2-year postoperative values. Lat, lateral.

Table 4. Tunnel widening between immediate and 2-year postoperative.

	AL Group (n = 48)	IF Group (n = 44)	p-Value *
Femur AP Proximal (mm)	0.76 ± 1.37	0.93 ± 1.59	0.574
Femur AP Middle (mm)	1.14 ± 1.48	1.36 ± 1.46	0.459
Femur AP Distal (mm)	1.27 ± 1.51	1.56 ± 1.45	0.355
Tibia AP Proximal (mm)	1.30 ± 1.33	1.33 ± 1.61	0.914
Tibia AP Middle (mm)	2.03 ± 1.45	1.32 ± 1.34	0.017
Tibia AP Distal (mm)	1.52 ± 1.41	0.84 ± 1.09	0.012
Femur Lat Proximal (mm)	0.98 ± 1.47	0.54 ± 1.73	0.198
Femur Lat Middle (mm)	0.29 ± 1.59	0.91 ± 1.46	0.244
Femur Lat Distal (mm)	1.23 ± 1.60	1.20 ± 1.16	0.905
Tibia Lat Proximal (mm)	1.85 ± 1.25	1.00 ± 1.19	**0.001**
Tibia Lat Middle (mm)	2.36 ± 1.46	1.03 ± 1.10	**<0.001**
Tibia Lat Distal (mm)	2.34 ± 1.25	0.85 ± 1.27	**<0.001**

Bold indicates statistical significance ($p < 0.05$). Values are presented as mean and standard deviation. * Comparisons between the AL and IF groups. Lat, lateral.

3.2. Clinical Outcomes

There were no significant differences in patient-reported outcomes (Lysholm score, 2000 IKDC subjective score, and Tegner activity level) between the two groups at 2 years after ACLR (Table 5).

Table 5. Clinical outcomes: 2-year postoperative patient-reported outcomes.

	AL Group (n = 48)	IF Group (n = 44)	p-Value *
Lysholm score	82.5 ± 14.5	83.5 ± 19.3	0.766
IKDC subjective score	75.3 ± 17.4	80.5 ± 13.6	0.121
Tegner activity level **	5	6	0.153

Values are presented as mean and standard deviation. * Comparisons between the AL and IF groups. ** Data are presented as a frequency distribution. IKDC, international knee documentation committee.

3.3. Second-Look Arthroscopic Evaluation

Twenty-four patients in each group underwent second-look arthroscopic evaluation, and the operation was performed at an average of 24.5 and 26.8 months after ACLR in the AL and IF groups, respectively. After the second-look arthroscopic examination, total graft maturation scores (KUMC score) were compared between the two groups. In patients undergoing second-look arthroscopy, there was no significant difference in the KUMC scores between the two groups (Table 6). All correlation coefficients ranged from 0.838 to 0.905, indicating good reliability. Regarding newly identified problems in group 1, two meniscal tears were identified. In group 2, two cyclops lesions and two meniscal tears were identified.

Table 6. Second-look arthroscopic evaluation: graft maturation scores (KUMC scores).

	AL Group (n = 24)	IF Group (n = 24)	p-Value *
Graft integrity **	2	2	1.000
Graft synovial coverage **	2	2	0.690
Graft tension **	2	2	0.931
Graft vascularization **	2	2	0.306
KUMC score **	8	7	0.741

* Comparisons between the AL and IF groups. ** Data are presented as a frequency distribution. KUMC, Korea University Medical Center.

4. Discussion

The main findings of this study were that ACLR using interference screw fixation was associated with less postoperative tibial tunnel widening than that using adjustable-loop femoral cortical suspensory fixation at the 2-year follow-up and that there were no significant differences between the two groups with regard to femoral tunnel widening or clinical outcomes. However, it was difficult to clearly explain the difference in tunnel widening between the two groups. The exact reason was not found, but various factors are presumed to be involved.

Several potential reasons for the differences between the two groups can be considered with regard to tibial tunnel widening. Interference screw fixation has the advantage of reducing micro-movements compared to adjustable-loop femoral cortical suspensory fixation. In a randomized controlled trial, Fauno and Kaalund [14] found that tunnel widening is influenced by the mechanical properties of the implants. They found that extracortical fixation of the graft was associated with more laxity than close-to-joint fixation. Similarly, Giorgio et al. [23] reported that the use of a more elastic fixation system (TightRope) is associated with more laxity and results in greater tunnel widening. They explained that graft motion, such as the bungee-cord and windshield-wiper effects, is caused by low-stiffness systems such as those using extracortical fixation. In the study by Sabat et al. [24], tunnel widening was significantly lesser in the transfix group than in the EndoButton group. They thought that this was because the fixation point was farther away from the aperture. Interestingly, Lind et al. [25] suggested that the femoral fixation technique could potentially affect the biomechanical and biological environment in the tibial tunnel, thus affecting tunnel widening in the tibia. Accordingly, we thought that the difference in the femoral fixation method in our study could have influenced the tunnel widening in the tibia.

However, unlike tibial tunnel widening, a significant difference in femoral tunnel widening was not seen in the present study. We attributed this to the difference between the characteristics of the distal femur and the proximal tibia. Chang et al. [26] reported the mechanical and structural properties of distal femur and proximal tibial bones in vivo. Their study showed that the stiffness of the distal femur was greater than that of the proximal tibia. Therefore, the widening of the femoral tunnel could be expected to be relatively small. Kuskucu [27] reported that a graft that becomes free because of fixation in the tunnel at a site distant from the tunnel opening in the joint will result in greater micro-movement with knee motion. Since micro-movement in the femoral tunnel was less than that in the tibial tunnel, the difference in the femoral tunnel width was not significant.

In contrast to the results of our study, some previous studies have reported that greater femoral tunnel widening occurred when using a suspensory device on the femoral side. Mayr et al. [5] reported that ACLR using adjustable-loop cortical button fixation was associated with greater femoral tunnel enlargement than that with biodegradable interference screw fixation. However, their study differed from our study in that they used an all-inside ACLR. In the suspensory group, patients were treated with all-side ACLR using adjustable-loop button fixation on both the femoral and tibial sides. Suspensory tibial fixation may have influenced whether tunnel widening occurred in the femur or tibia. In a similar study, Baumfeld et al. [15] reported a comparison between double cross-pin and suspensory graft fixation. Femoral tunnel widening associated with the use of the EndoButton suspensory fixation system was significantly greater than that with the use of double cross-pins for fixation within the tunnel. However, their results may be different from ours because they did not standardize the tibial fixation method.

In this study, both groups showed excellent overall clinical outcomes. Patient-reported outcomes, including the Lysholm score, 2000 IKDC subjective score, and Tegner activity level, improved over a postoperative period of 2 years. However, there were no significant differences between the two groups. In addition, in patients undergoing second-look arthroscopy, there was no significant difference in the graft maturation scoring system (KUMC) scores between the two groups. Raj et al. [28] evaluated the correlation between the bone tunnel diameter following ACLR using a hamstring-tendon autograft and functional outcomes. They concluded that neither the diameter nor widening of the bone tunnel during the follow-up period was correlated with functional outcomes. Several studies have reported that there were no clinical implications of tunnel widening after ACLR [12,29–32]. However, the absence of clinical differences may be attributed to the small difference in tunnel widening between the two groups. Therefore, the results of long-term follow-up may vary. Tunnel widening should be considered in revision ACLR, but a difference of approximately 1 mm will not have significant implications.

This study has several limitations. First, this study was designed retrospectively, and the operations were performed by two surgeons. Although the same outside-in technique was used, the difference between antegrade and retrograde drilling for the femoral tunnel could affect the results. Second, the use of an interference screw can affect the width of the tunnel. There was a risk of graft and tunnel damage during screw insertion. However, the analysis showed that there was no significant difference in tunnel widening by the interference screw in the present study. Third, the minimum follow-up period was only 2 years. Although there was no difference in clinical outcomes in this study, further studies are needed as outcomes may vary at the mid- to long-term follow-up.

5. Conclusions

In conclusion, tibial tunnel widening after ACLR using a hamstring-tendon autograft was significantly greater with adjustable-loop femoral cortical suspensory fixation than with interference screw fixation at the 2-year follow-up. However, the clinical outcomes in the two groups were comparable at the 2-year follow-up.

Author Contributions: T.-J.L.: study concepts/design, manuscript drafting/revision, K.-M.J.: data acquisition/analysis, manuscript revision, T.-J.K.: data acquisition/analysis, S.-M.L.: data acquisition/analysis, J.-H.B.: study concepts/design, manuscript drafting/revision. All authors have read and agreed to the published version of the manuscript.

Funding: This research received no external funding.

Institutional Review Board Statement: This study was approved by the institutional ethical review board (2021GR0105).

Informed Consent Statement: The informed consent was obtained from each patient.

Acknowledgments: Authors would like to acknowledge support from Sports Medical Center at our institution for obtaining clinical measurements and Medical Science Research Center for statistical analysis.

Conflicts of Interest: Each author certifies that he has no commercial associations (e.g., consultancies, stock ownership, equity interest, patent/licensing arrangements, etc.) that might pose a conflict of interest in connection with the submitted article.

References

1. Barrow, A.E.; Pilia, M.; Guda, T.; Kadrmas, W.R.; Burns, T.C. Femoral suspension devices for anterior cruciate ligament reconstruction: Do adjustable loops lengthen? *Am. J. Sports Med.* **2014**, *42*, 343–349. [CrossRef] [PubMed]
2. Mayr, R.; Heinrichs, C.H.; Eichinger, M.; Coppola, C.; Schmoelz, W.; Attal, R. Biomechanical comparison of 2 anterior cruciate ligament graft preparation techniques for tibial fixation: Adjustable-length loop cortical button or interference screw. *Am. J. Sports Med.* **2015**, *43*, 1380–1385. [CrossRef] [PubMed]
3. Rodeo, S.A.; Kawamura, S.; Kim, H.J.; Dynybil, C.; Ying, L. Tendon healing in a bone tunnel differs at the tunnel entrance versus the tunnel exit: An effect of graft-tunnel motion? *Am. J. Sports Med.* **2006**, *34*, 1790–1800. [CrossRef]
4. Lee, D.H.; Son, D.W.; Seo, Y.R.; Lee, I.G. Comparison of femoral tunnel widening after anterior cruciate ligament reconstruction using cortical button fixation versus transfemoral cross-pin fixation: A systematic review and meta-analysis. *Knee Surg. Relat. Res.* **2020**, *32*, 11. [CrossRef]
5. Mayr, R.; Smekal, V.; Koidl, C.; Coppola, C.; Fritz, J.; Rudisch, A.; Kranewitter, C.; Attal, R. Tunnel widening after ACL reconstruction with aperture screw fixation or all-inside reconstruction with suspensory cortical button fixation: Volumetric measurements on CT and MRI scans. *Knee* **2017**, *24*, 1047–1054. [CrossRef] [PubMed]
6. Pereira, V.L.; Medeiros, J.V.; Nunes, G.R.S.; de Oliveira, G.T.; Nicolini, A.P. Tibial-graft fixation methods on anterior cruciate ligament reconstructions: A literature review. *Knee Surg. Relat. Res.* **2021**, *33*, 7. [CrossRef]
7. Noonan, B.C.; Bachmaier, S.; Wijdicks, C.A.; Bedi, A. Intraoperative Preconditioning of Fixed and Adjustable Loop Suspensory Anterior Cruciate Ligament Reconstruction With Tibial Screw Fixation-An In Vitro Biomechanical Evaluation Using a Porcine Model. *Arthroscopy* **2018**, *34*, 2668–2674. [CrossRef]
8. Onggo, J.R.; Nambiar, M.; Pai, V. Fixed- Versus Adjustable-Loop Devices for Femoral Fixation in Anterior Cruciate Ligament Reconstruction: A Systematic Review. *Arthroscopy* **2019**, *35*, 2484–2498. [CrossRef]
9. Kamitani, A.; Hara, K.; Arai, Y.; Atsumi, S.; Takahashi, T.; Nakagawa, S.; Fuji, Y.; Inoue, H.; Takahashi, K. Adjustable-Loop Devices Promote Graft Revascularization in the Femoral Tunnel After ACL Reconstruction: Comparison With Fixed-Loop Devices Using Magnetic Resonance Angiography. *Orthop. J. Sports Med.* **2021**, *9*, 2325967121992134. [CrossRef]
10. Asif, N.; Khan, M.J.; Haris, K.P.; Waliullah, S.; Sharma, A.; Firoz, D. A prospective randomized study of arthroscopic ACL reconstruction with adjustable- versus fixed-loop device for femoral side fixation. *Knee Surg. Relat. Res.* **2021**, *33*, 42. [CrossRef]
11. Choi, N.H.; Yang, B.S.; Victoroff, B.N. Clinical and Radiological Outcomes After Hamstring Anterior Cruciate Ligament Reconstructions: Comparison Between Fixed-Loop and Adjustable-Loop Cortical Suspension Devices. *Am. J. Sports Med.* **2017**, *45*, 826–831. [CrossRef] [PubMed]
12. Sundararajan, S.R.; Sambandam, B.; Singh, A.; Rajagopalakrishnan, R.; Rajasekaran, S. Does Second-Generation Suspensory Implant Negate Tunnel Widening of First-Generation Implant Following Anterior Cruciate Ligament Reconstruction? *Knee Surg. Relat. Res.* **2018**, *30*, 341–347. [CrossRef] [PubMed]
13. Buelow, J.U.; Siebold, R.; Ellermann, A. A prospective evaluation of tunnel enlargement in anterior cruciate ligament reconstruction with hamstrings: Extracortical versus anatomical fixation. *Knee Surg. Sports Traumatol. Arthrosc.* **2002**, *10*, 80–85. [CrossRef]
14. Fauno, P.; Kaalund, S. Tunnel widening after hamstring anterior cruciate ligament reconstruction is influenced by the type of graft fixation used: A prospective randomized study. *Arthroscopy* **2005**, *21*, 1337–1341. [CrossRef] [PubMed]
15. Baumfeld, J.A.; Diduch, D.R.; Rubino, L.J.; Hart, J.A.; Miller, M.D.; Barr, M.S.; Hart, J.M. Tunnel widening following anterior cruciate ligament reconstruction using hamstring autograft: A comparison between double cross-pin and suspensory graft fixation. *Knee Surg. Sports Traumatol. Arthrosc.* **2008**, *16*, 1108–1113. [CrossRef]
16. Lind, M.; Feller, J.; Webster, K.E. Bone tunnel widening after anterior cruciate ligament reconstruction using EndoButton or EndoButton continuous loop. *Arthroscopy* **2009**, *25*, 1275–1280. [CrossRef]
17. Oh, J.Y.; Kim, K.T.; Park, Y.J.; Won, H.C.; Yoo, J.I.; Moon, D.K.; Cho, S.H.; Hwang, S.C. Biomechanical comparison of single-bundle versus double-bundle anterior cruciate ligament reconstruction: A meta-analysis. *Knee Surg. Relat. Res.* **2020**, *32*, 14. [CrossRef]
18. Chalmers, P.N.; Mall, N.A.; Moric, M.; Sherman, S.L.; Paletta, G.P.; Cole, B.J.; Bach, B.R., Jr. Does ACL reconstruction alter natural history?: A systematic literature review of long-term outcomes. *J. Bone Jt. Surg. Am.* **2014**, *96*, 292–300. [CrossRef]
19. Leiter, J.R.; Gourlay, R.; McRae, S.; de Korompay, N.; MacDonald, P.B. Long-term follow-up of ACL reconstruction with hamstring autograft. *Knee Surg. Sports Traumatol. Arthrosc.* **2014**, *22*, 1061–1069. [CrossRef]
20. Kim, S.G.; Jung, J.H.; Song, J.H.; Bae, J.H. Evaluation parameters of graft maturation on second-look arthroscopy following anterior cruciate ligament reconstruction: A systematic review. *Knee Surg. Relat. Res.* **2019**, *31*, 2. [CrossRef]
21. Kim, S.G.; Kim, S.H.; Kim, J.G.; Jang, K.M.; Lim, H.C.; Bae, J.H. Hamstring autograft maturation is superior to tibialis allograft following anatomic single-bundle anterior cruciate ligament reconstruction. *Knee Surg. Sports Traumatol. Arthrosc.* **2018**, *26*, 1281–1287. [CrossRef]
22. Fleiss, J.; levin, B.; Paik, M. The measurement of interrater agreement. In *Statistical Methods for Rates and Proportions*, 3rd ed.; Wiley Online Library: Hoboken, NJ, USA, 1987; Chapter 18. [CrossRef]
23. Giorgio, N.; Moretti, L.; Pignataro, P.; Carrozzo, M.; Vicenti, G.; Moretti, B. Correlation between fixation systems elasticity and bone tunnel widening after ACL reconstruction. *Muscles Ligaments Tendons J.* **2016**, *6*, 467–472. [CrossRef] [PubMed]

24. Sabat, D.; Kundu, K.; Arora, S.; Kumar, V. Tunnel widening after anterior cruciate ligament reconstruction: A prospective randomized computed tomography—Based study comparing 2 different femoral fixation methods for hamstring graft. *Arthroscopy* **2011**, *27*, 776–783. [CrossRef] [PubMed]
25. Lind, M.; Feller, J.; Webster, K.E. Tibial bone tunnel widening is reduced by polylactate/hydroxyapatite interference screws compared to metal screws after ACL reconstruction with hamstring grafts. *Knee* **2009**, *16*, 447–451. [CrossRef]
26. Chang, G.; Rajapakse, C.S.; Babb, J.S.; Honig, S.P.; Recht, M.P.; Regatte, R.R. In vivo estimation of bone stiffness at the distal femur and proximal tibia using ultra-high-field 7-Tesla magnetic resonance imaging and micro-finite element analysis. *J. Bone Miner Metab.* **2012**, *30*, 243–251. [CrossRef] [PubMed]
27. Kuskucu, S.M. Comparison of short-term results of bone tunnel enlargement between EndoButton CL and cross-pin fixation systems after chronic anterior cruciate ligament reconstruction with autologous quadrupled hamstring tendons. *J. Int. Med. Res.* **2008**, *36*, 23–30. [CrossRef]
28. Raj, M.A.V.; Ram, S.M.; Venkateswaran, S.R.; Manoj, J. Bone tunnel widening following arthroscopic reconstruction of anterior cruciate ligament (Acl) using hamstring tendon autograft and its functional consequences. *Int. J. Orthop. Sci.* **2018**, *4*, 160–163. [CrossRef]
29. Mayr, R.; Smekal, V.; Koidl, C.; Coppola, C.; Eichinger, M.; Rudisch, A.; Kranewitter, C.; Attal, R. ACL reconstruction with adjustable-length loop cortical button fixation results in less tibial tunnel widening compared with interference screw fixation. *Knee Surg. Sports Traumatol. Arthrosc.* **2020**, *28*, 1036–1044. [CrossRef] [PubMed]
30. Monaco, E.; Fabbri, M.; Redler, A.; Gaj, E.; De Carli, A.; Argento, G.; Saithna, A.; Ferretti, A. Anterior cruciate ligament reconstruction is associated with greater tibial tunnel widening when using a bioabsorbable screw compared to an all-inside technique with suspensory fixation. *Knee Surg. Sports Traumatol. Arthrosc.* **2019**, *27*, 2577–2584. [CrossRef]
31. Lopes, O.V., Jr.; de Freitas Spinelli, L.; Leite, L.H.C.; Buzzeto, B.Q.; Saggin, P.R.F.; Kuhn, A. Femoral tunnel enlargement after anterior cruciate ligament reconstruction using RigidFix compared with extracortical fixation. *Knee Surg. Sports Traumatol. Arthrosc.* **2017**, *25*, 1591–1597. [CrossRef]
32. Karikis, I.; Ejerhed, L.; Sernert, N.; Rostgard-Christensen, L.; Kartus, J. Radiographic Tibial Tunnel Assessment After Anterior Cruciate Ligament Reconstruction Using Hamstring Tendon Autografts and Biocomposite Screws: A Prospective Study with 5-Year Follow-Up. *Arthroscopy* **2017**, *33*, 2184–2194. [CrossRef] [PubMed]

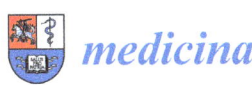

Article

Beneficial Effect of Curved Dilator System for Femoral Tunnel Creation in Preventing Femoral Tunnel Widening after Anterior Cruciate Ligament Reconstruction

O-Sung Lee [1], Joong Il Kim [2], Seok Hyeon Han [3] and Joon Kyu Lee [4,*]

1. Department of Orthopedic Surgery, Eulji University School of Medicine, Uijeongbu-si 11759, Republic of Korea; xixzeus@naver.com
2. Department of Orthopaedic Surgery, Hallym University Kangnam Sacred Heart Hospital, Seoul 07741, Republic of Korea; jungil@hanmail.net
3. Department of Orthopaedic Surgery, Konkuk University Medical Center, Seoul 05030, Republic of Korea; shh3892@naver.com
4. Department of Orthopaedic Surgery, Konkuk University Medical Center, Research Institute of Medical Science, Konkuk University School of Medicine, Seoul 05030, Republic of Korea
* Correspondence: ndfi@naver.com; Tel.: +82-10-3280-8129

Abstract: *Backgrounds and objectives:* A prevalent concern in anterior cruciate ligament (ACL) reconstruction is postoperative tunnel widening. We hypothesized that employing a curved dilator system (CDS) for femoral tunnel creation can reduce this widening after ACL reconstruction compared to the use of a conventional rigid reamer. *Materials and Methods:* A retrospective study was conducted involving 56 patients who underwent primary ACL reconstruction between January 2012 and July 2013. The patients were categorized into two groups: the reamer group ($n = 28$) and CDS group ($n = 28$). All participants were followed up for a minimum of 2 years. Clinical assessment included the Lachman test and pivot-shift test, and the Lysholm score and subjective International Knee Documentation Committee scores. Radiographic evaluation covered the tunnel widening rate, represented as the ratio of the tunnel diameter 2 years after surgery to the tunnel diameter immediately after surgery, and the ratio (A/B) of femoral tunnel (A) to tibial tunnel (B) diameters at respective time points. *Results:* No significant disparities were found between the two groups in terms of clinical outcomes. However, the reamer group exhibited a greater femoral tunnel widening rate compared to the CDS group (reamer group vs. CDS group: 142.7 ± 22.0% vs. 128.0 ± 19.0% on the anteroposterior (AP) radiograph and 140.8 ± 14.2% vs. 122.9 ± 13.4% on the lateral radiograph; all $p < 0.05$). Two years post-operation, the A/B ratio rose in the reamer group (0.96 ± 0.05→1.00 ± 0.05 on the AP radiograph and 0.94 ± 0.03→1.00 ± 0.0.04 on the lateral radiograph; all $p < 0.05$), while it decreased in the CDS group (0.99 ± 0.02→0.96 ± 0.05 on the AP radiograph and 0.97 ± 0.03→0.93 ± 0.06 on the lateral radiograph; all $p < 0.05$). *Conclusion:* The use of CDS for femoral tunnel creation in primary ACL reconstruction provides a potential advantage by limiting tunnel widening compared to the conventional rigid-reamer approach.

Keywords: bone tunnel widening; bone tunnel enlargement; anterior cruciate ligament; anterior cruciate ligament reconstruction

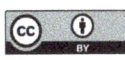

1. Introduction

The issue of tunnel widening following anterior cruciate ligament (ACL) reconstruction is a well-documented complication, which could potentially lead to surgical failure. [1–4]. It not only jeopardizes the graft success but also requires staged management in revision ACL reconstruction [5,6]. While the precise cause of tunnel widening remains elusive, contributing factors have been suggested to be biological, biomechanical, and mechanical [7–10]. Biological factors include healing at the graft–tunnel interface and increased cytokine levels leading to inflammatory responses, infection, and cell apoptosis. Biomechanical factors include foreign body reactions and necrosis due to heat during drilling for tunnel creation. And, mechanical factors include the graft fixation method, the graft motion within the tunnel, the position of the tunnel, and accelerated rehabilitation.

Among these mechanical factors, different outcomes related to tunnel widening have been reported with varying graft fixation methods, graft types, tunnel locations, and femoral tunnel creation methods [11–16]. However, the literature offers scarce comparative data on tunnel widening after using a dilator versus a conventional reamer in ACL reconstruction. We introduce the curved dilator system (CDS) in order to overcome the weakness of the anteromedial (AM) portal technique with a conventional reamer, which may hinder the attainment of an anatomical position for the femoral tunnel [17]. By using CDS for femoral tunnel creation, we theorize that it might condense the inner wall of the tunnel and hence mitigate tunnel widening. Consequently, we posit that utilizing the CDS in ACL reconstruction could potentially reduce both mechanical and biomechanical tunnel widening in comparison to the conventional rigid reamer. Therefore, this study aims to examine tunnel enlargement following ACL reconstruction conducted using the CDS versus the conventional reamer.

2. Materials and Methods

We examined individuals who underwent initial ACL reconstruction from January 2012 to July 2013. The inclusion criteria were primary ACL reconstruction using the allogenous tibialis tendon. Only those patients who underwent both clinical and radiological assessments at a 2-year postoperative follow-up were incorporated in the study. The exclusion criteria were as follows: (1) previous intra-articular ligament reconstruction, (2) multiple-ligament injury, and (3) previous osseous procedures. A concomitant meniscal injury was not an exclusion criterion. The institutional review board granted approval for this research.

2.1. Surgical Procedure

Surgical procedures exhibited no variations, with the exception of the technique employed for femoral tunnel creation between the groups. The portals utilized included anterolateral, AM, and accessory anteromedial (AAM). Notably, the AM portal was positioned slightly more proximal than the standard approach. In contrast, the AAM portal was created 10–15 mm medial to the medial border of the patellar tendon, representing a notably lateral shift from the usual AAM portal placement and situated distally at the level immediately proximal to the lateral meniscal superior surface [17].

In the reamer group, the procedure involved inserting a guide pin through a drill guide, targeting the center of the ACL footprint. A conventional rigid reamer with the same diameter as the graft was utilized to create the femoral tunnel. On the other hand, in the CDS group, a 4.5 mm-diameter curved guide trocar with a sharp end was introduced at the anatomical footprint of the ACL. Subsequently, another 4.5 mm-diameter curved guide trocar with a sharp end was carefully inserted at a marked point while the knee was flexed to slightly over 90°, which was the optimal angle to prevent damage to the medial condyle cartilage during trocar passage. The trocar was then gently hammered until it completely penetrated the far cortex of the lateral condyle. Afterward, the trocar was removed, and the tunnel was gradually widened in incremental steps, increasing by 1 mm in diameter at a time to match the graft's diameter.

For creating the tibial tunnel, the entry point was positioned at the level of the tibial tubercle, 2–3 cm medial to the tubercle, just above the attachment site of the pes anserinus. A guide pin was inserted at a 55° angle to the tibial plateau, guided by a tibial drill, aiming at the center of the ACL footprint. The tibial tunnel was then drilled along the guide pin using a standard reamer with a diameter that corresponded to that of the graft.

All patients in both groups conducted the same standardized home-based rehabilitation protocol. Routine follow ups were conducted at 2 weeks, 6 weeks, 3 months, 6 months, 1 year, and annually thereafter to ensure appropriate rehabilitation for each phase.

2.2. Clinical and Radiological Assessment

Clinical and radiological assessments were conducted prior to the surgery, at 3 months, 12 months after the operation, and annually thereafter. The clinical and radiological outcomes achieved 2 years after the operation were utilized for comparing the groups.

The assessment of knee joint stability included the Lachman test and pivot-shift test. The Lachman test measured anterior translation compared to the uninvolved side and was graded from 0 to 3 (0, <2 mm; 1, 2–5 mm; 2, 5–10 mm; 3, >10 mm). The pivot-shift test was evaluated against the uninvolved side and graded from 0 to 3 (0, same as uninvolved side; 1, gentle gliding; 2, clunk; 3, locking). Clinical status was evaluated 1 day before the surgery and annually thereafter using the Lysholm score and subjective International Knee Documentation Committee (IKDC) scores. A Lysholm score consists of eight items, including limping, locking, pain, stair climbing, the use of supports, instability, swelling, and squatting. Subjective IKDC scores include 18 items covering the domains of symptoms (7 items), sports activities (10 items), and function (1 item). The IKDC-SKF ranges from 0 to 100; higher scores indicate higher levels of function and fewer symptoms.

For radiological assessment, standardized anteroposterior (AP) and lateral knee radiographs were taken to evaluate tunnel widening. The diameter of the femoral and tibial tunnels was measured based on the method by L'Insalata et al. [2]. This involved measuring the length between the inner borders of the sclerotic margins perpendicular to the tunnel axis on the AP and lateral radiographs (Figure 1). Radiographs obtained immediately after the surgery and 2 years postoperatively were used for evaluation.

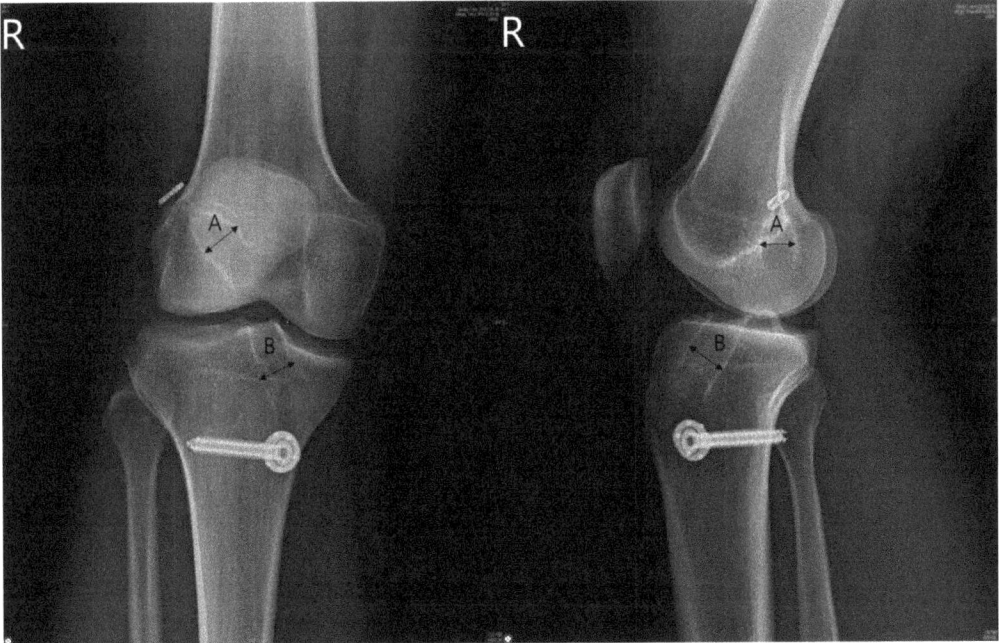

Figure 1. Tunnel diameter was determined as the widest distance between the sclerotic margins of the tunnel perpendicular to the axis of the tunnel based on the method by L'Insalata et al. The diameters were measured from the AP and lateral radiograph of the operated knee at 2 years post-operation.

All radiological parameters were measured twice, with a 2-week interval and using a Picture Archiving and Communication System, by two orthopedic surgeons who were not part of the surgical team. To assess tunnel widening, a tunnel widening rate was calculated, representing the ratio of the tunnel diameter after 2 years of surgery to the tunnel diameter immediately after surgery. Additionally, the ratio (A/B) of the diameter of the femoral tunnel (A) and tibial tunnel (B) was calculated at each point to account for slight differences in the graft diameter among cases.

2.3. Statistical Analysis

Continuous variables were expressed as means with standard deviations, and their comparison was conducted using Student's t-test. Categorical variables, on the other hand, were analyzed using the Pearson chi-square test. The inter- and intraobserver reliabilities of radiological measurements were determined to be acceptable based on the calculated intraclass correlation coefficients. Two orthopedic surgeons working in the knee division of the orthopedic department performed two measurements, at 1-week intervals, and the inter- and intra-observer reliability for the radiologic measurements were 0.89 (range, 0.87–0.97) and 0.91 (range, 0.85–0.96), respectively. A post hoc power analysis was conducted using G power calculator 3.1.9.2 to ensure that the sample size for this retrospective study was sufficient. All statistical analyses were carried out using SPSS software (ver. 25.0.0), and statistical significance was set at a p-value of less than 0.05.

3. Results

Among a total of 60 consecutive patients who underwent primary ACL reconstruction, 4 patients were excluded due to not meeting the selection criteria or inadequate follow up. These exclusions were based on the following reasons: less than 2 years of follow up for two patients, one patient experienced postoperative complications related to an infection, and one patient had missing clinical data or radiographs.

Ultimately, 56 patients with a minimum 2-year follow up were included in the study and divided into two groups based on the surgical instrument used for femoral tunneling: the reamer group (standard rigid reamer, n = 28), which involved a standard rigid reamer, and the CDS group (curved dilator system, n = 28), which involved a curved dilator system. Patients' demographic data, including age, sex, and body mass index, were retrieved from medical records and are presented in Table 1. Demographic characteristics showed no significant differences between the two groups.

Table 1. Demographic data of patients in the reamer and CDS groups.

	Reamer	CDS	p-Value
No. of knees	28	28	
Age, years	30.2 ± 11.1 (17~54)	28.6 ± 12.7 (17~57)	0.537 †
Male/Female	24/4	25/3	0.521 *
Right/Left	15/13	16/13	0.900 *
BMI, kg/m^2	24.1 ± 2.6	25.2 ± 3.4	0.215 †

BMI, body mass index; CDS, curved dilator system. The values are presented as the mean ± standard deviation with the range in parentheses. † Derived using Student's t-test. * Derived using the Pearson chi-square test.

Clinical and Radiological Results

Clinical evaluations of knee joint stability, including the Lachman test and pivot-shift test, revealed no significant differences between the two groups. Similarly, no significant differences were found in the Lysholm score and subjective IKDC score between groups (Table 2).

Table 2. Comparison of the clinical outcomes between the reamer and CDS groups 2 years after surgery.

	Reamer (n = 28)	CDS (n = 28)	p-Value
Lachman test (Grade, 0:1:2:3)	4:19:4:1	6:17:3:2	0.804 *
Pivot-shift test (Grade, 0:1:2:3)	9:15:3:1	7:16:4:1	0.833 *
Lysholm score	89.4 ± 10.9	91.8 ± 8.6	0.392 †
IKDC scores	80.2 ± 8.8	77.8 ± 10.1	0.427 †

CDS, curved dilator system; IKDC, International Knee Documentation Committee. The values are presented as the mean ± standard deviation with the range in parentheses. † Derived using Student's t-test. * Derived using the Pearson chi-square test.

The femoral tunnel widening rate on the AP radiograph was greater in the reamer group than in the CDS group (reamer group, 142.7 ± 22.0 vs. CDS group, 128.0 ± 19.0; $p = 0.014$). The femoral tunnel widening rate on the lateral radiograph was also larger in the reamer group than in the CDS group (reamer group, 140.8 ± 14.2 vs. CDS group, 122.9 ± 13.4; $p = 0.001$). However, the tibial tunnel widening rate on both the AP and lateral radiographs showed no statistically significant differences in both groups (Table 3).

Table 3. Comparison of tunnel widening rate (percent) between the reamer and CDS groups using the plain radiograph 2 years after surgery.

		Reamer (%)	CDS (%)	p-Value
Femoral tunnel	AP	142.7 ± 22.0	128.0 ± 19.0	0.014
	Lateral	140.8 ± 14.2	122.9 ± 13.4	0.001
Tibial tunnel	AP	133.9 ± 16.4	132.7 ± 19.7	0.821
	Lateral	131.7 ± 11.0	127.5 ± 13.0	0.246

CDS, curved dilator system. The tunnel widening rate from immediately to 2 years after surgery was calculated. The values are presented as the mean ± standard deviation. The statistical significance was set at $p < 0.05$ and derived using Student's t-test.

Regarding the ratio (A/B) of the diameters of the femoral tunnel (A) and tibial tunnel (B), the ratio increased in the reamer group from immediately after surgery to the last follow up (AP radiograph: 0.96 ± 0.05 to 1.00 ± 0.05, $p < 0.001$; lateral radiograph: 0.94 ± 0.03 to 1.00 ± 0.04, $p < 0.001$). Conversely, in the CDS group, the ratio decreased (AP radiograph: 0.99 ± 0.02 to 0.96 ± 0.05, $p = 0.001$; lateral radiograph: 0.97 ± 0.03 to 0.93 ± 0.06, $p = 0.020$) (Table 4).

Table 4. Ratio (A/B) of the femoral tunnel (A) and tibia tunnel (B) immediately and 2 years after surgery.

		Postoperative, Immediate	Postoperative, 2 Years	p-Value
Reamer	AP	0.96 ± 0.05	1.00 ± 0.05	<0.001
	Lateral	0.94 ± 0.03	1.00 ± 0.04	<0.001
CDS	AP	0.99 ± 0.02	0.96 ± 0.05	0.001
	Lateral	0.97 ± 0.03	0.93 ± 0.06	0.020

CDS, curved dilator system. The values are presented as the mean ± standard deviation. The statistical significance was set at $p < 0.05$ and derived using Student's t-test.

4. Discussion

The main findings of our investigation are as follows: (1) Femoral tunnel widening was significantly larger in the reamer group than in the CDS group 2 years following primary ACL reconstruction. (2) The diameter ratio of the femoral to tibial tunnel decreased in the CDS group but increased in the reamer group 2 years after surgery. These findings suggest that using a curved dilator system (CDS) to create the femoral tunnel in ACL reconstruction could be advantageous in preventing femoral tunnel widening, compared to the conventional rigid reamer.

Tunnel enlargement is a widely recognized complication after ACL surgery since the early 1990s [1,2,18]. The prevalence of tunnel widening has been documented, ranging in variability from 20% to 100% from several studies [11,13,14,19–21]. This complication is concerning as it can lead to ACL reconstruction failure due to unsuitable conditions for graft fixation. Moreover, it may necessitate complex, staged management for revision ACL surgery, including initial bone grafting procedures to fill the widened tunnels [10,22,23]. This complication is not only related to surgical techniques but also to the type of fixation devices, graft selection, and demographic factors [12,15,16,19,24,25]. The relation between tunnel widening and clinical outcomes remains uncertain. Some studies have hypothesized that tunnel widening potentially serves as an early finding of graft failure. However, many recent studies could not find any relationship between tunnel enlargement and the clinical results after surgery, and only a few have demonstrated the impact on the clinical outcome of tunnel widening [15,16,21,25–27].

While the precise causes of tunnel enlargement are very partially understood, it is generally agreed upon that multiple factors, including biological, biomechanical, and mechanical, contribute to its occurrence. Several studies reported which factors affect tunnel widening, such as the types of grafts, the type of fixation device, the position and size of the tunnel holes, the micro-motion of the graft in the tunnel, and altered cytokine levels in the synovial joint fluid [28–33]. Biological factors such as graft healing at the tunnel surface, inflammatory reactions, abnormal activity of the osteoclast, and infection are implicated in tunnel widening after ACL reconstruction. A biomechanical factor is heat necrosis from drilling and foreign bodies. A certain amount of heat by drilling may induce the necrosis of the bone and secondary inflammation. And, several studies have reported that various types of allogenic grafts may raise the risk for tunnel enlargement with the foreign-body immune response [1,20,34,35]. Several studies reported the graft type, cyclic loading of the knee joint, and motion of the graft within the tunnel as mechanical factors after ACL reconstruction [26,29,36]. The longitudinal motion of the graft along the tunnel, known as the bungee effect, and the transverse motion of the graft perpendicular to the axis of the tunnel known as the windshield-wiper effect may lead to subsequent bone resorption.

Recently, surgeons suggested some possible treatments in order to mitigate the tunnel widening. A preclinical study showed that the utilization of mesenchymal stem cells seeded in a collagen type-I scaffold enhanced the biological healing of ACL grafts in a rabbit model [37]. Additionally, Robinson J. et al. reported that a poly-L-lactic acid-hydroxyapatite-blended bio-absorbable screw reduced the tunnel widening after ACL surgery using the hamstring tendon [19]. Yamazaki S. et al. demonstrated in their study that the utilization of transforming growth factor-beta 1 substantially enhanced the production of collagen fibers linking the tendon graft to bone in dogs [38]. And, Hashimoto Y. et al. reported that recombinant BMP-2 treatment resulted in the successful regeneration of the tendon–bone junction in a rabbit model [5]. Additionally, hyperbaric oxygen significantly promoted the incorporation of bone to tendon, and rose the tensile strength of the graft by enhancing the amount of trabecular bone around the graft [17].

Our hypothesis is that continuous dilators for the creation of the femoral tunnel might reduce the tunnel widening compared to conventional drilling with a rigid reamer by creating a more condense tunnel wall. Previous studies have reported varying results regarding tunnel widening according to the type of reamer used for tunnel drilling [13,17]. Justin R. Knight et al. observed significantly greater tibial tunnel deformation when using the acorn reamer compared to the mono-fluted reamer [17]. However, Rainer Siebold et al. did not find a significant reduction in postoperative tunnel widening after ACL reconstruction using compaction drilling with a stepped router [17]. In our investigation, we sought to determine if the creation of the femoral tunnel using CDS could effectively decrease femoral bone tunnel widening following ACL reconstruction, and our hypothesis was strongly supported.

Despite these findings, our study has some limitations. Firstly, it was retrospective and lacked randomization, potentially leading to selection bias. However, we carefully compared the two groups, ensuring no significant differences in basic demographic data, thereby minimizing confounding factors. Secondly, the evaluation period was limited to 2 years after surgery, and further investigation is required to assess whether changes in tunnel diameter affect long-term clinical outcomes after ACL reconstruction. Thirdly, we did not employ three-dimensional imaging modalities like CT or MRI to evaluate tunnel diameters. Nonetheless, the method used in our study, as established by L'Insalata et al., has been widely accepted as a standard approach for measuring tunnel diameter after ACL reconstruction in numerous published studies.

5. Conclusions

The femoral tunnel widening rate was larger in the reamer group than in the CDS group on both the AP and lateral radiographs, and the ratio (A/B) of the diameter of the femoral tunnel (A) and tibial tunnel (B) decreased in the CDS group but increased in the reamer group 2 years after ACL reconstruction. These results suggest that using CDS in primary ACL reconstruction may help prevent femoral tunnel widening, compared to the conventional rigid reamer. Nevertheless, there were no notable disparities in clinical results among the two groups during the 2-year follow up. Additional investigations with extended follow-up durations are warranted to comprehensively understand the long-term implications of our findings.

Author Contributions: Conceptualization, J.K.L.; Methodology, J.K.L. and O.-S.L.; Formal Analysis, J.I.K. and O.-S.L.; Investigation, S.H.H.; Resources, J.K.L.; Data Curation, S.H.H. and J.I.K.; Writing—Original Draft Preparation, O.-S.L.; Writing—Review and Editing, J.K.L.; Visualization, O.-S.L.; Supervision, J.K.L. All authors have read and agreed to the published version of the manuscript.

Funding: This research received no external funding.

Institutional Review Board Statement: This study was approved by the Institutional Review Board of Hallym University Sacred Heart Hospital (IRB no.: 2016-I037 issued on the 8 March 2016).

Informed Consent Statement: Patient consent was waived due to anonymity of the data used in the study. It was approved by the Institutional Review Board of Seoul National University Hospital.

Data Availability Statement: The data presented in this study are available on request from the corresponding author. The data are not publicly available due to privacy.

Conflicts of Interest: The authors declare that they have no competing interest.

References

1. Peyrache, M.D.; Djian, P.; Christel, P.; Witvoet, J. Tibial tunnel enlargement after anterior cruciate ligament reconstruction by autogenous bone-patellar tendon-bone graft. *Knee Surg. Sport. Traumatol. Arthrosc.* **1996**, *4*, 2–8. [CrossRef]
2. L'Insalata, J.C.; Klatt, B.; Fu, F.H.; Harner, C.D. Tunnel expansion following anterior cruciate ligament reconstruction: A comparison of hamstring and patellar tendon autografts. *Knee Surg. Sport. Traumatol. Arthrosc.* **1997**, *5*, 234–238. [CrossRef]
3. Wilson, T.C.; Kantaras, A.; Atay, A.; Johnson, D.L. Tunnel enlargement after anterior cruciate ligament surgery. *Am. J. Sport. Med.* **2004**, *32*, 543–549. [CrossRef]

4. Yu, J.K.; Paessler, H.H. Relationship between tunnel widening and different rehabilitation procedures after ACL reconstruction with quadrupled hamstring tendons. *Chin. J. Surg.* **2004**, *42*, 984–988.
5. Inclan, P.M.; Brophy, R.H. Revision anterior cruciate ligament reconstruction. *Bone Jt. J.* **2023**, *105-B*, 474–480. [CrossRef]
6. Petrovic, K.; Vanhoenacker, F.M.; Nikolic, O.; Vandenberk, P. Tunnel enlargement and recurrent graft tear after ACL reconstruction. *J. Belg. Soc. Radiol.* **2012**, *95*, 370. [CrossRef] [PubMed]
7. Hoher, J.; Moller, H.D.; Fu, F.H. Bone tunnel enlargement after anterior cruciate ligament reconstruction: Fact or fiction? *Knee Surg. Sport. Traumatol. Arthrosc.* **1998**, *6*, 231–240. [CrossRef] [PubMed]
8. Silva, A.; Sampaio, R.; Pinto, E. Femoral tunnel enlargement after anatomic ACL reconstruction: A biological problem? *Knee Surg. Sport. Traumatol. Arthrosc.* **2010**, *18*, 1189–1194. [CrossRef]
9. de Padua, V.B.C.; Vilela, J.C.R.; Espindola, W.A.; Godoy, R.C.G. Bone Tunnel Enlargement with Non-Metallic Interference Screws in Acl Reconstruction. *Acta Ortop. Bras.* **2018**, *26*, 305–308. [CrossRef] [PubMed]
10. Yue, L.; DeFroda, S.F.; Sullivan, K.; Garcia, D.; Owens, B.D. Mechanisms of Bone Tunnel Enlargement Following Anterior Cruciate Ligament Reconstruction. *JBJS Rev.* **2020**, *8*, e0120. [CrossRef]
11. Fauno, P.; Kaalund, S. Tunnel widening after hamstring anterior cruciate ligament reconstruction is influenced by the type of graft fixation used: A prospective randomized study. *Arthroscopy* **2005**, *21*, 1337–1341. [CrossRef] [PubMed]
12. Jagodzinski, M.; Foerstemann, T.; Mall, G.; Krettek, C.; Bosch, U.; Paessler, H.H. Analysis of forces of ACL reconstructions at the tunnel entrance: Is tunnel enlargement a biomechanical problem? *J. Biomech.* **2005**, *38*, 23–31. [CrossRef]
13. Siebold, R.; Kiss, Z.S.; Morris, H.G. Effect of compaction drilling during ACL reconstruction with hamstrings on postoperative tunnel widening. *Arch. Orthop. Trauma Surg.* **2008**, *128*, 461–468. [CrossRef]
14. Gokce, A.; Beyzadeoglu, T.; Ozyer, F.; Bekler, H.; Erdogan, F. Does bone impaction technique reduce tunnel enlargement in ACL reconstruction? *Int. Orthop.* **2009**, *33*, 407–412. [CrossRef]
15. Lee, D.K.; Kim, J.H.; Lee, B.H.; Kim, H.; Jang, M.J.; Lee, S.S.; Wang, J.H. Influence of Graft Bending Angle on Femoral Tunnel Widening After Double-Bundle ACL Reconstruction: Comparison of Transportal and Outside-In Techniques. *Orthop. J. Sport. Med.* **2021**, *9*, 23259671211035780. [CrossRef]
16. Lee, T.J.; Jang, K.M.; Kim, T.J.; Lee, S.M.; Bae, J.H. Adjustable-Loop Cortical Suspensory Fixation Results in Greater Tibial Tunnel Widening Compared to Interference Screw Fixation in Primary Anterior Cruciate Ligament Reconstruction. *Medicina* **2022**, *58*, 1193. [CrossRef]
17. Lee, K.B.; Kwon, B.C.; Kim, J.I.; Lee, H.M.; Lee, J.K. Anatomic femoral tunnel creation during anterior cruciate ligament reconstruction using curved dilator system. *J. Orthop. Surg.* **2019**, *27*, 2309499019840822. [CrossRef] [PubMed]
18. Fahey, M.; Indelicato, P.A. Bone tunnel enlargement after anterior cruciate ligament replacement. *Am. J. Sport. Med.* **1994**, *22*, 410–414. [CrossRef]
19. Robinson, J.; Huber, C.; Jaraj, P.; Colombet, P.; Allard, M.; Meyer, P. Reduced bone tunnel enlargement post hamstring ACL reconstruction with poly-L-lactic acid/hydroxyapatite bioabsorbable screws. *Knee* **2006**, *13*, 127–131. [CrossRef] [PubMed]
20. Iorio, R.; Vadala, A.; Argento, G.; Di Sanzo, V.; Ferretti, A. Bone tunnel enlargement after ACL reconstruction using autologous hamstring tendons: A CT study. *Int. Orthop.* **2007**, *31*, 49–55. [CrossRef] [PubMed]
21. Mayr, R.; Smekal, V.; Koidl, C.; Coppola, C.; Eichinger, M.; Rudisch, A.; Kranewitter, C.; Attal, R. ACL reconstruction with adjustable-length loop cortical button fixation results in less tibial tunnel widening compared with interference screw fixation. *Knee Surg. Sport. Traumatol. Arthrosc.* **2020**, *28*, 1036–1044. [CrossRef]
22. Ugutmen, E.; Ozkan, K.; Guven, M.; Sener, N.; Altintas, F. Early tunnel enlargement after arthroscopic ACL reconstructions. *Acta Orthop. Belg.* **2007**, *73*, 625–629. [PubMed]
23. Mermerkaya, M.U.; Buyukdogan, K.; Hakyemez, O.S.; Birinci, M.; Avci, C.C. Editorial Commentary: Anatomic or Not, the Tunnel Will Get Wider! *Arthroscopy* **2020**, *36*, 1112–1113. [CrossRef]
24. Vadala, A.; Iorio, R.; De Carli, A.; Argento, G.; Di Sanzo, V.; Conteduca, F.; Ferretti, A. The effect of accelerated, brace free, rehabilitation on bone tunnel enlargement after ACL reconstruction using hamstring tendons: A CT study. *Knee Surg. Sport. Traumatol. Arthrosc.* **2007**, *15*, 365–371. [CrossRef]
25. Moran, T.E.; Ignozzi, A.J.; Taleghani, E.R.; Bruce, A.S.; Hart, J.M.; Werner, B.C. Flexible Versus Rigid Reaming Systems for Independent Femoral Tunnel Reaming During ACL Reconstruction: Minimum 2-Year Clinical Outcomes. *Orthop. J. Sport. Med.* **2022**, *10*, 23259671221083568. [CrossRef] [PubMed]
26. Cohen, S.B.; Pandarinath, R.; O'Hagan, T.; Marchetto, P.A.; Hyatt, A.; Wascher, J.; Deluca, P.F. Results of ACL reconstruction with tibial Retroscrew fixation: Comparison of clinical outcomes and tibial tunnel widening. *Physician Sportsmed.* **2015**, *43*, 138–142. [CrossRef]
27. Weber, A.E.; Delos, D.; Oltean, H.N.; Vadasdi, K.; Cavanaugh, J.; Potter, H.G.; Rodeo, S.A. Tibial and Femoral Tunnel Changes After ACL Reconstruction: A Prospective 2-Year Longitudinal MRI Study. *Am. J. Sport. Med.* **2015**, *43*, 1147–1156. [CrossRef] [PubMed]
28. Darabos, N.; Haspl, M.; Moser, C.; Darabos, A.; Bartolek, D.; Groenemeyer, D. Intraarticular application of autologous conditioned serum (ACS) reduces bone tunnel widening after ACL reconstructive surgery in a randomized controlled trial. *Knee Surg. Sport. Traumatol. Arthrosc.* **2011**, *19* (Suppl. S1), S36–S46. [CrossRef] [PubMed]

29. Biset, A.; Douiri, A.; Robinson, J.R.; Laboudie, P.; Colombet, P.; Graveleau, N.; Bouguennec, N. Tibial tunnel expansion does not correlate with four-strand graft maturation after ACL reconstruction using adjustable cortical suspensory fixation. *Knee Surg. Sport. Traumatol. Arthrosc.* **2023**, *31*, 1761–1770. [CrossRef]
30. Flury, A.; Wild, L.; Waltenspul, M.; Zindel, C.; Vlachopoulos, L.; Imhoff, F.B.; Fucentese, S.F. Tibial tunnel enlargement is affected by the tunnel diameter-screw ratio in tibial hybrid fixation for hamstring ACL reconstruction. *Arch. Orthop. Trauma Surg.* **2023**, *143*, 1923–1930. [CrossRef] [PubMed]
31. Lee, S.S.; Kim, I.S.; Shin, T.S.; Lee, J.; Lee, D.H. Femoral Tunnel Position Affects Postoperative Femoral Tunnel Widening after Anterior Cruciate Ligament Reconstruction with Tibialis Anterior Allograft. *J. Clin. Med.* **2023**, *12*, 1966. [CrossRef]
32. Okutan, A.E.; Gurun, E.; Surucu, S.; Kehribar, L.; Mahirogullari, M. Morphological Changes in the Tibial Tunnel After ACL Reconstruction With the Outside-In Technique and Adjustable Suspensory Fixation. *Orthop. J. Sport. Med.* **2023**, *11*, 23259671231155153. [CrossRef]
33. Tatrai, M.; Halasi, T.; Tallay, A.; Tatrai, A.; Pavlik, A. Low Femoral Tunnel Widening Incidence Rate After ACL Reconstruction Using Patellar Tendon Graft with Press-Fit Fixation. *Indian J. Orthop.* **2023**, *57*, 596–602. [CrossRef] [PubMed]
34. Zhang, Q.; Zhang, S.; Cao, X.; Liu, L.; Liu, Y.; Li, R. The effect of remnant preservation on tibial tunnel enlargement in ACL reconstruction with hamstring autograft: A prospective randomized controlled trial. *Knee Surg. Sport. Traumatol. Arthrosc.* **2014**, *22*, 166–173. [CrossRef] [PubMed]
35. Sauer, S.; Lind, M. Bone Tunnel Enlargement after ACL Reconstruction with Hamstring Autograft Is Dependent on Original Bone Tunnel Diameter. *Surg. J.* **2017**, *3*, e96–e100. [CrossRef]
36. Iorio, R.; Di Sanzo, V.; Vadala, A.; Conteduca, J.; Mazza, D.; Redler, A.; Bolle, G.; Conteduca, F.; Ferretti, A. ACL reconstruction with hamstrings: How different technique and fixation devices influence bone tunnel enlargement. *Eur. Rev. Med. Pharmacol. Sci.* **2013**, *17*, 2956–2961. [PubMed]
37. Knight, J.R.; Condie, D.; Querry, R.; Robertson, W.J. The use of a mono-fluted reamer results in decreased enlargement of the tibial tunnel when using a transtibial ACL reconstruction technique. *Knee Surg. Sport. Traumatol. Arthrosc.* **2014**, *22*, 357–362. [CrossRef] [PubMed]
38. Yamazaki, S.; Yasuda, K.; Tomita, F.; Tohyama, H.; Minami, A. The effect of transforming growth factor-beta1 on intraosseous healing of flexor tendon autograft replacement of anterior cruciate ligament in dogs. *Arthroscopy* **2005**, *21*, 1034–1041. [CrossRef]

Disclaimer/Publisher's Note: The statements, opinions and data contained in all publications are solely those of the individual author(s) and contributor(s) and not of MDPI and/or the editor(s). MDPI and/or the editor(s) disclaim responsibility for any injury to people or property resulting from any ideas, methods, instructions or products referred to in the content.

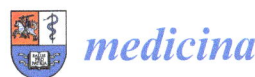

Article

Changes in Bone Marrow Lesions Following Root Repair Surgery Using Modified Mason–Allen Stitches in Medial Meniscus Posterior Root Tears

Kyu Sung Chung [1,*], Jeong Ku Ha [1], Jin Seong Kim [2] and Jin Goo Kim [3]

1. Department of Orthopedic Surgery and Sports Medical Center, Sports Medical Research Institute, Seoul Paik Hospital, College of Medicine, Inje University, Seoul 04551, Korea
2. Department of Sports Medical Center, Sports Medical Research Institute, Seoul Paik Hospital, College of Medicine, Inje University, Seoul 04551, Korea
3. Department of Orthopedic Surgery and Sports Center, Myong-Ji Hospital, Seoul 10475, Korea
* Correspondence: drokokboy@hanmail.net

Abstract: *Background and Objectives*: Root repair can prevent osteoarthritis (OA) by restoring hoop tension in medial meniscus posterior root tears (MMPRTs). This study aims to investigate bone marrow edema (BME) lesions known to be associated with OA following MMPRTs. *Methods*: Thirty patients with transtibial pull-out repair were recruited. Subchondral BME lesions were evaluated using magnetic resonance imaging (MRI) at 1-year follow-ups. Participants were categorized into three groups: no change of BME lesions (group one), improved BME lesions (group two) and worsened BME lesions (group three). Clinical scores and radiological outcomes, specifically Kellgren–Lawrence grade, medial joint space width and cartilage grade and meniscal extrusion were evaluated and compared between groups. *Results*: After surgery, twenty-three patients with no BME, three patients with BME lesions on the medial femoral condyle, one patient with BME lesions on the medial tibia plateau and three patients with BME lesions on both were investigated. A total of 20 patients in group one (66.7%) showed no change in BME lesions. In group two, seven patients (23.3%) presented with improved BME lesions. Only three patients (10%) showed worsened BME lesions (group three). Moreover, Lysholm scores and the rate of progression of cartilage grades were significantly worse in group three patients. Meniscal extrusion was significantly reduced in group two, whereas extrusion was significantly progressed in group three. *Conclusions*: Patients with worsened BME lesions showed less favorable outcomes than other patients. A decrease in meniscal extrusion can have a positive effect on BME lesions after root repair.

Keywords: bone marrow lesion; knee; meniscus; root tear; root repair

1. Introduction

Bone marrow edema (BME) is defined as an area of low signal intensity on T1-weighted images that is associated with intermediate or high signal intensity findings on T2-weighted images. BME lesions are a risk factor for structural deterioration in knee osteoarthritis and are strongly associated with the progression of osteoarthritis (OA) [1–3].

The meniscus is composed of an interconnecting network of collagen fibers, proteoglycans and glycoproteins [4,5]. Collagen fibers stretch under axial-load-increasing internal hoop stress which absorbs and redistributes forces transmitted to the joint [6–10]. Medial meniscus posterior root tears (MMPRTs) are defined as an avulsion injury or radial tear occurring in posterior bone attachment [11–16]. MMPRTs can predispose patients to degenerative OA due to the loss of hoop tension and load-sharing ability, which results in unsupportable peak pressures on the knee joint [14]. Root repair can restore the meniscal function; thus, it can prevent or delay osteoarthritic changes [17–19]. Root repair shows superior mid- [20] and long-term [21] clinical outcomes when compared with meniscectomy.

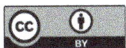

One of the main goals of root repair is the prevention and delay of the onset of osteoarthritic changes through the restoration of meniscal hoop tension. If root repair is not effective or successful, BME lesions will worsen following surgery. Several studies of both the clinical and radiological outcomes of root repair have reported favorable results [22–27]. However, there is little evidence or investigation into the change of BME lesions following root repair.

It has been shown that greater meniscus extrusion is a significant predictor of the progression of arthritic changes in osteoarthritic knees [18]. Therefore, it seems logical that if meniscus extrusion can be eliminated or reduced, the MMPRT will be successfully repaired, and the chance of subsequent degenerative arthritis will be reduced. However, there are no studies that have investigated the correlation between meniscus extrusion and BME lesions.

As such, this study aims to clarify the treatment effects of root repair through investigating the change of BME lesions following root repair and comparing these with both pre- and post-operative 1-year follow-up results in MMPRTs. In addition, this study aims to investigate the correlation of meniscus extrusion and BME lesions after root repair. We hypothesize that patients with worsened BME lesions will show less-favorable outcomes than other patients and that patients with more reduced meniscal extrusions can demonstrate positive effects on BME lesions after root repair.

2. Materials and Methods

2.1. Study Population

This study protocol was approved by our institutional review board (PAIK-08-003), and all patients signed an approved written consent form. Between 2017 and 2020, patients who consented underwent magnetic resonance imaging (MRI) scans both prior to surgery and 1-year following surgery. MMPRT was defined as a complete radial tear on the medial meniscus posterior bone. This was diagnosed by MRI scans (Intera Achieva; Philips, Eindhoven, Netherlands) indicated via an absence of an identifiable meniscus or a high-intensity signal replacing the normal dark meniscal signal (ghost sign) in the sagittal plane, a vertical linear defect at the root on the coronal plane, and a radial linear defect at the posterior insertion point in the axial plane [28,29].

The inclusion criteria for the study were: first, MMPRT shown on an MRI scan in a patient with persistent knee pain; second, patients who underwent arthroscopic pull-out fixation by modified Mason–Allen stitches; third, patients with a Kellgren–Lawrence (K-L) score of grade two or less. Study exclusion criteria were: first, patients whose MMPRT was combined with a high tibial osteotomy; second, patients with a concomitant ligament injury; and finally, patients who did not want an MRI scan follow-up 1-year after surgery (Figure 1).

Participants were identified using medical records. Prior to surgery, participants were interviewed in the outpatient department and their clinical histories were reviewed and collated in a database.

2.2. Evaluation of Bone Marrow Lesions

The MRI scans were evaluated both prior to surgery and 1-year following surgery. The evaluations of the BME lesions at both the medial femoral condyle (MFC) and medial tibial plateau (MTP) were conducted. Changes of the BME lesions were assessed by comparing the statuses of the BME lesions between MRI scans prior to surgery and 1-year post surgery. Participants were categorized into 3 groups: no change of BME lesions (group 1), improved BME lesions (group 2) and worsened BME lesions (group 3), through comparisons between pre- and post-operative BME lesion statuses (Figures 2 and 3). The cartilage grade in the medial compartment was graded according to the modified Outerbridge classification by MRI. The healing status was assessed by checking continuity between the bone bed and meniscus on post-operative 1-year follow-up MRI scans.

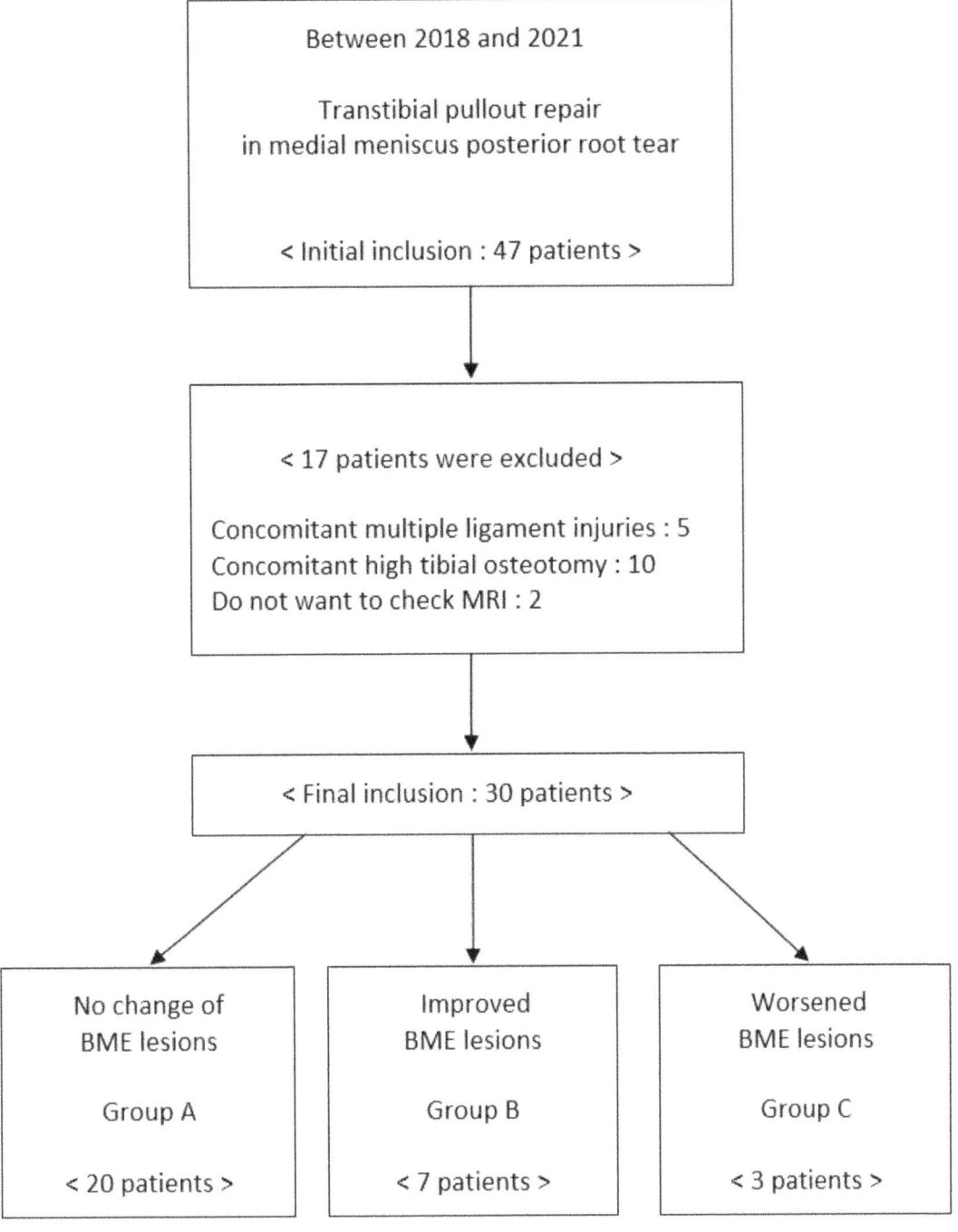

Figure 1. Flow chart of included participants.

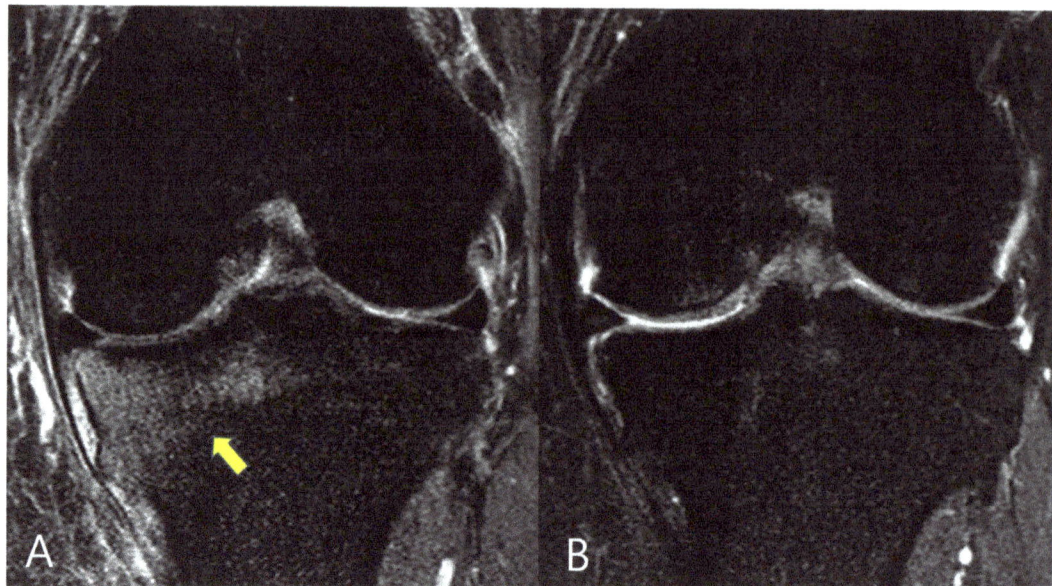

Figure 2. Magnetic resonance imaging (MRI) scans of a patient with a medial meniscus posterior root tear. (**A**) Pre-operative MRI view with a bone marrow edema lesion on the medial tibial plateau (yellow arrow). (**B**) One-year follow-up MRI view showing no bone marrow edema lesion on the medial tibial plateau.

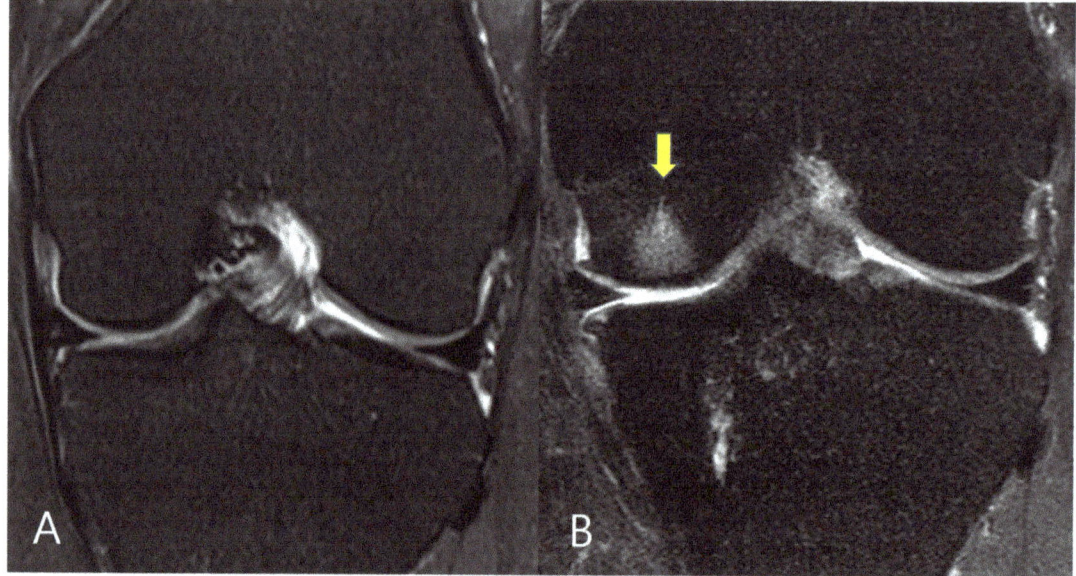

Figure 3. Magnetic resonance imaging (MRI) scans of a patient with a medial meniscus posterior root tear. (**A**) Pre-operative MRI view with no bone marrow edema lesion on the medial femoral condyle. (**B**) One-year follow-up MRI view showing a bone marrow edema lesion on the medial femoral condyle (yellow arrow).

2.3. Surgical Technique for Pullout Fixation

All surgical procedures were performed by one surgeon (K.S.C.) and involved transtibial pull-out repair using modified Mason–Allen stitches [30]. When MMPRT was confirmed on arthroscopic examination, the superficial medial collateral ligament (sMCL) was released by periosteal stripping on the distal attachment area of the sMCL. This created a sufficient working space depending on the patient's status [31]. A meniscus resector and shaver (Linvatec; Largo, FL, USA) was used to remove the fibrous tissue and obtain fresh meniscal tissue. A curette (Linvatec; Largo, FL, USA) was then inserted through the anteromedial (AM) portal, forming a bone bed at the native root insertion site. A suture hook (Linvatec; Largo, FL, USA) loaded with No. 1 polydioxanone (PDS; Ethicon; Somerville, NJ, USA) was then passed and PDS inserted at a point 5 mm medial to the torn edge in a vertical direction. One more PDS was placed in a position inside that of the first suture, in an identical manner. The shuttle relay method completed the horizontal loop. One or two simple vertical stitches were made which overlayed and crossed the horizontal suture. After making a suitable bone tunnel by anterior cruciate ligament reconstruction tibial tunnel guide (Linvatec; Largo, FL, USA), the ends of the sutures were pulled through the tibial tunnel. Finally, the meniscus was reduced and stabilized by tying the suture over an Endo-button (Smith & Nephew; Andover, MA, USA).

2.4. Postoperative Rehabilitation

After three weeks of immobilization, range of motion (ROM) exercises were started and progressed to up to 90° flexion until 6-weeks after surgery. Toe touch weight-bearing using crutches commenced immediately after surgery, with the brace locked to allow for full extension of the knee joint for the first 3-weeks after surgery. Progressive partial weight-bearing exercises commenced 3-weeks following surgery. Full weight-bearing and progressive closed kinetic chain strengthening exercises were permitted 6-weeks after surgery. Light running was permitted after 3-months and sports participation after 6-months. Permanent lifestyle modifications aimed at avoiding deep knee flexion were recommended

2.5. Clinical Outcomes

The Lysholm score, Western Ontario and McMaster Universities Osteoarthritis Index (WOMAC) and Knee injury and Osteoarthritis Outcome Score (KOOS) were evaluated as the clinical outcomes both prior to and 1-year after surgery.

2.6. Radiological Outcomes

The Rosenberg 45° posteroanterior standing view was used to assess the K-L arthritis grade and measure the medial joint space both prior to surgery and 1-year after surgery [32]. The K-L grade (0/1/2/3/4) was defined as follows: grade 0 indicated no degenerative change. Grade 1 indicated questionable osteophytes and no joint space narrowing. Grade 2 showed definite osteophytes with possible joint space narrowing. Grade 3 showed definite joint space narrowing with moderate multiple osteophytes and some sclerosis. Finally, grade 4 indicated severe joint space narrowing with cysts, osteophytes and sclerosis [33]. The medial joint space was measured from the center of the medial femoral condyle to the center of the medial tibial plateau using a picture-archiving and communication system (PACS, Marotech; Infinitti, Seoul, Korea).

Each MRI scan was checked and the BME lesion, cartilage grade, healing status and meniscal extrusion were evaluated both prior to surgery and 1-year following surgery. Extrusion of the medial meniscus (in mm) was defined as the amount of meniscal displacement from the superomedial aspect of the tibial plateau to the periphery of the meniscal body at the level of the medial collateral ligament (MCL) in the coronal plane.

Radiographic images were examined independently by two authors who were blinded to the procedures used, in consultation with a single experienced musculoskeletal radiologist. All radiographic measurements were documented three times at 2-week intervals using PACS. The averages of these measurements were used in our analyses. Intraclass correlation coefficients (ICCs) were calculated to determine the interobserver reliability of the differences in radiological outcome measurements. All measurements that allowed 1 decimal value were documented three times at 2-week intervals to assess their test–retest reliability.

2.7. Statistical Analysis

Statistical analyses were performed using SPSS software (ver. 20.0 for Windows; SPSS Inc., Chicago, IL, USA). Statistical significance was set at 5% ($p < 0.05$). The final clinical outcomes, clinical scores and radiological outcomes for each group were compared. The Kruskal–Wallis test was used to compare variables which were not normally distributed between groups and other non-parametric values. The chi-squared (χ^2) test was used to compare categorical data. If more than 20% of the expected frequencies were >5, Fisher's exact test was used.

The statistical power of the study was calculated retrospectively at 79% to compare the rate of progression of the cartilage grade between group 1 (25%) and group 3 (100%) at the 0.05 significance level using Fisher's exact test.

3. Results

In total, 30 patients were enrolled. The mean age of the patients was 58.7 ± 5.7 years (Table 1). Demographics and clinical characteristics prior to surgery are shown in Table 1. This was similar between all three groups, with no significant differences ($p > 0.05$).

Table 1. Pre-operative Demographics and Characteristics of Patients Included.

Demography (n = 30)	
Age, years	58.7 ± 5.7
Sex, male/female	2/27
Follow-up period, mo	12.2 ± 1.1
Body mass index, kg/m^2	26.6 ± 3.9
Duration between symptom onset & repair [a], weeks	4.9 ± 3.6
Clinical scores	
Lysholm score	47.8 ± 6.5
WOMAC score	54.6 ± 6.7
KOOS score	69.6 ± 6.1
Radiological status	
Mechanical axis (varus), degree	3.1 ± 2.0
Kellgren–Lawrence grade (0/1/2/3/4) [b], n	518/7/0/0
Medial joint space width [b], mm	3.6 ± 0.6
Outerbridge cartilage grade (0/1/2/3/4) [c], n	5/6/13/5/1

[a] The point of diagnosis was defined as the time when painful symptoms originally occurred. [b] The values were acquired through posteroanterior 45° flexion weight-bearing radiographs. [c] The values were acquired through magnetic resonance imaging. Data are presented as mean ± standard deviation.

The results of subchondral BME lesions after surgery are described in Table 2. A total of 20 patients had no change of BME lesion, 66.7% (group one). There were seven patients with improved BME lesion, 23.3% (group two). Finally, there were three patients with worsened BME lesions, 10% (group three). All ICCs ranged from 0.90 to 0.96, indicating an excellent reliability (ICCs > 0.9) of the current study [34,35]. The outcomes both before and after surgery in each group are shown in Table 3. All clinical scores following surgery were significantly improved in all groups compared with the pre-operative scores ($p < 0.001$).

Table 2. Bone Marrow Lesions (BME) of Included Participants.

BME Lesion (n = 30)	Pre-Operation (n)	Change of BME Lesions of Included Participants at Final Follow-Up (n)	Post-Operation (n)
No BME lesion	20	No BME: 17 BME on MFC: 1 BME on MTP: 1 BME on both: 1	23
BME lesion on MFC only	1	BME on MFC: 1	3
BME lesion on MTP only	6	No BME: 6	1
BME lesion on MFC and MTP both	3	BME on MFC: 1 BME on both: 2	3

MFC: medial femoral condyle. MTP: medial tibial plateau.

Table 3. Pre-operative and Post-operative Clinical and Radiological Outcomes in Each Group.

BME Lesion (n = 29)	No Change of BME Lesion (Group 1)		Improved BME Lesion (Group 2)		Worsened BME Lesion (Group 3)	
Number	20		7		3	
Clinical scores	Preoperation	Postoperation	Preoperation	Postoperation	Preoperation	Postoperation
Lysholm score	47.6 ± 6.8	81.7 ± 8.2	50.1 ± 6.3	86.9 ± 6.7	44.0 ± 3.5	73.7 ± 4.0
WOMAC score	53.1 ± 7.2	16.7 ± 8.7	57.3 ± 4.3	12.7 ± 4.5	58.7 ± 4.0	22.3 ± 6.8
KOOS score	68.8 ± 6.5	26.5 ± 9.6	69.7 ± 4.6	24.1 ± 5.8	75.0 ± 3.6	34.3 ± 10.7
Radiological status						
Kellgren–Lawrence grade (0/1/2/3/4) [a], n	4/12/4/0/0	2/11/5/2/0	0/5/2/0/0	0/4/3/0/0	1/1/1/0/0	1/0/2/0/0
Medial joint space width [a], mm	3.6 ± 0.6	3.3 ± 0.5	3.5 ± 0.8	3.4 ± 0.8	3.4 ± 0.5	3.0 ± 0.3
Meniscus extrusion [b], mm	3.4 ± 0.8	3.3 ± 1.1	3.7 ± 1.0	2.7 ± 0.8	2.8 ± 0.9	5.5 ± 1.5
Outerbridge cartilage grade (0/1/2/3/4) [b], n	4/4/10/2/0	3/4/9/4/0	0/1/3/2/1	2/2/2/1/0	1/1/0/1/0	0/1/1/0/1

[a] The values were acquired through posteroanterior 45o flexion weight-bearing radiographs. [b] The values were acquired through magnetic resonance imaging. Data are presented as mean ± standard deviation.

When comparing the post-operative clinical and radiological outcomes between groups, the overall clinical and radiological outcomes showed a tendency for group two to be higher than other groups (Table 4). Clinically, the Lysholm score of group three was significantly lower than those of the other groups. Regarding cartilage status, the number of patients with progression of cartilage grade after surgery was five (25%) in group one, zero (0%) in group two and three (100%) in group three, showing group three to have the worst cartilage grades following surgery.

In terms of meniscal extrusion, there was no significant difference in the results in group one. Meniscal extrusion was significantly reduced in group two, whereas extrusion significantly progressed in group three (Tables 3 and 4). Thus, a decrease in meniscal extrusion can have a positive effect on BME lesions after root repair in MMPRTs.

Table 4. Postoperative Clinical and Radiological Outcomes Between Groups [a].

Postoperative Outcomes	No Change of BME Lesion (n = 20)	Improved BME Lesion (n = 7)	Worsened BME Lesion (n = 3)	p Value
Clinical scores				
Lysholm score	81.7 ± 8.2	86.9 ± 6.7	73.7 ± 4.0	0.034 [b]
Difference of Lysholm between pre- and post-operation	34.1 ± 8.2	36.7 ± 11.2	29.7 ± 1.5	0.416 [b]
WOMAC score	16.7 ± 8.7	12.7 ± 4.5	22.3 ± 6.8	0.160 [b]
Difference of WOMAC between pre- and post-operation	36.4 ± 12.7	44.6 ± 2.7	36.3 ± 2.9	0.106 [b]
KOOS score	26.5 ± 9.6	24.1 ± 5.8	34.3 ± 10.7	0.291 [b]
Difference of KOOS between pre- and post-operation	42.3 ± 9.5	45.6 ± 8.0	40.7 ± 10.3	0.431 [b]
Radiological status				
Medial joint space, mm	3.3 ± 0.5	3.4 ± 0.8	3.0 ± 0.3	0.623 [b]
Progression of joint space narrowing, mm	0.4 ± 0.4	0.1 ± 0.2	0.4 ± 0.2	0.081 [b]
Kellgren–Lawrence grade (KL grade), 0/1/2/3/4	2/11/5/2/0	0/4/3/0/0	1/0/2/0/0	0.347 [c]
Progression of KL grade, no. (%)	7 (35%)	1 (14%)	1 (33%)	0.829 [c]
Continuity between bone bed and meniscus [d]	20 (100%)	7 (100%)	3 (100%)	1.000 [c]
Difference values of meniscus extrusion (pre-post) [d], mm	0.1 ± 1.3	0.9 ± 1.4	−2.7 ± 1.5	0.019 [b]
Cartilage grade (modified outerbridge), 0/1/2/3/4 [d]	3/4/9/4/0	2/2/2/1/0	0/1/1/0/1	0.548 [c]
Progression of Cartilage grade, no. (%) [d]	5 (25%)	0 (0%)	3 (100%)	0.006 [c]

[a] Values are expressed as mean ± standard deviation. [b] Kruskal–Wallis test. [c] Fisher exact test. [d] The value was taken from magnetic resonance imaging checked at postoperative 1-year follow-up.

4. Discussion

The study showed 90% of the included participants to have either no change in BME lesions or an improvement of BME lesions. Only 10% of participants had worsened BME lesions. Patients with worsened BME lesions showed less favorable outcomes than other patients. Patients with improved BME lesions showed more reduced extrusion after surgery, whereas patients with worsened BME lesions showed more progressed extrusion.

BME lesions are known to be associated with the progression of osteoarthritis and a potential risk factor for structural deterioration in knee osteoarthritis [1–3]. BME lesions can fluctuate in size within a short time, and are associated with the progression of arthritic changes and fluctuations of pain in knee OA [1–3]. Thus, non-functioning meniscus by loss of hoop tension can lead to progression of BME lesions on the tibiofemoral joint.

MMPRTs are defined as an avulsion injury or radial tear occurring in the posterior bony attachment [11–13], and they can lead to arthritic changes due to the loss of meniscal hoop tension and load-sharing ability on the tibiofemoral joint [14]. There are presently two surgical options for MMPRT: meniscectomy [26,36] and root repair [22–27]. The 'traditional' gold standard treatment for MMPRT is meniscectomy, which is widely used. However, meniscectomy cannot restore meniscal hoop tension; thus, most meniscectomized cases ultimately progress to degenerative arthritis [36–38]. However, this study shows that better outcomes are seen after meniscal repair compared with partial meniscectomy for MMRTs. This is demonstrated through greater improvements in Lysholm scores, lower rates of progression to knee OA and a lower re-operation rate [39]. In a recently published long-term study comparing meniscectomy and root repair surgery, root repair surgery was more effective than meniscectomy in terms of both clinical outcomes and survival rate. In terms of clinical failure, defined as conversion to TKA, the 10-year survival rate of meniscectomy patients was 44.4%, whereas that of root repair surgery patients was 79.6% [21]. Thus, management with restoring meniscal hoop tension is critical to delay arthritis in MMPRTs. Moreover, it can prevent further progression of both newly formed BME lesions or existing BME lesions in the tibiofemoral joint. However, to our knowledge, there is little existing evidence to clarify the treatment's effects of root repair through the investigation of BME lesion change following surgery.

In the current study, only three patients (10%) showed worsened BME lesions after surgery; thus, it is assumed that in almost all included participants, root repair surgery restored the meniscal hoop tension and load-bearing ability on tibiofemoral joints. This suggests root repair to be a favorable surgical procedure to prevent or delay the progression of osteoarthritis in MMPRTs, an aspect of BME lesions.

In this study, all clinical scores following surgery were significantly improved when compared with the pre-operative scores in all groups, even in worsened BME lesion patients. This suggests that root repair has better clinical outcomes following surgery in MMPRTs patients. Moreover, the overall clinical and radiological outcomes showed a tendency for group two to score higher than groups one and three. However, the Lysholm score was significantly lower in the worsened BME lesion group, group three. Radiologically, regarding cartilage status, the number of patients with a progression of cartilage grade after surgery was five patients (25%) in group one. In group two, this was 0 (0%). However, all patients with worsened BME lesions showed a worsened cartilage status after surgery, suggestive of a link between cartilage injury and BME lesions. In a previously reported study, Outerbridge grade $\geq$ three chondral lesions were found to be independent negative prognostic factors following root repair [23]. This suggests worsened BME lesions may be negative prognostic factors.

The results of the current study show worsened BME lesions to have a clinically unfavorable effect following root repair surgery. In MMPRTs, it is important to restore well-functioned meniscus by root repair. This study indicates that one of the goals of root repair surgery is to prevent BME lesions as much as feasibly possible. This is the clinical relevance of the study.

To our knowledge, there are no studies that have investigated the correlation between meniscus extrusion and the BME lesions. It would be worthwhile to note that this is the first study to investigate the correlation between meniscal extrusion and BME lesions. In this study, patients with improved BME lesions showed more reduced extrusion after surgery, whereas patients with worsened BME lesion showed more progressed extrusion. This means that reduced meniscal extrusion correlates with more favorable clinical outcomes compared with more progressed extrusion. Thus, more reduced meniscal extrusion after root repair can have a positive effect on BME lesions. Chung et al. reported that patients with a decreased meniscus extrusion at 1-year post-operative have more favorable clinical scores and radiographic findings at midterm follow-ups than those with increased extrusion at 1-year post-operative [40]. Meniscal extrusion has a critical impact on the results; thus, surgeons should reduce meniscus extrusion as much as possible when performing root repair. However, this result might be caused by the small sample size of this study. In the future, a larger cohort study will be needed to identify the role of meniscal extrusion in BME lesions.

This study has several limitations. First, it is a retrospective and non-randomized study; thus, there may be selection bias in the selection of participant enrollment. However, basic demographic and preoperative data were similar between groups. Therefore, any selection bias would not have any significant influence on BME lesions following surgery. Secondly, the present study performed was an in vivo study; thus, it has the potential weaknesses of an in silico study [41]. Thirdly, the sample size was relatively small, and the number of patients with worsened BME lesions was less than those of the other two groups. However, a good statistical power was achieved to compare the rates of progression of cartilage grade between groups one and three. Fourth, the follow-up duration was short at only 1-year. Finally, although the meniscal healing status was assessed by evaluating continuity between the bone bed and meniscus proper, the actual restoration of hoop tension and the healing status of the fixed meniscus was not assessed. This was due to patients not consenting to further arthroscopies.

5. Conclusions

Patients with worsened BME lesions have poor clinical outcomes compared with other patients. A decrease in meniscal extrusion can have a positive effect on BME lesions after root repair. Surgeons should reduce meniscus extrusion as much as possible when performing root repair. In the future, a larger prospective cohort study will be needed to identify the relevant role of meniscal extrusion in BME lesions.

Author Contributions: Conceptualization, K.S.C. and J.K.H.; methodology, K.S.C.; formal analysis, K.S.C.; investigation, J.S.K.; data curation, J.K.H. and J.S.K.; writing—original draft preparation, K.S.C.; writing—review and editing, J.S.K.; supervision, J.K.H. and J.G.K. All authors have read and agreed to the published version of the manuscript.

Funding: This work was supported by the National Research Foundation of Korea (NRF) grant funded by the Korea government (MSIT) (No. 2021R1G1A1014579).

Institutional Review Board Statement: The study was conducted in accordance with the Declaration of Helsinki and approved by the Institutional Review Board of Inje University Seoul Paik Hospital (PAIK 2022-08-003).

Informed Consent Statement: The Institutional Review Board waived the requirements of informed consent as all data were anonymous. Therefore, this study was performed without prior informed consent.

Data Availability Statement: The data presented in this study are available on request from the corresponding author.

Conflicts of Interest: The authors declare no conflict of interest.

References

1. Felson, D.; Chaisson, C.; Hill, C.L.; Totterman, S.M.; Gale, M.E.; Skinner, K.M.; Kazis, L.; Gale, D.R. The Association of Bone Marrow Lesions with Pain in Knee Osteoarthritis. *Ann. Intern. Med.* **2001**, *134*, 541–549. [CrossRef] [PubMed]
2. Link, T.M.; Steinbach, L.S.; Ghosh, S.; Ries, M.; Lu, Y.; Lane, N.; Majumdar, S. Osteoarthritis: MR Imaging Findings in Different Stages of Disease and Correlation with Clinical Findings. *Radiology* **2003**, *226*, 373–381. [CrossRef] [PubMed]
3. Felson, D.T.; McLaughlin, S.; Goggins, J.; LaValley, M.P.; Gale, M.E.; Totterman, S.; Li, W.; Hill, C.; Gale, D. Bone marrow edema and its relation to pro-gression of knee osteoarthritis. *Ann. Intern. Med.* **2003**, *139*, 330–336. [CrossRef] [PubMed]
4. Fithian, D.C.; Kelly, M.A.; Mow, V.C. Material properties and structure-function relationships in the menisci. *Clin. Orthop. Relat. Res.* **1990**, *252*, 19–31. [CrossRef]
5. Furumatsu, T.; Hiranaka, T.; Kintaka, K.; Okazaki, Y.; Higashihara, N.; Tamura, M.; Ozaki, T. A characteristic MRI finding to diagnose a partial tear of the medial meniscus posterior root: An ocarina sign. *Knee Surg. Relat. Res.* **2021**, *33*, 38. [CrossRef]
6. Papalia, R.; Vasta, S.; Franceschi, F.; D'Adamio, S.; Maffulli, N.; Denaro, V. Meniscal root tears: From basic science to ultimate surgery. *Br. Med. Bull.* **2013**, *106*, 91–115. [CrossRef]
7. Hiranaka, T.; Furuhashi, R.; Takashiba, K.; Kodama, T.; Michishita, K.; Inui, H.; Togashi, E. Agreement and accuracy of radiographic as-sessment using a decision aid for medial Oxford partial knee replacement: Multicentre study. *Knee Surg. Relat. Res.* **2022**, *34*, 13. [CrossRef]
8. Matthews, J.R.; Brutico, J.; Heard, J.; Chauhan, K.; Tucker, B.; Freedman, K.B. Comparison of clinical outcomes following osteochondral allograft transplantation for osteochondral versus chondral defects in the knee. *Knee Surg. Relat. Res.* **2022**, *34*, 23. [CrossRef]
9. Helito, C.P.; Da Silva, A.G.M.; Guimarães, T.M.; Sobrado, M.F.; Pécora, J.R.; Camanho, G.L. Functional results of multiple revision an-terior cruciate ligament with anterolateral tibial tunnel associated with anterolateral ligament reconstruction. *Knee Surg. Relat. Res.* **2022**, *34*, 24. [CrossRef]
10. Asif, N.; Khan, M.J.; Haris, K.P.; Waliullah, S.; Sharma, A.; Firoz, D. A prospective randomized study of arthroscopic ACL recon-struction with adjustable- versus fixed-loop device for femoral side fixation. *Knee Surg. Relat. Res.* **2021**, *33*, 42. [CrossRef]
11. Bhatia, S.; LaPrade, C.M.; Ellman, M.B.; LaPrade, R.F. Meniscal root tears: Significance, diagnosis, and treatment. *Am. J. Sports Med.* **2014**, *42*, 3016–3030. [CrossRef] [PubMed]
12. Kim, D.H.; Lee, G.C.; Kim, H.H.; Cha, D.H. Correlation between meniscal extrusion and symptom duration, alignment, and arthritic changes in medial meniscus posterior root tear: Research article. *Knee Surg. Relat. Res.* **2019**, *32*, 2. [CrossRef] [PubMed]
13. Kodama, Y.; Furumatsu, T.; Kamatsuki, Y.; Hiranaka, T.; Takahata, T.; Sadakane, M.; Ikuta, H.; Yasumitsu, M.; Ozaki, T. Preliminary diagnosis of medial meniscus posterior root tears using the Rosenberg radiographic view. *Knee Surg. Relat. Res.* **2019**, *31*, 9. [CrossRef] [PubMed]

14. Allaire, R.; Muriuki, M.; Gilbertson, L.; Harner, C.D. Biomechanical consequences of a tear of the posterior root of the medial me-niscus. Similar to total meniscectomy. *J. Bone Jt. Surg.* **2008**, *90*, 1922–1931. [CrossRef] [PubMed]
15. Kohli, S.; Schwenck, J.; Barlow, I. Failure rates and clinical outcomes of synthetic meniscal implants following partial meniscectomy: A systematic review. *Knee Surg. Relat. Res.* **2022**, *34*, 27. [CrossRef]
16. Matthews, J.R.; Wang, J.; Zhao, J.; Kluczynski, M.A.; Bisson, L.J. The influence of suture materials on the biomechanical behavior of suture-meniscal specimens: A comparative study in a porcine model. *Knee Surg. Relat. Res.* **2020**, *32*, 42. [CrossRef]
17. Chung, K.S.; Choi, C.H.; Bae, T.S.; Ha, J.K.; Jun, D.J.; Wang, J.H.; Kim, J.G. Comparison of Tibiofemoral Contact Mechanics After Various Transtibial and All-Inside Fixation Techniques for Medial Meniscus Posterior Root Radial Tears in a Porcine Model. *Arthrosc. J. Arthrosc. Relat. Surg.* **2018**, *34*, 1060–1068. [CrossRef]
18. Chung, K.S.; Ha, J.K.; Ra, H.J.; Kim, J.G. A meta-analysis of clinical and radiographic outcomes of posterior horn medial meniscus root repairs. *Knee Surg. Sports Traumatol. Arthrosc.* **2016**, *24*, 1455–1468. [CrossRef]
19. Feucht, M.J.; Kühle, J.; Bode, G.; Mehl, J.; Schmal, H.; Südkamp, N.P.; Niemeyer, P. Arthroscopic Transtibial Pullout Repair for Posterior Medial Meniscus Root Tears: A Systematic Review of Clinical, Radiographic, and Second-Look Arthroscopic Results. *Arthrosc. J. Arthrosc. Relat. Surg.* **2015**, *31*, 1808–1816. [CrossRef]
20. Chung, K.S.; Ha, J.K.; Yeom, C.H.; Ra, H.J.; Jang, H.S.; Choi, S.H.; Kim, J.G. Comparison of Clinical and Radiologic Results Between Partial Meniscectomy and Refixation of Medial Meniscus Posterior Root Tears: A Minimum 5-Year Follow-up. *Arthrosc. J. Arthrosc. Relat. Surg.* **2015**, *31*, 1941–1950. [CrossRef]
21. Chung, K.S.; Ha, J.K.; Ra, H.J.; Yu, W.J.; Kim, J.G. Root Repair Versus Partial Meniscectomy for Medial Meniscus Posterior Root Tears: Comparison of Long-term Survivorship and Clinical Outcomes at Minimum 10-Year Follow-up. *Am. J. Sports Med.* **2020**, *48*, 1937–1944. [CrossRef] [PubMed]
22. Jung, Y.-H.; Choi, N.-H.; Oh, J.-S.; Victoroff, B.N. All-Inside Repair for a Root Tear of the Medial Meniscus Using a Suture Anchor. *Am. J. Sports Med.* **2012**, *40*, 1406–1411. [CrossRef]
23. Moon, H.-K.; Koh, Y.-G.; Kim, Y.-C.; Park, Y.-S.; Jo, S.-B.; Kwon, S.-K. Prognostic Factors of Arthroscopic Pull-out Repair for a Posterior Root Tear of the Medial Meniscus. *Am. J. Sports Med.* **2012**, *40*, 1138–1143. [CrossRef] [PubMed]
24. Kim, J.-H.; Chung, J.-H.; Lee, D.-H.; Lee, Y.-S.; Kim, J.-R.; Ryu, K.-J. Arthroscopic Suture Anchor Repair Versus Pullout Suture Repair in Posterior Root Tear of the Medial Meniscus: A Prospective Comparison Study. *Arthrosc. J. Arthrosc. Relat. Surg.* **2011**, *27*, 1644–1653. [CrossRef] [PubMed]
25. Seo, H.-S.; Lee, S.-C.; Jung, K.-A. Second-Look Arthroscopic Findings After Repairs of Posterior Root Tears of the Medial Meniscus. *Am. J. Sports Med.* **2011**, *39*, 99–107. [CrossRef] [PubMed]
26. Kim, S.B.; Ha, J.K.; Lee, S.W.; Kim, D.W.; Shim, J.C.; Kim, J.G.; Lee, M.Y. Medial Meniscus Root Tear Refixation: Comparison of Clinical, Radiologic, and Arthroscopic Findings with Medial Meniscectomy. *Arthrosc. J. Arthrosc. Relat. Surg.* **2011**, *27*, 346–354. [CrossRef] [PubMed]
27. Lee, J.H.; Lim, Y.J.; Kim, K.B.; Kim, K.H.; Song, J.H. Arthroscopic Pullout Suture Repair of Posterior Root Tear of the Medial Meniscus: Radiographic and Clinical Results With a 2-Year Follow-up. *Arthrosc. J. Arthrosc. Relat. Surg.* **2009**, *25*, 951–958. [CrossRef]
28. Lee, Y.G.; Shim, J.C.; Choi, Y.S.; Kim, J.G.; Lee, G.J.; Kim, H.K. Magnetic resonance imaging findings of surgically proven medial meniscus root tear: Tear configuration and associated knee abnormalities. *J. Comput. Assist. Tomogr.* **2008**, *32*, 452–457. [CrossRef]
29. LaPrade, C.M.; James, E.W.; Cram, T.R.; Feagin, J.A.; Engebretsen, L.; LaPrade, R.F. Meniscal root tears: A classification system based on tear morphology. *Am. J. Sports Med.* **2015**, *43*, 363–369. [CrossRef]
30. Chung, K.S.; Ha, J.K.; Ra, H.J.; Kim, J.G. Arthroscopic Medial Meniscus Posterior Root Fixation Using a Modified Mason-Allen Stitch. *Arthrosc. Technol.* **2016**, *5*, e63–e66. [CrossRef]
31. Chung, K.S.; Ha, J.K.; Ra, H.J.; Kim, J.G. Does Release of the Superficial Medial Collateral Ligament Result in Clinically Harmful Effects After the Fixation of Medial Meniscus Posterior Root Tears? *Arthroscopy* **2017**, *33*, 199–208. [CrossRef] [PubMed]
32. Shelbourne, K.D.; Dickens, J.F. Digital Radiographic Evaluation of Medial Joint Space Narrowing after Partial Meniscectomy of Bucket-Handle Medial Meniscus Tears in Anterior Cruciate Ligament–Intact Knees. *Am. J. Sports Med.* **2006**, *34*, 1648–1655. [CrossRef] [PubMed]
33. Kellgren, J.H.; Lawrence, J.S. Radiological Assessment of Osteo-Arthrosis. *Ann. Rheum. Dis.* **1957**, *16*, 494–502. [CrossRef] [PubMed]
34. Walter, S.D.; Eliasziw, M.; Donner, A. Sample size and optimal designs for reliability studies. *Stat. Med.* **1998**, *17*, 101–110. [CrossRef]
35. Koo, T.K.; Li, M.Y. A Guideline of Selecting and Reporting Intraclass Correlation Coefficients for Reliability Research. *J. Chiropr. Med.* **2016**, *15*, 155–163. [CrossRef]
36. Han, S.B.; Shetty, G.M.; Lee, D.H.; Chae, D.J.; Seo, S.S.; Wang, K.H.; Yoo, S.H.; Nha, K.W. Unfavorable Results of Partial Meniscectomy for Complete Posterior Medial Meniscus Root Tear with Early Osteoarthritis: A 5- to 8-Year Follow-Up Study. *Arthrosc. J. Arthrosc. Relat. Surg.* **2010**, *26*, 1326–1332. [CrossRef]
37. Ozkoc, G.; Circi, E.; Gonc, U.; Irgit, K.; Pourbagher, A.; Tandogan, R.N. Radial tears in the root of the posterior horn of the medial meniscus. *Knee Surg. Sports Traumatol. Arthrosc.* **2008**, *16*, 849–854. [CrossRef]

38. Krych, A.J.; Johnson, N.R.; Mohan, R.; Dahm, D.L.; Levy, B.A.; Stuart, M.J. Partial meniscectomy provides no benefit for symptomatic degenerative medial meniscus posterior root tears. *Knee Surg. Sports Traumatol. Arthrosc.* **2018**, *26*, 1117–1122. [CrossRef]
39. Ro, K.-H.; Kim, J.-H.; Heo, J.-W.; Lee, D.-H. Clinical and Radiological Outcomes of Meniscal Repair Versus Partial Meniscectomy for Medial Meniscus Root Tears: A Systematic Review and Meta-analysis. *Orthop. J. Sports Med.* **2020**, *8*, 2325967120962078. [CrossRef]
40. Chung, K.S.; Ha, J.K.; Ra, H.J.; Nam, G.W.; Kim, J.G. Pullout fixation of posterior medial meniscus root tears: Correlation between meniscus extrusion and midterm clinical results. *Am. J. Sport. Med.* **2017**, *45*, 42–49. [CrossRef]
41. Jamari, J.; Ammarullah, M.I.; Santoso, G.; Sugiharto, S.; Supriyono, T.; Heide, E. In Silico Contact Pressure of Metal-on-Metal Total Hip Implant with Different Materials Subjected to Gait Loading. *Metals* **2022**, *12*, 1241. [CrossRef]

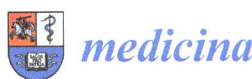

Review

Medial Meniscus Posterior Root Tear: How Far Have We Come and What Remains?

Hyun-Soo Moon [1,2], Chong-Hyuk Choi [1,3], Min Jung [1,3], Kwangho Chung [1,4], Se-Han Jung [1,5], Yun-Hyeok Kim [3] and Sung-Hwan Kim [1,5,*]

1. Arthroscopy and Joint Research Institute, Yonsei University College of Medicine, Seoul 03722, Republic of Korea
2. Department of Orthopedic Surgery, Hallym University Sacred Heart Hospital, Hallym University College of Medicine, Anyang 14068, Republic of Korea
3. Department of Orthopedic Surgery, Severance Hospital, Yonsei University College of Medicine, Seoul 03722, Republic of Korea
4. Department of Orthopedic Surgery, Yongin Severance Hospital, Yonsei University College of Medicine, Yongin 16995, Republic of Korea
5. Department of Orthopedic Surgery, Gangnam Severance Hospital, Yonsei University College of Medicine, Seoul 06273, Republic of Korea
* Correspondence: orthohwan@gmail.com or orthohwan@yonsei.ac.kr; Tel.: +82-2-2019-3415 or 82-10-4705-4262; Fax: +82-2-573-5393

Abstract: Medial meniscus posterior root tears (MMRTs), defined as tears or avulsions that occur within 1 cm of the tibial attachment of the medial meniscus posterior root, lead to biomechanically detrimental knee conditions by creating a functionally meniscal-deficient status. Given their biomechanical significance, MMRTs have recently been gaining increasing interest. Accordingly, numerous studies have been conducted on the anatomy, biomechanics, clinical features, diagnosis, and treatment of MMRTs, and extensive knowledge has been accumulated. Although a consensus has not yet been reached on several issues, such as surgical indications, surgical techniques, and rehabilitation protocols, this article aimed to comprehensively review the current knowledge on MMRTs and to introduce the author's treatment strategies.

Keywords: meniscus root; medial meniscus posterior root; root tear; medial meniscus posterior root tear; meniscus root repair; transtibial pull-out repair

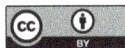

1. Introduction

Over the past few decades, perceptions of the clinical importance of menisci have changed [1]. The meniscus was once considered a functionless remnant vestige [2]; however, as a result of extensive research over a long time, it is now accepted as one of the most important structures of the knee joint. The meniscus is responsible for approximately 40–80% of the load transmission in the knee joint [3], and damage to this structure increases the peak contact pressure and decreases the contact area of the articular surface of the knee [4]. In addition, the meniscus plays several vital biomechanical roles, such as shock absorption, joint stabilization, lubrication, and proprioception [5]. Accordingly, a paradigm of treatment for meniscus tears has changed from resection to preservation [1,6].

There are various types of meniscus tears based on their location and patterns, each with different characteristics [7–9]. Among these, a medial meniscus posterior root tear (MMRT) is considered a detrimental injury because it causes conditions similar to those of total meniscectomy [10]. Although an MMRT was not well known until approximately a decade ago, numerous studies conducted with increasing attention to its biomechanical and clinical importance have been reported [11]. MMRTs account for approximately 10% of all types of meniscus tears and 22–28% of medial meniscus tears [12–16]. Given that MMRTs commonly precede advanced knee osteoarthritis [17], the actual incidence is considered higher than the reported one. Although much remains to be studied and understood, the multifaceted findings on MMRTs currently form the basis of their treatment strategies. Several review papers have been published on meniscus root tears; however, only a few articles have provided a comprehensive summary of the latest knowledge specifically focusing on MMRTs. Therefore, we aimed to comprehensively review the current knowledge on MMRTs, including their anatomy, biomechanics, clinical presentation, treatment options, and clinical outcomes, and we provide our treatment strategies.

2. Medial Meniscus Posterior Root Tear

2.1. Anatomy

The medial meniscus posterior root (MMPR), the tibial attachment of the medial meniscus posterior horn, is a ligamentous structure that anchors the meniscus to the tibia. The structural transition from a fibrocartilaginous meniscus body to a ligament-like structure facilitates the load transmission from the meniscus to the bone [18]. The MMPR is mainly composed of collagen fibers running parallel to the longitudinal axis of the meniscus, which also contributes to resisting the tensile force applied to the meniscus [19]. Owing to these mechanical characteristics, the MMPR stabilizes the meniscus between the femoral condyle and tibial plateau and allows effective load transmission [10]. The MMPR is located approximately 9.6 mm posterior and 0.7 mm lateral from the medial tibial eminence apex, with an area of the attachment site of approximately 30.4 mm^2 [20] (Figure 1A). In addition, the MMPR has diagonally-oriented posterior fibrous expansions called shiny white fibers, which increase the attachment area of the MMPR to the tibial plateau [20,21]. Shiny white fibers are used as anatomical landmarks during surgical procedures, involving the MMPR or posterior cruciate ligament [21,22].

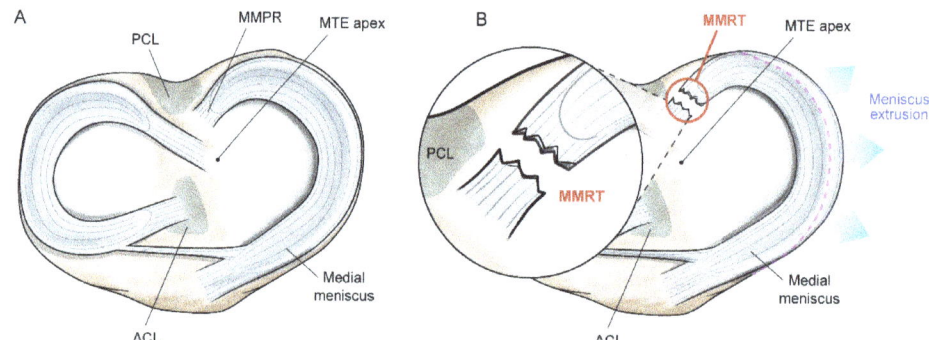

Figure 1. (**A**) An illustration showing the medial meniscus posterior root and its surrounding anatomical structures. (**B**) The occurrence of a medial meniscus posterior root tear leads to the loss of hoop tension in the meniscus, resulting in meniscus extrusion. PCL: posterior cruciate ligament; MMPR: medial meniscus posterior root; MTE: medial tibial eminence; MMRT: medial meniscus posterior root tear; ACL: anterior cruciate ligament.

2.2. Definition and Classification

An MMRT is defined as a tear or avulsion that occurs within 1 cm of the tibial attachment of the MMPR [23] (Figure 1B). This type of meniscal injury can be classified according to the system by LaPrade et al. as follows: (1) type 1, partial stable tear; (2) type 2, complete radial tear; (3) type 3, bucket-handle tear with meniscus root detachment; (4) type 4, complex oblique tear extending into the root attachment; and (5) type 5, avulsion fracture of the root attachment [23]. This concise classification system is clinically beneficial because it provides criteria for distinguishing MMRTs from other types of meniscus tears and helps determine treatment options. Furthermore, this classification system provides potential criteria for predicting the chronicity of an MMRT. Types 1, 2, and 4 are associated with acute or chronic tears, whereas types 3 and 5 are usually found in acute traumatic tears [23,24]. Among the five types of MMRTs, type 2 is the most common [23,24].

3. Biomechanics

The MMPR plays an important role in transmitting and distributing the load applied to the meniscus, thereby preserving the adjacent articular cartilage. The hoop tension generated by the collagen fibers that make up the meniscus and its root attachment counteracts the compressive forces applied to the knee joint while maintaining the meniscus between the femur and tibia [5]. A radial tear of these structures disrupts hoop tension. This disruption pushes the meniscus out between the two bones, eventually causing the meniscus to lose its function (Figure 1B). In a cadaveric study, Allaire et al. reported that an MMRT increased the contact pressure in the medial compartment of the knee by 25%, equivalent to that after total medial meniscectomy [10]. Subsequent biomechanical studies have consistently shown that an MMRT increases contact pressure while decreasing the contact area in the medial compartment of the knee [25–27]. On the other hand, the repair of an MMRT restores joint mechanics to a condition similar to that of an intact knee under time-zero conditions [10,25–27]. However, the non-anatomical repair may not restore the native biomechanics of the knee [28]. In addition to loading profiles, MMRTs have been reported to directly affect knee stability by causing rotation and translation of the joint [10].

4. Clinical Presentation

4.1. Pathophysiology and Clinical Features

MMRTs are caused by acute traumatic events or degenerative changes [29]. Although there are no clear criteria for differentiating them, degenerative MMRTs are thought to occur during light daily activities or without accompanying acute injuries to other knee structures.

Most traumatic MMRTs occur in association with ligament injuries of the knee. Anterior cruciate ligament injuries can accompany MMRTs [30]. In particular, MMRTs can be observed in cases of multi-ligament injuries [31–33], and varus injury patterns may further increase the possibility of MMRTs [32]. The incidence of traumatic MMRTs associated with ligament injuries of the knee ranges from 3% to 14% [31–33].

Degenerative MMRTs are relatively more common than traumatic MMRTs and are more susceptible to tears than root tears in other locations [29]. The medial meniscus posterior horn carries a large portion of the load applied to the knee joint, including compressive and shear forces [3]. Furthermore, the MMPR shows the lowest mobility of all meniscus roots, making it vulnerable to degenerative tears [34]. Park et al. reported that the degree of MMPR degeneration was highly associated with the degree of an MMRT and that degeneration, accompanied by fibrocartilage metaplasia or calcification, may precede an MMRT [35]. Possible risk factors for these types of MMRTs include older age, female sex, increased body mass index (BMI), increased varus alignment of the lower extremity, and decreased sports activity levels [14]. MMRTs tend to occur during light daily activities, such as squatting, rising from a chair, or going up or down stairs [12,36]. Interestingly, compared with other meniscus tears, MMRTs showed a relatively clear onset of symptoms. The onset of acute symptoms is commonly expressed as painful popping [13], and approximately 85–91% of patients state that they clearly recall the time of symptom onset [37,38]. According to Bae et al., a single painful popping sensation could be a highly predictive clinical sign for identifying MMRTs, with a positive predictive value of 96.5% [13]. In terms of physical examination, several parameters, such as pain on full flexion, joint line tenderness, and the McMurray test, can be used; however, there are no specific physical findings to diagnose MMRTs [12,39]. The Akmese sign, with severe medial joint line tenderness in near extension and minimal or no tenderness in knee hyperflexion, has recently been proposed as a possible physical examination to distinguish MMRTs from other medial meniscus pathologies, with high sensitivity and specificity [40].

4.2. Imaging

Magnetic resonance imaging (MRI) is the gold standard for diagnosing MMRTs. Although the quality of imaging and the ability of the observer may affect the accuracy of image interpretation, MRI is known to have a high accuracy in identifying MMRTs. According to Lee et al., the sensitivity, specificity, and accuracy of MRI for the detection of MMRTs are 86–90%, 94–95%, and 94%, respectively [41]. MMRTs show characteristic radiographic findings in each plane on MRI, which are as follows: (1) vertical high signal at the MMPR on the coronal image (truncation or cleft sign), (2) vertical high signal at the MMPR on the axial plane, and (3) absence of identifiable MMPR on the sagittal plane, but the meniscus reappears immediately in adjacent images (ghost sign) (Figure 2A–C) [42–44]. In addition, medial meniscus extrusion in the coronal plane, a medial displacement of the medial meniscus with respect to the outer border of the medial tibial plateau, can be used to predict MMRTs (Figure 2D) [45–47]. Choi et al. reported that a medial meniscus extrusion >3 mm could be associated with the occurrence of an MMRT [47]. The comprehensive use of the abovementioned radiographic findings can facilitate the accurate diagnosis of MMRTs [42,43]. In addition, T2-weighted sequences are considered most useful for identifying MMRTs [41].

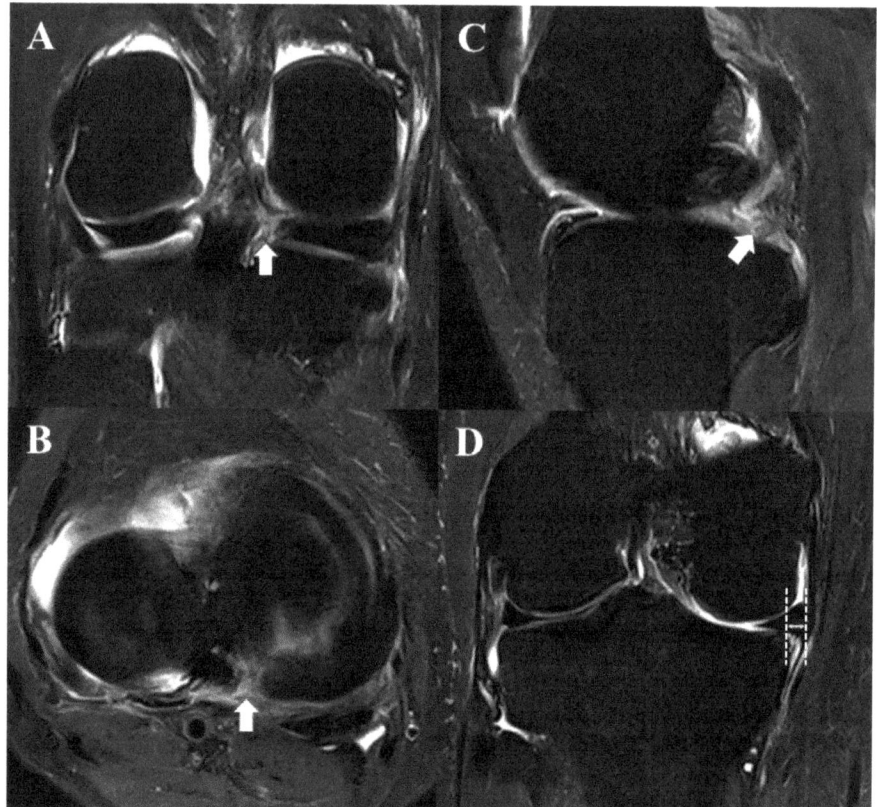

Figure 2. Characteristic magnetic resonance imaging findings, suggestive of a medial meniscus posterior root tear. (**A**) Vertical high signal on the coronal image (truncation or cleft sign; white arrow). (**B**) Vertical high signal on the axial image (white arrow). (**C**) Loss of identifiable medial meniscus posterior root on the sagittal image (ghost sign; white arrow). (**D**) Meniscus extrusion on the coronal image (the length of the white arrow).

Plain radiography or ultrasonography can be used as screening tools for diagnosing MMRTs. Patients with MMRTs reportedly show a relatively decreased medial joint space of the knee on weight-bearing knee radiographs, possibly attributable to osteoarthritis and medial meniscus subluxation [48–50]. The peripheral medial joint space-width ratio, which compares the peripheral medial joint space width between the affected and unaffected knees, may be smaller in patients with MMRTs than in those without MMRTs on standing knee radiographs [49]. Similarly, Kodama et al. found that patients with MMRTs showed decreased medial joint space width and increased distance between the medial tibial eminence and medial femoral condyle on weight-bearing posterior-anterior knee radiographs [50]. In the ultrasound examination, medial meniscus extrusion is used to predict the occurrence of MMRTs. Although medial meniscus extrusion is not a pathognomonic sign of MMRTs, parameters indicating the degree of extrusion and the amount of change can be used to predict these tears. On ultrasonographic evaluation, patients with MMRTs have greater medial meniscus extrusion than those without MMRTs [51]. Furthermore, dynamic medial meniscus extrusion, in accordance with changes in weight-bearing conditions, is reduced in patients with MMRTs [52].

5. Treatment

Treatment options for MMRTs include non-operative treatment, meniscectomy, surgical repair, and high tibial osteotomy. Although non-operative treatment and partial meniscectomy were the most commonly used treatment options for MMRTs until a decade ago, the frequency of surgical repair has increased as the biomechanical importance of the MMPR has been elucidated [10,25–27]. Surgical repair is not appropriate for some cases of MMRTs, and non-operative treatment and meniscectomy remain available in some situations. However, based on the findings of numerous clinical studies, surgical repair has become the treatment of choice for MMRTs.

5.1. Non-Operative Treatment

Non-operative treatments include medication, intra-articular injection, and unloader knee braces primarily aimed at relieving the symptoms and also include lifestyle modification and supervised exercise for long-term results [53–56]. These kinds of treatments can be applied to the following patients who are not suitable for surgical treatments: (1) older patients, (2) those with significant comorbidities, (3) those with advanced knee osteoarthritis (Kellgren-Lawrence grade ≥ 3), and (4) those unwilling to comply with a strict postoperative rehabilitation protocol. In certain groups of patients, symptomatic and functional improvements can be achieved with non-operative treatment [53,54]. However, since meniscal pathology remains unresolved in these cases, clinical improvement is mostly limited to the short term, and degenerative changes in the knee joint are reported to progress [53–55,57,58].

5.2. Meniscectomy

A torn MMRT tissue can cause impingement between the tibiofemoral joints, leading to pain and mechanical symptoms [12]. Meniscectomy can be a treatment option to relieve these symptoms. Arthroscopic partial meniscectomy for MMRTs can lead to clinical improvement and is reported to show a particularly good prognosis in patients with well aligned non-arthritic knees [12,59,60]. However, the mid-to-long-term clinical results of partial meniscectomy for MMRTs are generally poor, and degenerative changes in the knee joint also progress [61,62]. In addition, arthritic changes in the knee after partial meniscectomy for MMRTs have been reported to be more severe than those after non-operative treatment and surgical repair [58,63,64]. According to a recent study by Yang et al., meniscectomy for MMRTs results in a more significant stress concentration in the tibial cartilage compared with that in untreated MMRTs under dynamic loading conditions [65]. Therefore, owing to its limited clinical benefit, meniscectomy should be performed cautiously in selective cases [29].

5.3. Surgical Repair

MMRTs lead to biomechanically detrimental conditions in the knee by creating a functionally meniscal-deficient status, but surgical repair is reported to normalize it [10,25–27]. According to a cadaveric study by Padalecki et al., the repair of MMRTs could restore the loading profiles of the knee, being indistinguishable from those conditions with an intact meniscus [26]. Although this finding is based on a time-zero study, it provides a rationale for surgical repair of an MMRT. Along with scientific evidence, unsatisfactory clinical outcomes of meniscectomy have led to increasing interest in performing surgical repair for MMRTs [61–64].

5.3.1. Indication and Prognostic Factors

The indications for surgical repair of MMRTs are continuously expanding on the basis of numerous studies. Although a consensus has not yet been reached, patients who are suitable for surgical repair of MMRTs are those who meet most of the following conditions: (1) young and physically active, (2) without severe arthritic changes in the knee, (3) without severe varus malalignment of the lower extremity, (4) without high BMI, and (5) willingness to comply with a strict postoperative rehabilitation program [66–73]. In general, older age, high-grade cartilage lesions of the tibiofemoral joint, and varus alignment of the lower extremities are typical poor prognostic factors for surgical repair of MMRTs [66–69]. Since chronological age differs from biological age, no clear criteria exist for age-related surgical indications. Although 65 years of age is sometimes used as a criterion [38,56,74], several patient characteristics, such as activity level and comorbidities, should be comprehensively considered when deciding on surgery. Arthritic knee changes can be evaluated by plain radiography, MRI, or arthroscopy. It has been reported that radiographic osteoarthritis grade ≥ 3, according to the Kellgren-Lawrence grade system, and cartilage lesions in the medial tibiofemoral joint of grade ≥ 3, according to the Outerbridge classification system, are associated with unfavorable prognoses [66–70,75]. Concerning the lower limb alignment, varus >5° is known to be a poor prognostic factor [66–69]. However, findings from a recent study suggest that the surgical outcomes of patients with a hip-knee-ankle angle between 5° and 10° varus were not inferior to those of patients with a hip-knee-ankle angle <5° varus [74]. Therefore, rather than taking the angle of the lower limb alignment as an absolute criterion, evaluating whether the varus alignment is due to constitutional varus or pathological causes may also be required. High BMI is also reported to be a risk factor for poor outcomes after the surgical repair of MMRTs [70,71]. As in severe varus alignment of the lower extremities, a high BMI may adversely affect the repaired MMRT by increasing its load [75]. In addition, given the relatively low failure load of suture fixation and the limited healing rate of MMRTs [70,72,73], patients should comply with strict postoperative rehabilitation programs to obtain an optimal healing environment [76]. Furthermore, the preoperative symptom duration was found to affect surgical outcomes [38]. A careful patient selection process that considers the aforementioned factors may lead to relatively favorable surgical outcomes. Further research is required to establish optimal surgical indications for the repair of MMRTs.

5.3.2. Surgical Techniques

The repair methods for MMRTs include two techniques: one uses a suture anchor (suture anchor repair), and the other uses a transosseous tunnel (transtibial pull-out repair). Suture anchor repair is performed by placing the suture anchor on the region of an MMRT above the posterior tibial plateau [36,77–80]. This method has the advantage of reducing the risk of the bungee effect, micromotion between the meniscus-suture complex, and abrasion of the suture material, which may be found in long meniscus-suture constructs, resulting from transtibial pull-out repair [81,82]. However, this surgical method is technically demanding and requires an additional high posteromedial working portal and specialized instruments. It also involves the risk of damaging the cartilage and neurovascular structures [75]. In transtibial pull-out repair, after the suture strands stitched on the torn edge of an MMRT are pulled out through a transosseous tunnel, created from the footprint of the MMRT, to the tibia outer cortex, fixation is made above the anterior tibial cortex. As mentioned, this surgical method may have potential disadvantages, such as micromotion and suture abrasion [81,82]. However, this method is technically less challenging and has a relatively low risk of damage to the vital structures of the knee joint [75]. It also avoids potential complications caused by the loosening of the suture anchor [29]. Therefore, most surgeons use transtibial pullout repair for MMRTs [83]. Although there are few related studies, a paper reported that there are no differences in surgical outcomes between the two surgical techniques for MMRTs [36]. In addition to these two representative techniques, various additional procedures have been used to minimize meniscal extrusion that may persist after surgical repair, including peripheral release, centralization suture, and whip-running suture [84–87]. However, no well designed clinical study has demonstrated a method that reliably reduces residual meniscus extrusion [88].

Regardless of the surgical method chosen for the repair of MMRTs, it is of utmost importance to ensure that the repair occurs within the anatomical footprint of the MMPR. Unlike anatomical repair, non-anatomical repair cannot restore the loading profile of the knee joint, including the tibiofemoral contact area and pressure [28]. Additionally, complex suture configurations, such as the modified Kessler stitch or modified Mason-Allen stitch, have been reported to show better biomechanical properties than those with simple suture configurations [72,73]. Accordingly, efforts to perform surgical repairs using complex suture configurations at the anatomical footprint with a more familiar surgical technique would be paramount.

5.3.3. Postoperative Rehabilitation

Almost all surgeons apply a rehabilitation program to their patients after the surgical repair of MMRTs. Biomechanically, the load applied to the meniscus generated by weight bearing can affect the repair site [3]. In addition, displacement of the repair construct has been reported after cyclic loading [89]. This displacement may lead to repair loosening and surgical failure. Indeed, the successful healing rate after the surgical repair of MMRTs is approximately 70% [70]. Therefore, well organized postoperative rehabilitation programs are required to provide an optimal healing environment for the repaired MMRT by minimizing the potential effects of harmful stimuli. There are no standardized rehabilitation protocols yet, but most consist of protective strategies, such as limited weight-bearing, range of motion exercises, and brace application [76,90]. The details of the protocols varied greatly among studies. According to a systematic study by Kim et al., range of motion exercises were initiated immediately after surgery or two to three weeks after surgery, and partial weight-bearing was started from one to six weeks after surgery [76]. A knee brace or splint was applied in a fully extended position two to six weeks after surgery [76]. This was followed by progressive muscle-strengthening exercises, and a return to sports is usually allowed six months after surgery [76,90]. Because meniscus-to-bone healing after surgical repair is reported to progress for up to approximately 12 weeks [91], a certain period of protection for the repair construct is necessary to promote healing. However, prolonged protection also carries the risk of developing complications, such as muscle weakness and joint stiffness. Therefore, systematic rehabilitation should be applied under close monitoring, depending on the patient. In addition, accompanying lesions or concomitant surgical procedures should be considered.

5.3.4. Surgical Outcomes

Surgical repair of MMRTs provides both subjective and objective clinical benefits. The literature has consistently reported significant functional improvement, which could persist over the mid- to long-term after surgical repair of MMRTs [83,92,93]. Although surgical repair cannot prevent degenerative changes in the knee joint, the progression of osteoarthritis is less severe compared to that in non-operative treatment or meniscectomy [57,58,94,95]. Additionally, a paper reported that surgical repair is an economically superior treatment approach compared with other treatment modalities [58]. Therefore, although further multidisciplinary studies are required, surgical repair should be recommended for MMRTs, rather than other treatment methods, unless contraindicated [95].

5.4. High Tibial Osteotomy

High tibial osteotomy may be a treatment option for MMRTs. Because most MMRTs are degenerative in nature, it is not uncommon for them to be accompanied by cartilage lesions or varus deformities of the lower extremities [96]. As high-grade cartilage lesions in the medial tibiofemoral joint and severe varus malalignment are poor prognostic factors for the surgical repair of MMRTs [66–69], high tibial osteotomy can be an alternative to the surgical repair of MMRTs for patients with medial compartment osteoarthritis in a varus knee by redistributing the load applied to the knee. High tibial osteotomy has been reported to show favorable clinical outcomes for patients regardless of the healing of MMRTs [97,98]. Furthermore, although it would theoretically be ideal to perform concurrent surgical repair of MMRTs during high tibial osteotomy, it has been reported that there are no clinical benefits in combined surgical procedures compared to isolated high tibial osteotomy [99–101].

6. Author's Treatment Strategies for MMRTs

For patients diagnosed with MMRTs, we attempted to perform surgical repair as much as possible, avoiding meniscectomy. If patients with MMRTs do not meet the indications for surgical repair, non-operative treatment or high tibial osteotomy can be suggested by comprehensively considering not only the underlying knee pathology, but also the patient's characteristics, comorbidities, and willingness for treatment. Our indications for surgical repair of MMRTs are when all of the following are satisfied: (1) not older patients (usually by age 65 years); (2) radiographic osteoarthritis grade ≤ 2, according to the Kellgren-Lawrence grading system; (3) no pathologic varus alignment of the lower extremity (hip-knee-ankle angle $\leq 10°$ and $<5°$ greater compared to the hip-knee-ankle angle of the contralateral lower extremity); and (4) willingness to comply with a strict postoperative rehabilitation program (Figure 3). For the lower limb alignment, we aimed to avoid excluding patients with MMRTs from surgical candidates simply because the hip-knee-ankle angle is $>5°$, given that constitutional varus is present in a significant portion of the normal population [102,103]. Indeed, we recently found that the short-term clinical outcomes of surgical repair of MMRTs in patients with mild-to-moderate varus alignment were comparable to those in patients with neutral alignment [74]. Treatment plans for cartilage lesions in the medial tibiofemoral joint, which frequently accompany MMRTs, were determined using MRI and arthroscopic findings during surgery. The severity of cartilage lesions was assessed according to the International Cartilage Repair Society (ICRS) grading system [104]. In general, cartilage restoration procedures were not performed when cartilage lesions corresponded to the ICRS grade $\leq 3a$, but were performed for cartilage lesions of the ICRS grade 3b to 3d (if the calcified cartilage layer was exposed). For patients with ICRS grade 4 cartilage lesions, surgical repair of MMRTs, combined with cartilage restoration procedures, was conducted only if they did not want alternative treatment strategies.

The surgical repair of MMRTs is performed through arthroscopic transtibial pull-out repair using a modified reverse Mason-Allen stitch (Figure 4) [38,74]. First, diagnostic arthroscopy is performed via the parapatellar high anterolateral portal, and the accompanying lesions are thoroughly evaluated. When an MMRT is identified, the frayed portion of the torn edge of the MMRT is gently debrided using an arthroscopic shaver, followed by surgical repair. Before the repair process, the medial joint space width is measured using a 5-mm hook on an arthroscopic probe. If the medial gap is considered narrow enough to perform meniscal procedures, a percutaneous pie-crusting release of the superficial medial collateral ligament is performed using a 19-gauge intravenous catheterization needle. This additional procedure reduces the risk of iatrogenic articular cartilage damage and facilitates the surgical procedure without affecting the surgical outcomes and residual valgus laxity of the knee [105]. Subsequently, a crescent-shaped suture hook (Conmed Linvatec) or Knee Scorpion Suture Passer (Arthrex) is inserted into the joint through the anteromedial working portal, followed by making the stitch at approximately 3–5 mm medial to the posterior portion of the torn edge of the MMPR. This process is repeated on the anterior portion of the first stitch, and then a modified reverse Mason-Allen stitch with an ultra-high molecular weight polyethylene (UHMWPE) suture is made (Figure 5) [38,74,106]. We expect this horizontal loop stitch to increase the contact area of the meniscus-to-bone interface by pulling the meniscus, including its peripheral margin, from above. Additionally, using a No. 1 polydioxanone suture (PDS; Ethicon), an overlaid vertical stitch crossing the horizontal loop is created to produce a locking effect [107]. After suturing, an additional anteromedial portal is created. Subsequently, a posteromedial portal is created using the field of view provided by the arthroscope inserted through an additional anteromedial portal. The anatomical footprint of the MMPR is identified under observation through the posteromedial portal, and the bone bed of the footprint is decorticated using an arthroscopic rasp or curette to promote meniscus-to-bone healing. A tibial tunnel guide (Conmed Linvatec) is then inserted into the joint through an additional anteromedial portal and placed over the footprint of the MMPR with reference to the remnant stump and posterior cruciate ligament. A tibial transosseous tunnel is created, and a wire loop is inserted into the joint through the tibial tunnel. Next, the sutures stitched to the meniscus are passed through the wire loop and pulled out through the tibial tunnel by pulling the wire loop. Finally, sutures are tied over the EndoButton (Smith & Nephew), which is placed on the anterior tibial cortex just above the pes anserinus. With the knee fully extended, the PDS suture is tied first using a sliding knot while maintaining adequate tension by pulling the UHMWPE suture, and the UHMWPE suture is tied.

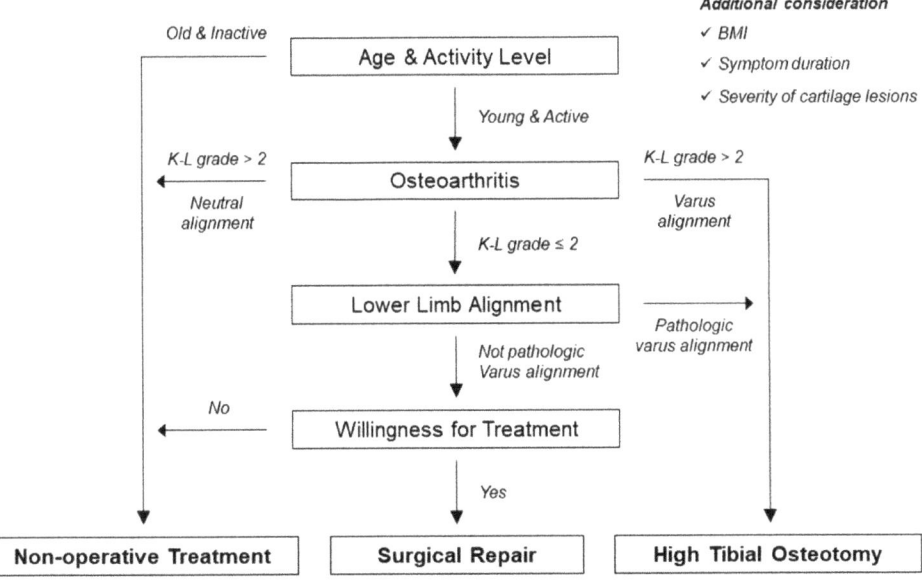

Figure 3. Flowchart of authors' treatment strategies for medial meniscus posterior root tear. K-L: Kellgren-Lawrence.

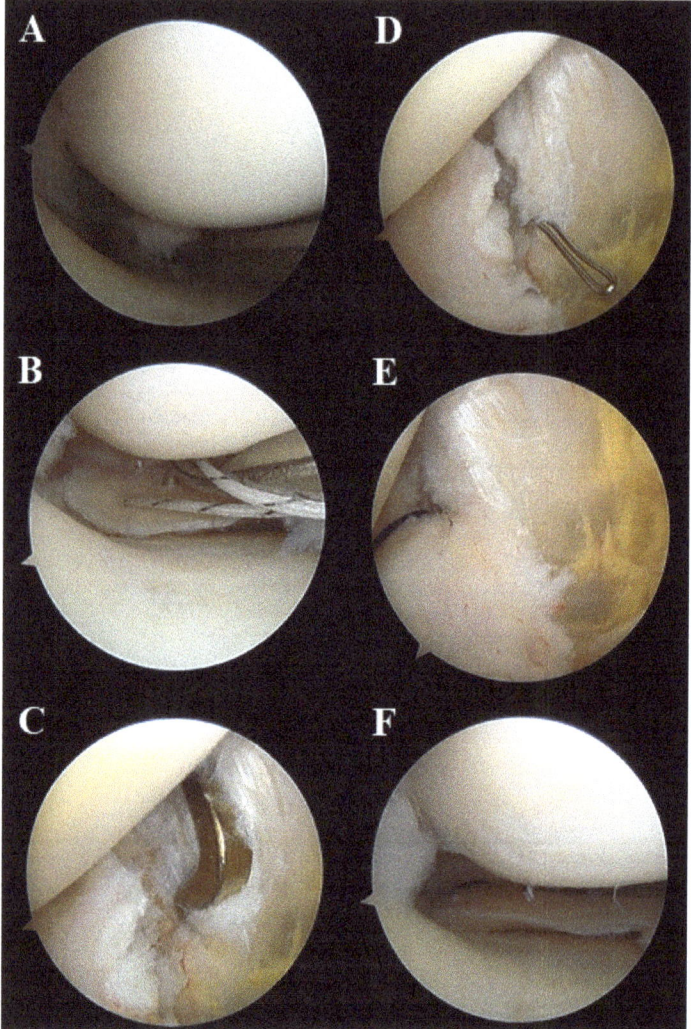

Figure 4. The process of arthroscopic transtibial pull-out repair of a medial meniscus posterior root tear (MMRT). (**A,B**) MMRT is confirmed, and a modified reverse Mason-Allen stitch is made (view from the parapatellar high anterolateral portal). (**C,D**) After identification of the anatomical footprint of the medial meniscus posterior root and decorticating the bone bed, a transosseous tibial tunnel is created, and a wire loop is inserted into the joint (view from the posteromedial portal). (**E**) Suture strands are pulled out through a tibial tunnel (view from the posteromedial portal) and (**F**) tied (view from the parapatellar high anterolateral portal). Reprinted with permission from Ref. [74]. Copyright 2021, copyright with permission from Moon and Kim.

Postoperatively, the patients are instructed to adhere to a strict rehabilitation program to ensure optimal conditions for MMRT healing. With the use of crutches and a hinged knee brace in the fully extended position, patients are restricted to toe-touch weight-bearing for four weeks postoperatively, followed by partial weight-bearing (<50% of their body weight) for six weeks. The crutches and brace are discontinued 10 weeks after surgery, and the patients are allowed to have a full weight-bearing gait. Passive range of motion exercises are initiated two weeks postoperatively and gradually increased. Similar to weight bearing, active range of motion exercises are allowed from 10 weeks postoperatively. For muscle strengthening, closed kinetic chain exercises are initiated 10 weeks postoperatively, gradually increasing the exercise intensity [108]. Deep knee flexion should be avoided during daily activities and exercise.

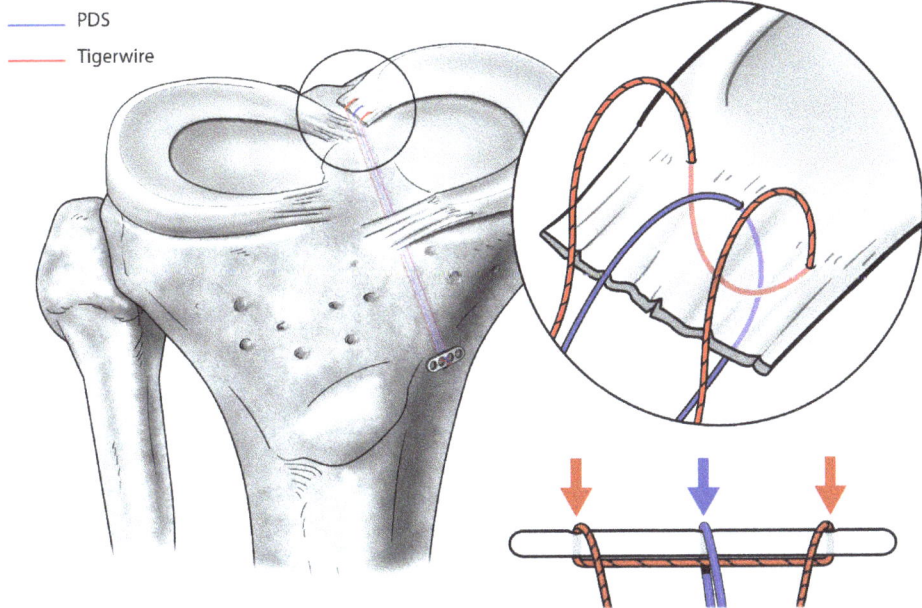

Figure 5. Pictorial illustration of the transtibial pull-out repair of a medial meniscus posterior root tear using a modified reverse Mason-Allen stitch. The stitch consists of the horizontal loop stitch (red thread; ultra-high molecular weight polyethylene suture [Tigerwire suture]) and the overlaid simple vertical stitch (blue thread; No. 1 PDS). Reprinted with permission from Ref. [38]. Copyright 2020, copyright with permission from Moon and Kim.

7. Summary and Future Direction

MMPR plays a vital biomechanical role in transmitting and distributing the load applied to the meniscus, thereby reducing the impact on the adjacent articular cartilage and preserving the knee joint. Damage to this structure can lead to functional meniscal deficiency, followed by a poor clinical course and rapid progression of osteoarthritis. Most MMRTs are degenerative in nature and usually occur during light daily activities with clinical symptoms, such as painful popping. MMRTs are usually diagnosed based on several characteristic MRI findings. Although there are several treatment options for MMRTs, surgical repair should be prioritized as much as possible to restore the biomechanical function of MMPR, which is supported by the favorable clinical outcomes reported in several clinical studies. However, consensus has yet to be reached regarding the optimal surgical indications, surgical techniques, and rehabilitation protocols for MMRTs. Addressing these issues necessitates further multidisciplinary research. Furthermore, unresolved challenges persist, such as residual meniscus extrusion, the limited healing rate of MMRTs, and the progression of osteoarthritis [38,70,109,110]. Tissue engineering and regenerative medicine may offer potential solutions for these matters. In particular, cell-based tissue regeneration, utilizing various cell sources, is particularly promising as a novel strategy to improve meniscus repair [111,112]. Several aspects in this field also need to be addressed, such as the recruitment and adhesion of cells to the site of meniscus tears, their differentiation into the appropriate cell phenotype, proliferation, and manipulation methods for clinical application [111]. Nonetheless, considering their reparative potential and mounting preclinical evidence, it is expected that most of these issues will be resolved in the near future.

Collaboration and joint research with these innovative fields are anticipated to potentially delay the progression of osteoarthritis by overcoming several existing limitations and optimizing the treatment strategies for MMRTs.

Author Contributions: Conceptualization, H.-S.M. and S.-H.K.; resources, H.-S.M., C.-H.C., M.J. and S.-H.K.; data curation, H.-S.M., K.C., S.-H.J. and Y.-H.K.; writing—original draft preparation, H.-S.M.; writing—review and editing, C.-H.C., M.J., K.C., S.-H.J. and S.-H.K.; supervision, S.-H.K.; project administration, S.-H.K.; funding acquisition, S.-H.K. All authors have read and agreed to the published version of the manuscript.

Funding: This research was supported by a faculty research grant from the Yonsei University College of Medicine (6-2021-0230).

Institutional Review Board Statement: Not applicable.

Informed Consent Statement: Not applicable.

Data Availability Statement: Not applicable.

Acknowledgments: MID (Medical Illustration & Design), as a member of the Medical Research Support Services of Yonsei University College of Medicine, providing excellent support with medical illustration.

Conflicts of Interest: The authors declare no conflict of interest.

References

1. Becker, R.; Kopf, S.; Seil, R.; Hirschmann, M.T.; Beaufils, P.; Karlsson, J. From meniscal resection to meniscal repair: A journey of the last decade. *Knee Surg. Sport. Traumatol. Arthrosc.* **2020**, *28*, 3401–3404. [CrossRef] [PubMed]
2. Sutton, J.B. The Nature of Certain Ligaments. *J. Anat. Physiol.* **1884**, *18*, i2–i238.
3. Walker, P.S.; Arno, S.; Bell, C.; Salvadore, G.; Borukhov, I.; Oh, C. Function of the medial meniscus in force transmission and stability. *J. Biomech.* **2015**, *48*, 1383–1388. [CrossRef] [PubMed]
4. Beamer, B.S.; Walley, K.C.; Okajima, S.; Manoukian, O.S.; Perez-Viloria, M.; DeAngelis, J.P.; Ramappa, A.J.; Nazarian, A. Changes in Contact Area in Meniscus Horizontal Cleavage Tears Subjected to Repair and Resection. *Arthroscopy* **2017**, *33*, 617–624. [CrossRef] [PubMed]
5. Fox, A.J.; Bedi, A.; Rodeo, S.A. The basic science of human knee menisci: Structure, composition, and function. *Sport. Health* **2012**, *4*, 340–351. [CrossRef]
6. Seil, R.; Becker, R. Time for a paradigm change in meniscal repair: Save the meniscus! *Knee Surg. Sport. Traumatol. Arthrosc.* **2016**, *24*, 1421–1423. [CrossRef]
7. Anderson, A.F.; Irrgang, J.J.; Dunn, W.; Beaufils, P.; Cohen, M.; Cole, B.J.; Coolican, M.; Ferretti, M.; Glenn, R.E., Jr.; Johnson, R.; et al. Interobserver reliability of the International Society of Arthroscopy, Knee Surgery and Orthopaedic Sports Medicine (ISAKOS) classification of meniscal tears. *Am. J. Sport. Med.* **2011**, *39*, 926–932. [CrossRef]
8. Kopf, S.; Beaufils, P.; Hirschmann, M.T.; Rotigliano, N.; Ollivier, M.; Pereira, H.; Verdonk, R.; Darabos, N.; Ntagiopoulos, P.; Dejour, D.; et al. Management of traumatic meniscus tears: The 2019 ESSKA meniscus consensus. *Knee Surg. Sport. Traumatol. Arthrosc.* **2020**, *28*, 1177–1194. [CrossRef]
9. Beaufils, P.; Becker, R.; Kopf, S.; Englund, M.; Verdonk, R.; Ollivier, M.; Seil, R. Surgical management of degenerative meniscus lesions: The 2016 ESSKA meniscus consensus. *Knee Surg. Sport. Traumatol. Arthrosc.* **2017**, *25*, 335–346. [CrossRef]
10. Allaire, R.; Muriuki, M.; Gilbertson, L.; Harner, C.D. Biomechanical consequences of a tear of the posterior root of the medial meniscus. Similar to total meniscectomy. *J. Bone Jt. Surg. Am.* **2008**, *90*, 1922–1931. [CrossRef]
11. Wang, Y.; Huang, C.; Qi, Y.; Bao, H.; Xu, Y. Global research status and hotspot analysis of meniscal root tears based on the WOS database. *Front. Surg.* **2022**, *9*, 944566. [CrossRef]
12. Bin, S.I.; Kim, J.M.; Shin, S.J. Radial tears of the posterior horn of the medial meniscus. *Arthroscopy* **2004**, *20*, 373–378. [CrossRef]
13. Bae, J.H.; Paik, N.H.; Park, G.W.; Yoon, J.R.; Chae, D.J.; Kwon, J.H.; Kim, J.I.; Nha, K.W. Predictive value of painful popping for a posterior root tear of the medial meniscus in middle-aged to older Asian patients. *Arthroscopy* **2013**, *29*, 545–549. [CrossRef]
14. Hwang, B.Y.; Kim, S.J.; Lee, S.W.; Lee, H.E.; Lee, C.K.; Hunter, D.J.; Jung, K.A. Risk factors for medial meniscus posterior root tear. *Am. J. Sport. Med.* **2012**, *40*, 1606–1610. [CrossRef]
15. Moon, H.S.; Choi, C.H.; Jung, M.; Lee, D.Y.; Eum, K.S.; Kim, S.H. Medial Meniscal Posterior Horn Tears Are Associated With Increased Posterior Tibial Slope: A Case-Control Study. *Am. J. Sport. Med.* **2020**, *48*, 1702–1710. [CrossRef]

16. Ozkoc, G.; Circi, E.; Gonc, U.; Irgit, K.; Pourbagher, A.; Tandogan, R.N. Radial tears in the root of the posterior horn of the medial meniscus. *Knee Surg. Sport. Traumatol. Arthrosc.* **2008**, *16*, 849–854. [CrossRef]
17. Lerer, D.B.; Umans, H.R.; Hu, M.X.; Jones, M.H. The role of meniscal root pathology and radial meniscal tear in medial meniscal extrusion. *Skelet. Radiol.* **2004**, *33*, 569–574. [CrossRef]
18. Andrews, S.H.; Rattner, J.B.; Jamniczky, H.A.; Shrive, N.G.; Adesida, A.B. The structural and compositional transition of the meniscal roots into the fibrocartilage of the menisci. *J. Anat.* **2015**, *226*, 169–174. [CrossRef]
19. Villegas, D.F.; Donahue, T.L. Collagen morphology in human meniscal attachments: A SEM study. *Connect Tissue Res.* **2010**, *51*, 327–336. [CrossRef]
20. Johannsen, A.M.; Civitarese, D.M.; Padalecki, J.R.; Goldsmith, M.T.; Wijdicks, C.A.; LaPrade, R.F. Qualitative and quantitative anatomic analysis of the posterior root attachments of the medial and lateral menisci. *Am. J. Sport. Med.* **2012**, *40*, 2342–2347. [CrossRef]
21. Anderson, C.J.; Ziegler, C.G.; Wijdicks, C.A.; Engebretsen, L.; LaPrade, R.F. Arthroscopically pertinent anatomy of the anterolateral and posteromedial bundles of the posterior cruciate ligament. *J. Bone Jt. Surg Am.* **2012**, *94*, 1936–1945. [CrossRef] [PubMed]
22. Yoon, H.K.; Park, S.H.; Oh, H.C.; Ha, J.W.; Choi, H. Combined PCL and PLC Reconstruction Improves Residual Laxity in PCL Injury Patients with Posterolateral Knee Laxity Less Than Grade III. *Yonsei. Med. J.* **2023**, *64*, 313–319. [CrossRef] [PubMed]
23. LaPrade, C.M.; James, E.W.; Cram, T.R.; Feagin, J.A.; Engebretsen, L.; LaPrade, R.F. Meniscal root tears: A classification system based on tear morphology. *Am. J. Sport. Med.* **2015**, *43*, 363–369. [CrossRef]
24. Moon, H.S.; Choi, C.H.; Jung, M.; Lee, D.Y.; Hong, S.P.; Kim, S.H. Early Surgical Repair of Medial Meniscus Posterior Root Tear Minimizes the Progression of Meniscal Extrusion: Response. *Am. J. Sport. Med.* **2021**, *49*, Np3–Np5. [CrossRef] [PubMed]
25. Marzo, J.M.; Gurske-DePerio, J. Effects of medial meniscus posterior horn avulsion and repair on tibiofemoral contact area and peak contact pressure with clinical implications. *Am. J. Sport. Med.* **2009**, *37*, 124–129. [CrossRef]
26. Padalecki, J.R.; Jansson, K.S.; Smith, S.D.; Dornan, G.J.; Pierce, C.M.; Wijdicks, C.A.; Laprade, R.F. Biomechanical consequences of a complete radial tear adjacent to the medial meniscus posterior root attachment site: In situ pull-out repair restores derangement of joint mechanics. *Am. J. Sport. Med.* **2014**, *42*, 699–707. [CrossRef]
27. Seo, J.H.; Li, G.; Shetty, G.M.; Kim, J.H.; Bae, J.H.; Jo, M.L.; Kim, J.S.; Lee, S.J.; Nha, K.W. Effect of repair of radial tears at the root of the posterior horn of the medial meniscus with the pullout suture technique: A biomechanical study using porcine knees. *Arthroscopy* **2009**, *25*, 1281–1287. [CrossRef]
28. LaPrade, C.M.; Foad, A.; Smith, S.D.; Turnbull, T.L.; Dornan, G.J.; Engebretsen, L.; Wijdicks, C.A.; LaPrade, R.F. Biomechanical consequences of a nonanatomic posterior medial meniscal root repair. *Am. J. Sport. Med.* **2015**, *43*, 912–920. [CrossRef]
29. Bhatia, S.; LaPrade, C.M.; Ellman, M.B.; LaPrade, R.F. Meniscal root tears: Significance, diagnosis, and treatment. *Am. J. Sport. Med.* **2014**, *42*, 3016–3030. [CrossRef]
30. Brody, J.M.; Lin, H.M.; Hulstyn, M.J.; Tung, G.A. Lateral meniscus root tear and meniscus extrusion with anterior cruciate ligament tear. *Radiology* **2006**, *239*, 805–810. [CrossRef]
31. Ra, H.J.; Ha, J.K.; Jang, H.S.; Kim, J.G. Traumatic posterior root tear of the medial meniscus in patients with severe medial instability of the knee. *Knee Surg. Sport. Traumatol. Arthrosc.* **2015**, *23*, 3121–3126. [CrossRef]
32. Kosy, J.D.; Matteliano, L.; Rastogi, A.; Pearce, D.; Whelan, D.B. Meniscal root tears occur frequently in multi-ligament knee injury and can be predicted by associated MRI injury patterns. *Knee Surg. Sport. Traumatol. Arthrosc.* **2018**, *26*, 3731–3737. [CrossRef]
33. Kim, Y.J.; Kim, J.G.; Chang, S.H.; Shim, J.C.; Kim, S.B.; Lee, M.Y. Posterior root tear of the medial meniscus in multiple knee ligament injuries. *Knee* **2010**, *17*, 324–328. [CrossRef]
34. Vedi, V.; Williams, A.; Tennant, S.J.; Spouse, E.; Hunt, D.M.; Gedroyc, W.M. Meniscal movement. An in-vivo study using dynamic MRI. *J. Bone Jt. Surg. Br.* **1999**, *81*, 37–41. [CrossRef]
35. Park, D.Y.; Min, B.H.; Choi, B.H.; Kim, Y.J.; Kim, M.; Suh-Kim, H.; Kim, J.H. The Degeneration of Meniscus Roots Is Accompanied by Fibrocartilage Formation, Which May Precede Meniscus Root Tears in Osteoarthritic Knees. *Am. J. Sport. Med.* **2015**, *43*, 3034–3044. [CrossRef]
36. Kim, J.H.; Chung, J.H.; Lee, D.H.; Lee, Y.S.; Kim, J.R.; Ryu, K.J. Arthroscopic suture anchor repair versus pullout suture repair in posterior root tear of the medial meniscus: A prospective comparison study. *Arthroscopy* **2011**, *27*, 1644–1653. [CrossRef]
37. Habata, T.; Uematsu, K.; Hattori, K.; Takakura, Y.; Fujisawa, Y. Clinical features of the posterior horn tear in the medial meniscus. *Arch. Orthop. Trauma. Surg.* **2004**, *124*, 642–645. [CrossRef]
38. Moon, H.S.; Choi, C.H.; Jung, M.; Lee, D.Y.; Hong, S.P.; Kim, S.H. Early Surgical Repair of Medial Meniscus Posterior Root Tear Minimizes the Progression of Meniscal Extrusion: 2-Year Follow-up of Clinical and Radiographic Parameters After Arthroscopic Transtibial Pull-out Repair. *Am. J. Sport. Med.* **2020**, *48*, 2692–2702. [CrossRef]
39. Lee, J.H.; Lim, Y.J.; Kim, K.B.; Kim, K.H.; Song, J.H. Arthroscopic pullout suture repair of posterior root tear of the medial meniscus: Radiographic and clinical results with a 2-year follow-up. *Arthroscopy* **2009**, *25*, 951–958. [CrossRef]
40. Akmese, R.; Malatyalı, B.; Kocaoglu, H.; Akkaya, Z.; Kalem, M. A New Clinical Sign for Diagnosing Medial Meniscus Posterior Root Tear. *Orthop. J. Sport. Med.* **2021**, *9*, 2325967120975511. [CrossRef]

41. Lee, S.Y.; Jee, W.H.; Kim, J.M. Radial tear of the medial meniscal root: Reliability and accuracy of MRI for diagnosis. *AJR Am. J. Roentgenol.* **2008**, *191*, 81–85. [CrossRef] [PubMed]
42. Choi, S.H.; Bae, S.; Ji, S.K.; Chang, M.J. The MRI findings of meniscal root tear of the medial meniscus: Emphasis on coronal, sagittal and axial images. *Knee Surg. Sport. Traumatol. Arthrosc.* **2012**, *20*, 2098–2103. [CrossRef] [PubMed]
43. Lee, Y.G.; Shim, J.C.; Choi, Y.S.; Kim, J.G.; Lee, G.J.; Kim, H.K. Magnetic resonance imaging findings of surgically proven medial meniscus root tear: Tear configuration and associated knee abnormalities. *J. Comput. Assist. Tomogr.* **2008**, *32*, 452–457. [CrossRef] [PubMed]
44. Harper, K.W.; Helms, C.A.; Lambert, H.S., 3rd; Higgins, L.D. Radial meniscal tears: Significance, incidence, and MR appearance. *AJR Am. J. Roentgenol.* **2005**, *185*, 1429–1434. [CrossRef] [PubMed]
45. Costa, C.R.; Morrison, W.B.; Carrino, J.A. Medial meniscus extrusion on knee MRI: Is extent associated with severity of degeneration or type of tear? *AJR Am. J. Roentgenol.* **2004**, *183*, 17–23. [CrossRef]
46. Furumatsu, T.; Kintaka, K.; Higashihara, N.; Tamura, M.; Kawada, K.; Xue, H.; Ozaki, T. Meniscus extrusion is a predisposing factor for determining arthroscopic treatments in partial medial meniscus posterior root tears. *Knee Surg. Relat. Res.* **2023**, *35*, 8. [CrossRef]
47. Choi, C.J.; Choi, Y.J.; Lee, J.J.; Choi, C.H. Magnetic resonance imaging evidence of meniscal extrusion in medial meniscus posterior root tear. *Arthroscopy* **2010**, *26*, 1602–1606. [CrossRef]
48. Gale, D.R.; Chaisson, C.E.; Totterman, S.M.; Schwartz, R.K.; Gale, M.E.; Felson, D. Meniscal subluxation: Association with osteoarthritis and joint space narrowing. *Osteoarthr. Cartil.* **1999**, *7*, 526–532. [CrossRef]
49. Asawatreratanakul, P.; Boonriong, T.; Parinyakhup, W.; Chuaychoosakoon, C. Screening for or diagnosing medial meniscal root injury using peripheral medial joint space width ratio in plain radiographs. *Sci. Rep.* **2023**, *13*, 4982. [CrossRef]
50. Kodama, Y.; Furumatsu, T.; Kamatsuki, Y.; Hiranaka, T.; Takahata, T.; Sadakane, M.; Ikuta, H.; Yasumitsu, M.; Ozaki, T. Preliminary diagnosis of medial meniscus posterior root tears using the Rosenberg radiographic view. *Knee Surg. Relat. Res.* **2019**, *31*, 9. [CrossRef]
51. Chiba, D.; Sasaki, T.; Ishibashi, Y. Greater medial meniscus extrusion seen on ultrasonography indicates the risk of MRI-detected complete medial meniscus posterior root tear in a Japanese population with knee pain. *Sci. Rep.* **2022**, *12*, 4756. [CrossRef]
52. Karpinski, K.; Diermeier, T.; Willinger, L.; Imhoff, A.B.; Achtnich, A.; Petersen, W. No dynamic extrusion of the medial meniscus in ultrasound examination in patients with confirmed root tear lesion. *Knee Surg. Sport. Traumatol. Arthrosc.* **2019**, *27*, 3311–3317. [CrossRef]
53. Neogi, D.S.; Kumar, A.; Rijal, L.; Yadav, C.S.; Jaiman, A.; Nag, H.L. Role of nonoperative treatment in managing degenerative tears of the medial meniscus posterior root. *J. Orthop. Traumatol.* **2013**, *14*, 193–199. [CrossRef]
54. Lim, H.C.; Bae, J.H.; Wang, J.H.; Seok, C.W.; Kim, M.K. Non-operative treatment of degenerative posterior root tear of the medial meniscus. *Knee Surg. Sport. Traumatol. Arthrosc.* **2010**, *18*, 535–539. [CrossRef]
55. Krych, A.J.; Reardon, P.J.; Johnson, N.R.; Mohan, R.; Peter, L.; Levy, B.A.; Stuart, M.J. Non-operative management of medial meniscus posterior horn root tears is associated with worsening arthritis and poor clinical outcome at 5-year follow-up. *Knee Surg. Sport. Traumatol. Arthrosc.* **2017**, *25*, 383–389. [CrossRef]
56. Lee, D.W.; Ha, J.K.; Kim, J.G. Medial meniscus posterior root tear: A comprehensive review. *Knee Surg. Relat. Res.* **2014**, *26*, 125–134. [CrossRef]
57. Bernard, C.D.; Kennedy, N.I.; Tagliero, A.J.; Camp, C.L.; Saris, D.B.F.; Levy, B.A.; Stuart, M.J.; Krych, A.J. Medial Meniscus Posterior Root Tear Treatment: A Matched Cohort Comparison of Nonoperative Management, Partial Meniscectomy, and Repair. *Am. J. Sport. Med.* **2020**, *48*, 128–132. [CrossRef]
58. Faucett, S.C.; Geisler, B.P.; Chahla, J.; Krych, A.J.; Kurzweil, P.R.; Garner, A.M.; Liu, S.; LaPrade, R.F.; Pietzsch, J.B. Meniscus Root Repair vs Meniscectomy or Nonoperative Management to Prevent Knee Osteoarthritis After Medial Meniscus Root Tears: Clinical and Economic Effectiveness. *Am. J. Sport. Med.* **2019**, *47*, 762–769. [CrossRef]
59. Lee, B.S.; Bin, S.I.; Kim, J.M.; Park, M.H.; Lee, S.M.; Bae, K.H. Partial Meniscectomy for Degenerative Medial Meniscal Root Tears Shows Favorable Outcomes in Well-Aligned, Nonarthritic Knees. *Am. J. Sport. Med.* **2019**, *47*, 606–611. [CrossRef]
60. Hong, S.Y.; Han, W.; Jang, J.; Lee, J.; Ro, D.H.; Lee, M.C.; Han, H.S. Prognostic Factors of Mid- to Long-term Clinical Outcomes after Arthroscopic Partial Meniscectomy for Medial Meniscal Tears. *Clin. Orthop. Surg.* **2022**, *14*, 227–235. [CrossRef]
61. Han, S.B.; Shetty, G.M.; Lee, D.H.; Chae, D.J.; Seo, S.S.; Wang, K.H.; Yoo, S.H.; Nha, K.W. Unfavorable results of partial meniscectomy for complete posterior medial meniscus root tear with early osteoarthritis: A 5- to 8-year follow-up study. *Arthroscopy* **2010**, *26*, 1326–1332. [CrossRef] [PubMed]
62. Krych, A.J.; Johnson, N.R.; Mohan, R.; Dahm, D.L.; Levy, B.A.; Stuart, M.J. Partial meniscectomy provides no benefit for symptomatic degenerative medial meniscus posterior root tears. *Knee Surg. Sport. Traumatol. Arthrosc.* **2018**, *26*, 1117–1122. [CrossRef]
63. Lee, N.H.; Seo, H.Y.; Sung, M.J.; Na, B.R.; Song, E.K.; Seon, J.K. Does meniscectomy have any advantage over conservative treatment in middle-aged patients with degenerative medial meniscus posterior root tear? *BMC Musculoskelet. Disord.* **2021**, *22*, 742. [CrossRef] [PubMed]

64. Chung, K.S.; Ha, J.K.; Yeom, C.H.; Ra, H.J.; Jang, H.S.; Choi, S.H.; Kim, J.G. Comparison of Clinical and Radiologic Results Between Partial Meniscectomy and Refixation of Medial Meniscus Posterior Root Tears: A Minimum 5-Year Follow-up. *Arthroscopy* **2015**, *31*, 1941–1950. [CrossRef] [PubMed]
65. Yang, Q.; Zhu, X.Y.; Bao, J.Y.; Zhang, J.; Xue, A.Q.; Wang, D.Y.; Mao, Z.M.; Tang, J.W.; Jiang, D.; Fan, Y.; et al. Medial meniscus posterior root tears and partial meniscectomy significantly increase stress in the knee joint during dynamic gait. *Knee Surg. Sport. Traumatol. Arthrosc.* **2022**, *31*, 2289–2298. [CrossRef]
66. Moon, H.K.; Koh, Y.G.; Kim, Y.C.; Park, Y.S.; Jo, S.B.; Kwon, S.K. Prognostic factors of arthroscopic pull-out repair for a posterior root tear of the medial meniscus. *Am. J. Sport. Med.* **2012**, *40*, 1138–1143. [CrossRef]
67. Ahn, J.H.; Jeong, H.J.; Lee, Y.S.; Park, J.H.; Lee, J.W.; Park, J.H.; Ko, T.S. Comparison between conservative treatment and arthroscopic pull-out repair of the medial meniscus root tear and analysis of prognostic factors for the determination of repair indication. *Arch. Orthop. Trauma. Surg.* **2015**, *135*, 1265–1276. [CrossRef]
68. Chung, K.S.; Ha, J.K.; Ra, H.J.; Kim, J.G. Prognostic Factors in the Midterm Results of Pullout Fixation for Posterior Root Tears of the Medial Meniscus. *Arthroscopy* **2016**, *32*, 1319–1327. [CrossRef]
69. Jiang, E.X.; Abouljoud, M.M.; Everhart, J.S.; DiBartola, A.C.; Kaeding, C.C.; Magnussen, R.A.; Flanigan, D.C. Clinical factors associated with successful meniscal root repairs: A systematic review. *Knee* **2019**, *26*, 285–291. [CrossRef]
70. Lee, S.S.; Ahn, J.H.; Kim, J.H.; Kyung, B.S.; Wang, J.H. Evaluation of Healing After Medial Meniscal Root Repair Using Second-Look Arthroscopy, Clinical, and Radiological Criteria. *Am. J. Sport. Med.* **2018**, *46*, 2661–2668. [CrossRef]
71. Brophy, R.H.; Wojahn, R.D.; Lillegraven, O.; Lamplot, J.D. Outcomes of Arthroscopic Posterior Medial Meniscus Root Repair: Association With Body Mass Index. *J. Am. Acad. Orthop. Surg.* **2019**, *27*, 104–111. [CrossRef]
72. Feucht, M.J.; Grande, E.; Brunhuber, J.; Burgkart, R.; Imhoff, A.B.; Braun, S. Biomechanical evaluation of different suture techniques for arthroscopic transtibial pull-out repair of posterior medial meniscus root tears. *Am. J. Sport. Med.* **2013**, *41*, 2784–2790. [CrossRef]
73. Kopf, S.; Colvin, A.C.; Muriuki, M.; Zhang, X.; Harner, C.D. Meniscal root suturing techniques: Implications for root fixation. *Am. J. Sport. Med.* **2011**, *39*, 2141–2146. [CrossRef]
74. Moon, H.S.; Choi, C.H.; Yoo, J.H.; Jung, M.; Lee, T.H.; Jeon, B.H.; Kim, S.H. Mild to Moderate Varus Alignment in Relation to Surgical Repair of a Medial Meniscus Root Tear: A Matched-Cohort Controlled Study With 2 Years of Follow-up. *Am. J. Sport. Med.* **2021**, *49*, 1005–1016. [CrossRef]
75. Lee, D.R.; Reinholz, A.K.; Till, S.E.; Lu, Y.; Camp, C.L.; DeBerardino, T.M.; Stuart, M.J.; Krych, A.J. Current Reviews in Musculoskeletal Medicine: Current Controversies for Treatment of Meniscus Root Tears. *Curr. Rev. Musculoskelet. Med.* **2022**, *15*, 231–243. [CrossRef]
76. Kim, J.S.; Lee, M.K.; Choi, M.Y.; Kong, D.H.; Ha, J.K.; Kim, J.G.; Chung, K.S. Rehabilitation after Repair of Medial Meniscus Posterior Root Tears: A Systematic Review of the Literature. *Clin. Orthop. Surg.* **2022**, *14*, e87. [CrossRef]
77. Jung, W.H.; Kim, D.H.; Chun, C.W.; Lee, J.H.; Ha, J.H.; Jeong, J.H. Arthroscopic, suture anchor repair through a novel medial quadriceptal portal for medial meniscal root tear. *Knee Surg. Sport. Traumatol. Arthrosc.* **2012**, *20*, 2391–2394. [CrossRef]
78. Jung, Y.H.; Choi, N.H.; Oh, J.S.; Victoroff, B.N. All-inside repair for a root tear of the medial meniscus using a suture anchor. *Am. J. Sport. Med.* **2012**, *40*, 1406–1411. [CrossRef]
79. Choi, N.H.; Son, K.M.; Victoroff, B.N. Arthroscopic all-inside repair for a tear of posterior root of the medial meniscus: A technical note. *Knee Surg. Sport. Traumatol. Arthrosc.* **2008**, *16*, 891–893. [CrossRef]
80. Lee, S.K.; Yang, B.S.; Park, B.M.; Yeom, J.U.; Kim, J.H.; Yu, J.S. Medial Meniscal Root Repair Using Curved Guide and Soft Suture Anchor. *Clin. Orthop. Surg.* **2018**, *10*, 111–115. [CrossRef]
81. Feucht, M.J.; Grande, E.; Brunhuber, J.; Rosenstiel, N.; Burgkart, R.; Imhoff, A.B.; Braun, S. Biomechanical comparison between suture anchor and transtibial pull-out repair for posterior medial meniscus root tears. *Am. J. Sport. Med.* **2014**, *42*, 187–193. [CrossRef] [PubMed]
82. Cerminara, A.J.; LaPrade, C.M.; Smith, S.D.; Ellman, M.B.; Wijdicks, C.A.; LaPrade, R.F. Biomechanical evaluation of a transtibial pull-out meniscal root repair: Challenging the bungee effect. *Am. J. Sport. Med.* **2014**, *42*, 2988–2995. [CrossRef] [PubMed]
83. Chang, P.S.; Radtke, L.; Ward, P.; Brophy, R.H. Midterm Outcomes of Posterior Medial Meniscus Root Tear Repair: A Systematic Review. *Am. J. Sport. Med.* **2022**, *50*, 545–553. [CrossRef] [PubMed]
84. Leafblad, N.D.; Smith, P.A.; Stuart, M.J.; Krych, A.J. Arthroscopic Centralization of the Extruded Medial Meniscus. *Arthrosc. Tech.* **2021**, *10*, e43–e48. [CrossRef]
85. Kim, J.H.; Ryu, D.J.; Park, J.S.; Shin, T.S.; Wang, J.H. Arthroscopic Transtibial Pull-Out Repair of Medial Meniscus Posterior Root Tear With a Whip Running Suture Technique. *Arthrosc. Tech.* **2021**, *10*, e1017–e1024. [CrossRef]
86. DePhillipo, N.N.; Kennedy, M.I.; Chahla, J.; LaPrade, R.F. Type II Medial Meniscus Root Repair With Peripheral Release for Addressing Meniscal Extrusion. *Arthrosc. Tech.* **2019**, *8*, e941–e946. [CrossRef]
87. Koga, H.; Watanabe, T.; Horie, M.; Katagiri, H.; Otabe, K.; Ohara, T.; Katakura, M.; Sekiya, I.; Muneta, T. Augmentation of the Pullout Repair of a Medial Meniscus Posterior Root Tear by Arthroscopic Centralization. *Arthrosc. Tech.* **2017**, *6*, e1335–e1339. [CrossRef]

88. Makiev, K.G.; Vasios, I.S.; Georgoulas, P.; Tilkeridis, K.; Drosos, G.; Ververidis, A. Clinical significance and management of meniscal extrusion in different knee pathologies: A comprehensive review of the literature and treatment algorithm. *Knee Surg. Relat. Res.* **2022**, *34*, 35. [CrossRef]
89. LaPrade, R.F.; LaPrade, C.M.; Ellman, M.B.; Turnbull, T.L.; Cerminara, A.J.; Wijdicks, C.A. Cyclic displacement after meniscal root repair fixation: A human biomechanical evaluation. *Am. J. Sport. Med.* **2015**, *43*, 892–898. [CrossRef]
90. Mueller, B.T.; Moulton, S.G.; O'Brien, L.; LaPrade, R.F. Rehabilitation Following Meniscal Root Repair: A Clinical Commentary. *J. Orthop. Sport. Phys.* **2016**, *46*, 104–113. [CrossRef]
91. Cui, P.; Sun, B.H.; Dai, Y.F.; Cui, T.Y.; Sun, J.L.; Shen, K.; Zhang, L.S.; Shi, C.X.; Wang, X.F. Healing of the Torn Anterior Horn of Rabbit Medial Meniscus to Bone after Transtibial Pull-Out Repair and Autologous Platelet-Rich Plasma Gel Injection. *Orthop. Surg.* **2023**, *15*, 617–627. [CrossRef]
92. Chung, K.S.; Ha, J.K.; Ra, H.J.; Yu, W.J.; Kim, J.G. Root Repair Versus Partial Meniscectomy for Medial Meniscus Posterior Root Tears: Comparison of Long-term Survivorship and Clinical Outcomes at Minimum 10-Year Follow-up. *Am. J. Sport. Med.* **2020**, *48*, 1937–1944. [CrossRef]
93. Chung, K.S.; Noh, J.M.; Ha, J.K.; Ra, H.J.; Park, S.B.; Kim, H.K.; Kim, J.G. Survivorship Analysis and Clinical Outcomes of Transtibial Pullout Repair for Medial Meniscus Posterior Root Tears: A 5- to 10-Year Follow-up Study. *Arthroscopy* **2018**, *34*, 530–535. [CrossRef]
94. Eseonu, K.C.; Neale, J.; Lyons, A.; Kluzek, S. Are Outcomes of Acute Meniscus Root Tear Repair Better Than Debridement or Nonoperative Management? A Systematic Review. *Am. J. Sport. Med.* **2022**, *50*, 3130–3139. [CrossRef]
95. Krivicich, L.M.; Kunze, K.N.; Parvaresh, K.C.; Jan, K.; DeVinney, A.; Vadhera, A.; LaPrade, R.F.; Chahla, J. Comparison of Long-term Radiographic Outcomes and Rate and Time for Conversion to Total Knee Arthroplasty Between Repair and Meniscectomy for Medial Meniscus Posterior Root Tears: A Systematic Review and Meta-analysis. *Am. J. Sport. Med.* **2022**, *50*, 2023–2031. [CrossRef]
96. Choi, E.S.; Park, S.J. Clinical Evaluation of the Root Tear of the Posterior Horn of the Medial Meniscus in Total Knee Arthroplasty for Osteoarthritis. *Knee Surg. Relat. Res.* **2015**, *27*, 90–94. [CrossRef]
97. Nha, K.W.; Lee, Y.S.; Hwang, D.H.; Kwon, J.H.; Chae, D.J.; Park, Y.J.; Kim, J.I. Second-look arthroscopic findings after open-wedge high tibia osteotomy focusing on the posterior root tears of the medial meniscus. *Arthroscopy* **2013**, *29*, 226–231. [CrossRef]
98. Itou, J.; Kuwashima, U.; Itoh, M.; Okazaki, K. High tibial osteotomy for medial meniscus posterior root tears in knees with moderate varus alignment can achieve favorable clinical outcomes. *J. Exp. Orthop.* **2022**, *9*, 65. [CrossRef]
99. Ke, X.; Qiu, J.; Chen, S.; Sun, X.; Wu, F.; Yang, G.; Zhang, L. Concurrent arthroscopic meniscal repair during open-wedge high tibial osteotomy is not clinically beneficial for medial meniscus posterior root tears. *Knee Surg. Sport. Traumatol. Arthrosc.* **2021**, *29*, 955–965. [CrossRef]
100. Kyun-Ho, S.; Hyun-Jae, R.; Ki-Mo, J.; Seung-Beom, H. Effect of concurrent repair of medial meniscal posterior root tears during high tibial osteotomy for medial osteoarthritis during short-term follow-up: A systematic review and meta-analysis. *BMC Musculoskelet. Disord.* **2021**, *22*, 623. [CrossRef]
101. Lee, D.W.; Lee, S.H.; Kim, J.G. Outcomes of Medial Meniscal Posterior Root Repair During Proximal Tibial Osteotomy: Is Root Repair Beneficial? *Arthroscopy* **2020**, *36*, 2466–2475. [CrossRef] [PubMed]
102. Bellemans, J.; Colyn, W.; Vandenneucker, H.; Victor, J. The Chitranjan Ranawat award: Is neutral mechanical alignment normal for all patients? The concept of constitutional varus. *Clin. Orthop. Relat. Res.* **2012**, *470*, 45–53. [CrossRef] [PubMed]
103. Song, M.H.; Yoo, S.H.; Kang, S.W.; Kim, Y.J.; Park, G.T.; Pyeun, Y.S. Coronal alignment of the lower limb and the incidence of constitutional varus knee in korean females. *Knee Surg. Relat. Res.* **2015**, *27*, 49–55. [CrossRef] [PubMed]
104. Brittberg, M.; Winalski, C.S. Evaluation of cartilage injuries and repair. *J. Bone Jt. Surg. Am.* **2003**, *85-A* (Suppl. S2), 58–69. [CrossRef] [PubMed]
105. Jeon, S.W.; Jung, M.; Chun, Y.M.; Lee, S.K.; Jung, W.S.; Choi, C.H.; Kim, S.J.; Kim, S.H. The percutaneous pie-crusting medial release during arthroscopic procedures of the medial meniscus does neither affect valgus laxity nor clinical outcome. *Knee Surg. Sport. Traumatol. Arthrosc.* **2018**, *26*, 2912–2919. [CrossRef]
106. Hiranaka, T.; Furumatsu, T.; Okazaki, Y.; Kintaka, K.; Kamatsuki, Y.; Zhang, X.; Xue, H.; Hamada, M.; Ozaki, T. Clinical evaluation of suture materials for transtibial pullout repair of medial meniscus posterior root tear. *Knee Surg. Relat. Res.* **2022**, *34*, 39. [CrossRef]
107. Ma, C.B.; MacGillivray, J.D.; Clabeaux, J.; Lee, S.; Otis, J.C. Biomechanical evaluation of arthroscopic rotator cuff stitches. *J. Bone Jt. Surg. Am.* **2004**, *86*, 1211–1216. [CrossRef]
108. Park, J.; Kim, M.; Park, J.H. Promoting Adherence to Joint Exercise Using the Donation Model: Proof via a Motion-Detecting Mobile Exercise Coaching Application. *Yonsei. Med. J.* **2022**, *63*, 1050–1057. [CrossRef]
109. Chung, K.S.; Ha, J.K.; Ra, H.J.; Kim, J.G. A meta-analysis of clinical and radiographic outcomes of posterior horn medial meniscus root repairs. *Knee Surg. Sport. Traumatol. Arthrosc.* **2016**, *24*, 1455–1468. [CrossRef]
110. Feucht, M.J.; Kühle, J.; Bode, G.; Mehl, J.; Schmal, H.; Südkamp, N.P.; Niemeyer, P. Arthroscopic Transtibial Pullout Repair for Posterior Medial Meniscus Root Tears: A Systematic Review of Clinical, Radiographic, and Second-Look Arthroscopic Results. *Arthroscopy* **2015**, *31*, 1808–1816. [CrossRef]

111. Bilgen, B.; Jayasuriya, C.T.; Owens, B.D. Current Concepts in Meniscus Tissue Engineering and Repair. *Adv. Health Mater.* **2018**, *7*, e1701407. [CrossRef]
112. Cucchiarini, M.; McNulty, A.L.; Mauck, R.L.; Setton, L.A.; Guilak, F.; Madry, H. Advances in combining gene therapy with cell and tissue engineering-based approaches to enhance healing of the meniscus. *Osteoarthr. Cartil.* **2016**, *24*, 1330–1339. [CrossRef]

Disclaimer/Publisher's Note: The statements, opinions and data contained in all publications are solely those of the individual author(s) and contributor(s) and not of MDPI and/or the editor(s). MDPI and/or the editor(s) disclaim responsibility for any injury to people or property resulting from any ideas, methods, instructions or products referred to in the content.

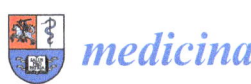

Article

Anatomical Study of the Lateral Tibial Spine as a Landmark for Weight Bearing Line Assessment during High Tibial Osteotomy

Tae Woo Kim * and June Seok Won

Department of Orthopedic Surgery, Seoul National University College of Medicine, Seoul National University Boramae Medical Center, Seoul 07061, Republic of Korea; chris9906@naver.com
* Correspondence: orthopassion@naver.com

Abstract: *Background:* Accurate pre-operative planning is essential for successful high tibial osteotomy (HTO). The lateral tibial spine is a commonly used anatomical landmark for weight-bearing line assessment. However, studies on the mediolateral (M-L) position of the lateral tibial spine on the tibial plateau and its variability are limited. *Purpose:* This study aimed to (1) analyze the M-L position of the lateral tibial spine on the tibial plateau and its variability, (2) investigate radiologic parameters that affect the position of the lateral tibial spine, and (3) determine whether the lateral tibial spine can be a useful anatomical landmark for weight-bearing line assessment during HTO. *Materials and Methods:* Radiological evaluation was performed on 200 participants (64% female, mean age 42.3 ± 13.2 years) who had standing anterior–posterior plain knee radiographs with a patellar facing forward orientation. The distances from the medial border of the tibial plateau to the lateral spine peak (dLSP) and lateral spine inflection point (dLSI) were measured using a picture archiving and communication system. The medial–lateral inter-spine distance (dISP) was also measured. All parameters were presented as percentages of the entire tibial plateau width. The relationships between the parameters were also investigated. *Results:* The mean value of dLSP was 56.9 ± 2.5 (52.4–64.5)%, which was 5% lower than the Fujisawa point (62%). The mean value of dLSI was 67.9 ± 2.2 (63.4–75.8)%, which was approximately 5% higher than the Fujisawa point. The values of the dLSP and dLSI were variable among patients, and the upper and lower 10% groups showed significantly higher and lower dLSP and dLSI, respectively, than the middle 10% group. The mean value of dISP was 16.5 ± 2.4%, and it was positively correlated with dLSP and dLSI. *Conclusions:* On average, the dLSP and dLSI were located −5% and +5% laterally from the conventional Fujisawa point, and they may be useful landmarks for correction amount adjustment during HTO. However, it should be noted that correction based on the lateral tibial spine can be affected by anatomical variations, especially in patients with small or large inter-spine distances.

Keywords: high tibial osteotomy; planning; landmark; lateral tibial spine; anatomy

Citation: Kim, T.W.; Won, J.S. Anatomical Study of the Lateral Tibial Spine as a Landmark for Weight Bearing Line Assessment during High Tibial Osteotomy. *Medicina* 2023, 59, 1571. https://doi.org/10.3390/medicina59091571

Academic Editors: Yong In and In Jun Koh

Received: 21 July 2023
Revised: 25 August 2023
Accepted: 26 August 2023
Published: 29 August 2023

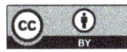

Copyright: © 2023 by the authors. Licensee MDPI, Basel, Switzerland. This article is an open access article distributed under the terms and conditions of the Creative Commons Attribution (CC BY) license (https://creativecommons.org/licenses/by/4.0/).

1. Introduction

High tibial osteotomy (HTO) is an efficient surgical option for treating middle-aged patients with medial knee osteoarthritis (OA) and varus alignment [1–5]. Accurate alignment correction is essential for successful HTO in patients with OA [6–11]. Under-correction can result in residual knee pain and shorten the longevity of the effects of this procedure [12]. Over-correction can induce lateral and patellofemoral arthritis and cause dissatisfaction associated with excessive valgus deformity [13–15].

To reduce the correction error during HTO, pre-operative planning based on weight-bearing line assessment plays an important role, and the first step in HTO pre-operative planning is the determination of the appropriate target point on the tibial plateau [16–21]. Since it was first documented in 1979, the Fujisawa point (62–63%) has been commonly used as an ideal realignment target during HTO, and the outcome of HTO has also been evaluated using this reference point [22–24]. However, some authors recommend adjusting the correction target depending on the severity of osteoarthritis and the reason for surgery [2,25].

The lateral tibial spine can also be used as an anatomical landmark for weight-bearing line assessment during HTO. Lee et al. reported that medial opening-wedge HTOs aimed at the lateral tibial spine showed comparable clinical outcomes to those of HTOs targeting the conventional Fujisawa point [26]. The lateral tibial spine is a bony eminence on the tibial plateau to which the anterior cruciate ligament attaches, which varies anatomically between individuals [27,28]. However, it is unclear whether the lateral tibial spine can be a constant anatomical landmark for HTO in the mediolateral dimension of the tibial plateau.

Therefore, this study aimed to (1) analyze the M-L position of the lateral tibial spine on the tibial plateau and its variability, (2) investigate the radiological parameters that affect the position of the lateral tibial spine, and (3) determine whether the lateral tibial spine can be a useful anatomical landmark for weight-bearing line assessment during HTO. We hypothesized that the lateral tibial spine can be a useful anatomical landmark for HTO and that it can also show anatomical variation correlated with specific radiologic parameters.

2. Materials and Methods

2.1. Study Population

A total of 517 consecutive standing knee anteroposterior (AP) radiographs of 517 patients diagnosed with medial compartment knee osteoarthritis at Seoul National University Boramae Medical Center between January 2019 and March 2020 were retrospectively reviewed. Of these, 317 radiographs were excluded, and the remaining 200 knee AP radiographs were examined. The exclusion criteria were as follows: (1) Kellgren–Lawrence grade IV with a large osteophyte; (2) bone deformity of the knee due to previous surgery or trauma; (3) rheumatoid arthritis; (4) infection; and (5) absence of a standing knee AP radiograph with proper lower extremity rotation (i.e., with the patella facing forward). In patients with bilateral knee OA, only the side with the more progressed knee OA was evaluated. Patient demographic data, including age and sex, and data on laterality were also collected. This study was approved by the Institutional Review Board (IRB No.20-2021-22), and the requirement for informed consent was waived due to the retrospective study design.

2.2. Radiologic Assessment

Standing knee AP radiographs were obtained using a UT 2000 X-ray machine (Philips Research, Eindhoven, The Netherlands) set at 90 Kv and 50 mA. Knee rotation was controlled using our standard protocol to locate the patella at the center of the femoral condyle during the examination. All radiographs were digitally acquired using a picture archiving and communication system (PACS), and radiographic assessments were performed using the PACS (INFINITT, Seoul, Republic of Korea). The standard knee AP view was marked with a digital ruler, and each value was calibrated automatically on the PACS system.

The peak and inflection points of the lateral tibial spine were determined as the most prominent points and the intersection point between the tibial spine slope and the tibial plateau, respectively. The distance between the medial tibial border and lateral spine peak point (dLSP), the distance between the medial tibial border and lateral spine inflection point (dLSI), and the mediolateral inter-spine distance (dISP) were measured and presented as a percentage of the entire tibial plateau width (Figure 1).

For the interobserver reliability test, two orthopedic surgeons independently measured the radiographic parameters. Each observer was blinded to the measurements of the other observer. For the intra-observer reliability test, each observer measured the radiological parameters twice at 8-week intervals.

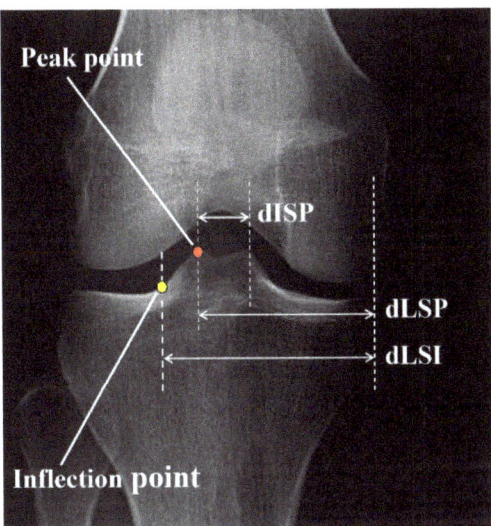

Figure 1. Radiographic measurements of the lateral tibial spine. Peak point: the most prominent point of the lateral tibial spine, inflection point: the intersection point between the tibial spine slope and tibial plateau, dLSP: distance between the tibial medial border and lateral spine peak point, dLSI: distance between the tibial medial border and lateral spine inflection point; dISP: medio-lateral inter-spine distance.

2.3. Analysis of Radiologic Parameters

To quantitatively analyze the location of the lateral tibial spine on the tibial plateau, the dLSP and dLSI were measured. To evaluate the variability in each parameter statistically, the upper 10% and lower 10% groups were compared with the middle 10% group, respectively. To determine whether other radiologic parameters could predict the amount of dLSP or dLSI, correlations between dLSP, dLSI, tibial plateau M-L width, and dISP were analyzed.

2.4. Statistical Analysis

All statistical analyses were performed using SPSS version 25.0 (IBM, Armonk, NY, USA). An a priori power analysis was performed with the assumption that a 2.0% M-L dimension was radiologically significant, with a standard deviation of 2.4% mm. It was found that 20 knees in each group were sufficient for all parameters ($\alpha = 0.05$, $\beta = 0.8$). p-values of <0.05 were considered statistically significant. All data are presented as mean and standard deviation. Student's t-test was used for intergroup comparisons. Correlation analyses between radiological parameters were performed using Pearson's correlation coefficients. Inter- and intra-observer reliabilities were evaluated using the intra-class correlation coefficient (ICC).

3. Results

In total, 200 standing AP knee radiographs (115 right and 85 left) from 200 patients (92 males, 108 females) were evaluated. The mean age of the patients was 56.2 ± 7.2 years, and the severity of knee OA was K-L grades I, II, and III in 14, 76, and 110 patients, respectively (Table 1). For all radiological parameters, the inter- and intra-observer ICC were >0.8 (Table 2).

Table 1. Patient demographics and measurements of radiologic parameters.

	Mean	SD (Min–Max)
Patient demographics		
age	56.2	7.2 (40–72)
gender	male (46%)	
laterality	right (57.5%)	
K-L grade	grade I: 14 grade II: 76 grade III: 110	
Radiologic parameters		
Tibial width (mm)	65.3	3.4 (60.1–73.4)
dLSP (%)	56.9	2.5 (52.4–64.5)
dLSI (%)	67.9	2.2 (63.4–75.8)
dISP (%)	16.5	2.4 (12.4–23.1)

K-L, Kellgren–Lawrence; dLSP, the distance between the tibial medial border and lateral spine peak point; dLSI, the distance between the tibial medial border and lateral spine inflection point; dISP, medio-lateral inter-spine distance.

Table 2. Intra-observer and inter-observer reliability of radiographic measurements.

	Intra-Observer Reliability	Inter-Observer Reliability
Tibial width (mm)	0.971 (0.966–0.979)	0.936 (0.946–0.952)
dLSP	0.995 (0.991–0.997)	0.996 (0.992–0.998)
dLSI	0.981 (0.966–0.989)	0.991 (0.984–0.995)
dISP	0.988 (0.980–0.993)	0.997 (0.995–0.998)

dLSP, the distance between the tibial medial border and lateral spine peak point; dLSI, the distance between the tibial medial border and lateral spine inflection point; dISP, medio-lateral inter-spine distance.

In the quantitative analysis of the lateral tibial spine position, the mean values of dLSP, dLSI, and dISP were 56.9 ± 2.5%, 67.9 ± 2.2%, and 16.5 ± 2.4%, respectively. The peak point and inflection point of the lateral tibial spine were located approximately 5% lower and 5% higher, respectively, than the conventional Fujisawa point (62–63%). However, both dLSP and dLSI varied broadly between individuals. The maximum and minimum values of dLSP were 64.5% and 52.4%, respectively, and the maximum and minimum values of dLSI were 75.8% and 63.4%, respectively. The upper 10% group showed significantly higher dLSP and dLSI than the middle 10% group ($p = 0.001$, $p = 0.002$); the lower 10% group also showed significantly lower dLSP and dLSI than the middle 10% group ($p = 0.001$, $p = 0.001$) (Figures 2 and 3).

In the correlation analysis, the dISP showed significant positive correlations with the dLSP ($r = 0.787$, $p = 0.001$) and dLSI ($r = 0.756$, $p = 0.001$) (Figure 4). In patients with larger inter-spine distances, the peak and inflection points of the lateral tibial spine were located more laterally. Similarly, in patients with a narrow inter-spine distance, the peak and inflection points of the lateral tibial spine were located more medially. However, the tibial plateau M-L width, sex, and laterality did not affect the dLSP or dLSI ($p > 0.05$) (Table 3).

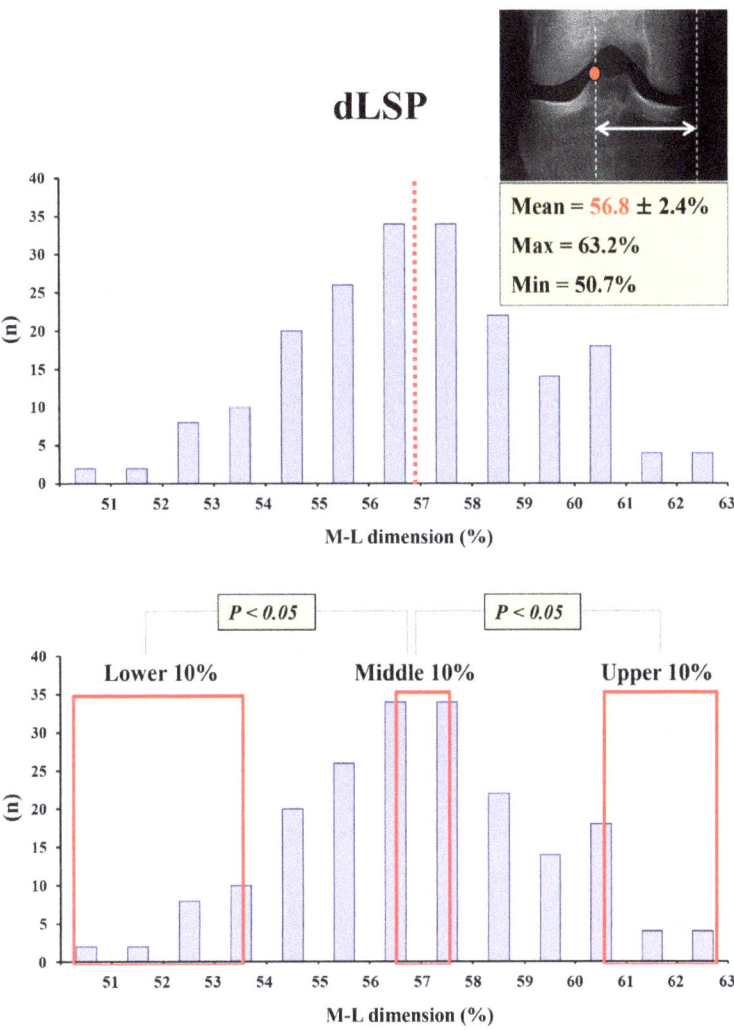

Figure 2. The mean and maximum/minimum values for dLSP and its variation. Red dot: peak point of lateral tibial spine, red dotted line and red font: mean value of dLSP, red frame: lower, middle, and upper 10% groups.

The mean value of dLSP was 56.9 ± 2.5%, and the maximum and minimum values of dLSP were 64.5% and 52.4%, respectively. The upper 10% and lower 10% groups showed significantly higher and lower dLSP than the middle 10% group, respectively.

The mean value of dLSI was 67.9 ± 2.2%, and the maximum and minimum values of dLSI were 75.8% and 63.4%, respectively. The upper 10% and lower 10% groups showed significantly higher and lower dLSP than the middle 10% group, respectively.

In the correlation analysis, dISP showed a significantly positive correlation with dLSP (r = 0.787, $p < 0.05$) and dLSI (r = 0.756, $p < 0.05$). In patients with large and small dISP, dLSP and dLSI also showed increasing and decreasing tendency, respectively.

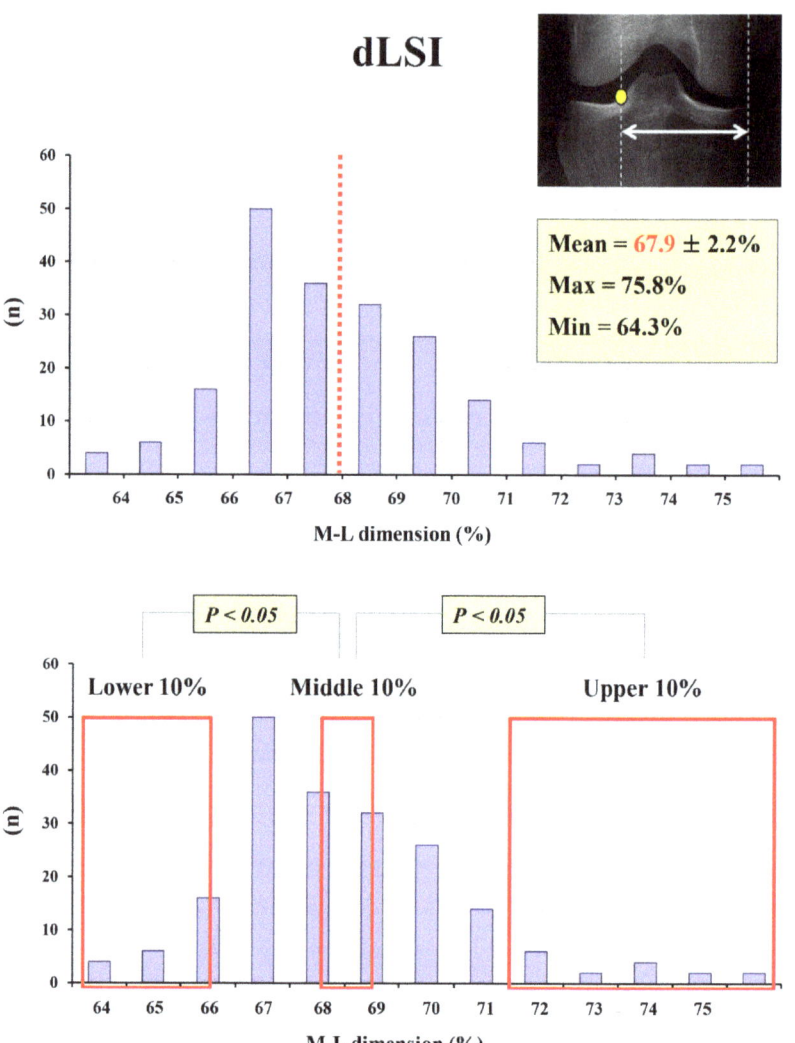

Figure 3. The mean and maximum/minimum values of dLSI and its variation. Yellow dot: inflection point of lateral tibial spine, red dotted line and red font: mean value of dLSI, red frame: lower, middle, and upper 10% groups.

Table 3. Comparison of radiologic parameters depending on gender and laterality.

	dLSI (%)	dLSP (%)	dISP (%)
Male	68.0 ± 2.2	57.0 ± 2.7	16.7 ± 2.3
Female	67.7 ± 2.3	56.8 ± 2.5	16.4 ± 2.3
p-value	0.352	0.512	0.241
Right	67.9 ± 2.1	56.7 ± 2.3	16.5 ± 2.2
Left	67.8 ± 2.2	56.8 ± 2.1	16.6 ± 2.1
p-value	0.671	0.490	0.540

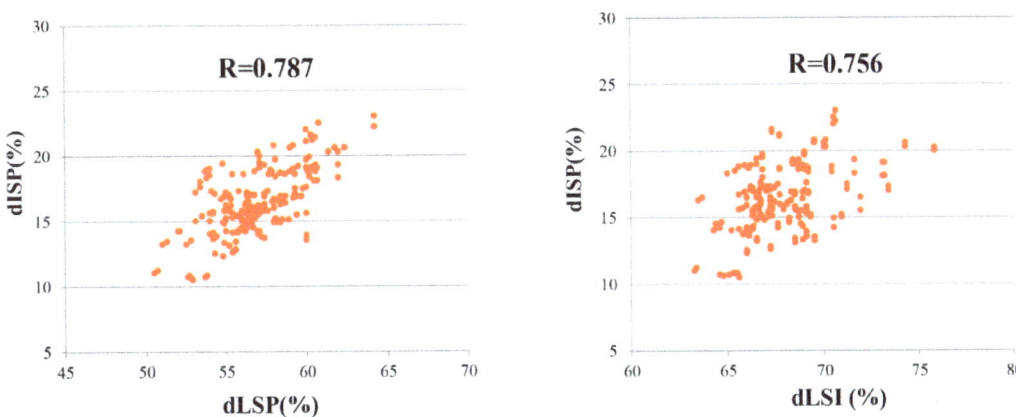

Figure 4. Correlation analysis between radiologic parameters. Yellow dot: inflection point of lateral tibial spine, red dot: peak point of lateral tibial spine, yellow arrow: dISP, shorter white arrow: dLSP, longer white arrow: dLSI.

4. Discussion

The principal finding of this study was that the lateral tibial spine could be a useful anatomical landmark for weight-bearing line assessment during HTO. The mean values of the peak and inflection points of the lateral tibial spine were located approximately −5% and +5% laterally from the conventional Fujisawa point, and it could be easily used for adjustment of the amount of correction. However, the values of the dLSP and dLSI varied among patients, and dISP correlated with dLSP and dLSI. Therefore, the hypothesis of this study was fully supported.

Previous studies on HTO that used the lateral tibial spine as a landmark for alignment correction reported results similar to those of the present study. Lee et al.'s study that compared HTOs aiming at either the peak of the lateral tibial spine or the Fujisawa point showed that the lateral spine peak point was located at 57.4 ± 1.6% from the medial border of the tibia [26]. Jiang et al.'s study also showed that the mean WBL percentage of the top of the tibial spine was 57.7 ± 2.1% [29]. However, the inflection point of the lateral tibial spine in our study was quite different from that of Jiang et al. (67.9 ± 2.2% vs. 74.6 ± 3.3%). In this study, the lateral end of the lateral tibial spine was defined as the inflection point where the tibial spine slope and tibial plateau intersect. On the other hand, in Jiang et al.'s study, the bottom point of the lateral slope was defined as the intersection point between the lateral slope of the lateral tibial spine and the joint line of the tibia. Since the lateral tibial slope and tibial plateau intersect in a round shape rather than an acute angle, the bottom point is located further to the lateral side than the inflection point. This discrepancy can be attributed to the different measurement methods of the intersection point between the tibial spine slope and the tibial plateau.

Quantitative analysis of the lateral tibial spine can be helpful in adjusting the amount of correction during HTO. Jakob et al. suggested that correction of the mechanical axis should differ based on the thickness of cartilage loss in the medial compartment (1/3 cartilage loss: WBL 55–57.5%, 2/3 cartilage loss: WBL 60–62.5%, full thickness cartilage loss: WBL 65–67.5%) [25]. Based on our results, the location of the peak, mid, and inflection points of the lateral tibial spine correspond well with Jakob et al.'s suggestion, depending on different arthroses of the medial compartment. Recent studies have also shown that HTO targeting the peak point of the lateral tibial spine showed clinical outcomes comparable to those of HTO targeting the conventional Fujisawa point [26]. Adjustment of the correction angle may also be necessary depending on the purpose of HTO. When anterior cruciate ligament (ACL) or posterior cruciate ligament (PCL) reconstruction fails in patients with varus deformity, neutral or slight varus alignment is usually targeted during HTO. Even during protective realignment surgery combined with cartilage regeneration procedures, the WBL target is a little more medial than the conventional Fujisawa point. In these cases, the peak point of the lateral tibial spine can be a more useful anatomical landmark than the conventional Fujisawa point.

Another remarkable finding of our study was that the dLSP and dLSI varied among patients. The discrepancy between maximum and minimum values in dLSP, and dLSI were more than 10%, respectively. Also, the upper 10% group showed significantly higher dLSP and dLSI than the middle 10% group; the lower 10% group also showed significantly lower dLSP and dLSI than the middle 10% group. These results can be explained by anatomical variation in the location and size of the lateral tibial spine. Anatomical studies that indicate variable tibial footprint sizes of the ACL among individuals may also indirectly support the variability in the inter-spine distance [27,28].

In the correlation analysis, dLSP and dLSI were significantly correlated with inter-spine distance in this study. Although the dLSP and dLSI were located −5%, and +5% laterally from the conventional Fujisawa point on average, anatomical variation can be an obstacle that reduces the accuracy and efficiency of dLSP or dLSI as an anatomical landmark for HTO. The inter-spine distance can be easily used to predict large or small dLSP or dLSI and to avoid over- or under-correction without direct measurement of each point. To the best of our knowledge, this is the first study to document anatomical variation in the lateral tibial spine and the radiologic predictor for anatomical variance in the lateral tibial spine.

This study had some limitations. First, this study investigated osteoarthritic knees in an Asian population, and the results may be different from those of a Western population. However, the location of the peak and inflection points in the lateral tibial spine was presented as a percentage of the entire tibial plateau width in this study, which may remove the effect of individual size differences in the tibial plateau and tibial spine. Further anatomical studies in different races are necessary to generalize the results of this study. Second, in contrast to the peak point method, the method used to define the intersection point between the lateral tibial spine and the tibial plateau can differ between examiners. The different values of the intersection point in the lateral tibial spine and tibial plateau between Jiang et al.'s study (bottom point) and this study (inflection point) may be related to different measurement methods, and more effort to reach a consensus is required. Third, in this study, the correlation between dLSP and dLSI and diverse radiologic parameters was not investigated. The femoral notch width, which is known to be related to the size of the ACL footprint, can also be a predictor for dLSP and dLSI. Thus, it is an interesting topic for future study. Fourth, this study was conducted using a standing knee AP image, which may be different from the actual situation in which HTO planning is performed in the long leg view. However, in our hospital, a patient's posture is identical between the standing knee AP view and the long leg view, and we believe that radiologic parameters related to the lateral tibial spine may not be different between the standing knee AP view and the long leg view.

5. Conclusions

On average, the dLSP and dLSI were located −5%, and +5% laterally from the conventional Fujisawa point, and they may be useful landmarks for correction amount adjustment during HTO. However, it should be noted that correction based on the lateral tibial spine can be affected by anatomical variations, especially in patients with small or large inter-spine distances.

Author Contributions: Conceptualization, methodology, writing-review and editing, supervision, funding acquisition: T.W.K., Data collection, data analysis, writing-original draft preparation, revision: J.S.W. All authors have read and agreed to the published version of the manuscript.

Funding: This research was funded by a grant No. HI22C1879 from the Korea Health Industry Development Institution.

Institutional Review Board Statement: This study was conducted in accordance with the Declaration of Helsinki, and approved by the Institutional Review Board of Seoul National University Boramae Medical Center (IRB No.20-2021-22).

Informed Consent Statement: Informed consent was waived due to the retrospective study design.

Data Availability Statement: The data presented in this study are available on request from the corresponding author. The data are not publicly available due to privacy.

Conflicts of Interest: The authors declare that they have no conflict of interest.

References

1. Brinkman, J.M.; Lobenhoffer, P.; Agneskirchner, J.D.; Staubli, A.E.; Wymenga, A.B.; van Heerwaarden, R.J. Osteotomies around the knee: Patient selection, stability of fixation and bone healing in high tibial osteotomies. *J. Bone Jt. Surg. Br.* **2008**, *90*, 1548–1557. [CrossRef] [PubMed]
2. Lee, D.C.; Byun, S.J. High tibial osteotomy. *Knee Surg. Relat. Res.* **2012**, *24*, 61–69. [CrossRef]
3. Yabuuchi, K.; Kondo, E.; Onodera, J.; Onodera, T.; Yagi, T.; Iwasaki, N.; Yasuda, K. Clinical Outcomes and Complications During and After Medial Open-Wedge High Tibial Osteotomy Using a Locking Plate: A 3- to 7-Year Follow-up Study. *Orthop. J. Sport. Med.* **2020**, *8*, 2325967120922535. [CrossRef] [PubMed]
4. Kanakamedala, A.C.; Hurley, E.T.; Manjunath, A.K.; Jazrawi, L.M.; Alaia, M.J.; Strauss, E.J. High Tibial Osteotomies for the Treatment of Osteoarthritis of the Knee. *JBJS Rev.* **2022**, *10*, e21. [CrossRef] [PubMed]
5. Na, B.R.; Yang, H.Y.; Seo, J.W.; Lee, C.H.; Seon, J.K. Effect of medial open wedge high tibial osteotomy on progression of patellofemoral osteoarthritis. *Knee Surg. Relat. Res.* **2022**, *34*, 42. [CrossRef] [PubMed]
6. Yoon, S.D.; Zhang, G.; Kim, H.J.; Lee, B.J.; Kyung, H.S. Comparison of Cable Method and Miniaci Method Using Picture Archiving and Communication System in Preoperative Planning for Open Wedge High Tibial Osteotomy. *Knee Surg. Relat. Res.* **2016**, *28*, 283–288. [CrossRef] [PubMed]
7. Kim, S.H.; Ro, D.H.; Lee, Y.M.; Cho, Y.; Lee, S.; Lee, M.C. Factors associated with discrepancies between preoperatively planned and postoperative alignments in patients undergoing closed-wedge high tibial osteotomy. *Knee* **2017**, *24*, 1129–1137. [CrossRef]
8. Kim, Y.T.; Choi, J.Y.; Lee, J.K.; Lee, Y.M.; Kim, J.I. Coronal tibiofemoral subluxation is a risk factor for postoperative overcorrection in high tibial osteotomy. *Knee* **2019**, *26*, 832–837. [CrossRef]
9. So, S.Y.; Lee, S.S.; Jung, E.Y.; Kim, J.H.; Wang, J.H. Difference in joint line convergence angle between the supine and standing positions is the most important predictive factor of coronal correction error after medial opening wedge high tibial osteotomy. *Knee Surg. Sports Traumatol. Arthrosc.* **2020**, *28*, 1516–1525. [CrossRef]
10. Na, Y.G.; Lee, B.K.; Choi, J.U.; Lee, B.H.; Sim, J.A. Change of joint-line convergence angle should be considered for accurate alignment correction in high tibial osteotomy. *Knee Surg. Relat. Res.* **2021**, *33*, 4. [CrossRef] [PubMed]
11. Ryu, D.J.; Lee, S.S.; Jung, E.Y.; Kim, J.H.; Shin, T.S.; Wang, J.H. Reliability of Preoperative Planning Method That Considers Latent Medial Joint Laxity in Medial Open-Wedge Proximal Tibial Osteotomy. *Orthop. J. Sports Med.* **2021**, *9*, 23259671211034151. [CrossRef] [PubMed]
12. Song, J.H.; Bin, S.I.; Kim, J.M.; Lee, B.S.; Choe, J.S.; Cho, H.K. Insufficient correction and preoperative medial tightness increases the risk of varus recurrence in open-wedge high tibial Osteotomy. *Arthroscopy* **2022**, *38*, 1547–1554. [CrossRef] [PubMed]
13. Ogawa, H.; Matsumoto, K.; Ogawa, T.; Takeuchi, K.; Akiyama, H. Preoperative varus laxity correlates with overcorrection in medial opening wedge high tibial osteotomy. *Arch. Orthop. Trauma. Surg.* **2016**, *136*, 1337–1342. [CrossRef] [PubMed]
14. Goshima, K.; Sawaguchi, T.; Shigemoto, K.; Iwai, S.; Fujita, K.; Yamamuro, Y. Comparison of Clinical and Radiologic Outcomes between Normal and Overcorrected Medial Proximal Tibial Angle Groups after Open-Wedge High Tibial Osteotomy. *Arthroscopy* **2019**, *35*, 2898–2908. [CrossRef] [PubMed]

15. Lee, S.S.; Kim, J.H.; Kim, S.; Jung, E.Y.; Ryu, D.J.; Lee, D.K.; Wang, J.H. Avoiding Overcorrection to Increase Patient Satisfaction after Open Wedge High Tibial Osteotomy. *Am. J. Sports Med.* **2022**, *50*, 2453–2461. [CrossRef]
16. Dugdale, T.W.; Noyes, F.R.; Styer, D. Preoperative planning for high tibial osteotomy. The effect of lateral tibiofemoral separation and tibiofemoral length. *Clin. Orthop. Relat. Res.* **1992**, *274*, 248–264. [CrossRef]
17. Schröter, S.; Ihle, C.; Mueller, J.; Lobenhoffer, P.; Stöckle, U.; van Heerwaarden, R. Digital planning of high tibial osteotomy. Interrater reliability by using two different software. *Knee Surg. Sports Traumatol. Arthrosc.* **2013**, *21*, 189–196. [CrossRef]
18. Elson, D.W.; Petheram, T.G.; Dawson, M.J. High reliability in digital planning of medial opening wedge high tibial osteotomy, using Miniaci's method. *Knee Surg. Sports Traumatol. Arthrosc.* **2015**, *23*, 2041–2048. [CrossRef]
19. Kim, H.J.; Park, J.; Shin, J.Y.; Park, I.H.; Park, K.H.; Kyung, H.S. More accurate correction can be obtained using a three-dimensional printed model in open-wedge high tibial osteotomy. *Knee Surg. Sports Traumatol. Arthrosc.* **2018**, *26*, 3452–3458. [CrossRef]
20. Bockmann, B.; Nebelung, W.; Boese, C.K.; Schulte, T.L.; Venjakob, A.J. Planning Results for High Tibial Osteotomies in Degenerative Varus Osteoarthritis Using Standing and Supine Whole Leg Radiographs. *Orthop. Surg.* **2021**, *13*, 77–82. [CrossRef]
21. Matsushita, T.; Watanabe, S.; Araki, D.; Nagai, K.; Hoshino, Y.; Kanzaki, N.; Matsumoto, T.; Niikura, T.; Kuroda, R. Differences in preoperative planning for high-tibial osteotomy between the standing and supine positions. *Knee Surg. Relat. Res.* **2021**, *33*, 8. [CrossRef] [PubMed]
22. Fujisawa, Y.; Masuhara, K.; Shiomi, S. The effect of high tibial osteotomy on osteoarthritis of the knee. An arthroscopic study of 54 knee joints. *Orthop. Clin. N. Am.* **1979**, *10*, 585–608. [CrossRef]
23. Yin, Y.; Li, S.; Zhang, R.; Guo, J.; Hou, Z.; Zhang, Y. What is the relationship between the "Fujisawa point" and postoperative knee valgus angle? A theoretical, computer-based study. *Knee* **2020**, *27*, 183–191. [CrossRef]
24. Kobayashi, H.; Saito, S.; Akamatsu, Y.; Kumagai, K.; Nejima, S.; Inaba, Y. The relationship between the "Fujisawa point" and anatomical femorotibial angle following simulated open wedge high tibial osteotomy. *BMC Musculoskelet. Disord.* **2022**, *23*, 776. [CrossRef] [PubMed]
25. Jakob, R.P.; Jacobi, M. Closing wedge osteotomy of the tibial head in treatment of single compartment arthrosis. *Orthopade* **2004**, *33*, 143–152. [CrossRef]
26. Lee, S.S.; Lee, H.I.; Cho, S.T.; Cho, J.H. Comparison of the outcomes between two different target points after open wedge high tibial osteotomy: The Fujisawa point versus the lateral tibial spine. *Knee* **2020**, *27*, 915–922. [CrossRef] [PubMed]
27. Zhang, L.; Li, C.; Zhang, J.; Zou, D.; Dimitriou, D.; Xing, X.; Tsai, T.Y.; Li, P. Significant race and gender differences in anterior cruciate ligament tibial footprint location: A 3D-based analysis. *J. Orthop. Traumatol.* **2023**, *24*, 33. [CrossRef]
28. Colombet, P.; Robinson, J.; Christel, P.; Franceschi, J.P.; Djian, P.; Bellier, G.; Sbihi, A. Morphology of anterior cruciate ligament attachments for anatomic reconstruction: A cadaveric dissection and radiographic study. *Arthroscopy* **2006**, *22*, 984–992. [CrossRef]
29. Jiang, X.; Li, B.; Xie, K.; Ai, S.; Hu, X.; Gao, L.; Wang, L.; Yan, M. Lateral tibial intercondylar eminence is a reliable reference for alignment correction in high tibial osteotomy. *Knee Surg. Sports Traumatol. Arthrosc.* **2023**, *31*, 1515–1523. [CrossRef]

Disclaimer/Publisher's Note: The statements, opinions and data contained in all publications are solely those of the individual author(s) and contributor(s) and not of MDPI and/or the editor(s). MDPI and/or the editor(s) disclaim responsibility for any injury to people or property resulting from any ideas, methods, instructions or products referred to in the content.

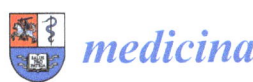

Article

Comparison of Anatomical Conformity between TomoFix Anatomical Plate and TomoFix Conventional Plate in Open-Wedge High Tibial Osteotomy

Sung-Sahn Lee [1], Jaesung Park [2] and Dae-Hee Lee [2],*

[1] Department of Orthopedic Surgery, Ilsan Paik Hospital, School of Medicine, Inje University, 170 Juwha Street, Goyangsi 10380, Korea; sungsahnlee@gmail.com
[2] Department of Orthopedic Surgery, Samsung Medical Center, School of Medicine, Sungkyunkwan University, 81 Irwon Street, Seoul 06351, Korea; jspark3168@gmail.com
* Correspondence: eoak22@empal.com; Tel.: +82-2-3410-3509

Abstract: *Background and Objectives*: The TomoFix anatomical plate was developed to improve plate position, proximal screw direction, and post-correction tibial contouring. The purpose of this study was to compare postoperative configurations between the TomoFix anatomical plate and the TomoFix conventional plate. It was hypothesized that the new modified plate provides a better fixative coaptation than the conventional plate. *Materials and Methods*: A total of 116 cases (112 patients) were enrolled in this study from March 2015 to February 2021. Among them, 63 patients underwent surgery using the TomoFix conventional plate, and 53 underwent surgery using the TomoFix anatomical plate. The radiographic outcomes, including the hip–knee–ankle (HKA) angle, medial proximal tibial angle (MPTA), tibial slope, plate angle, proximal screw angles, and plate-to-cortex distance at #1 hole (just below the osteotomy site) were compared between the two groups. *Results*: Patients with the TomoFix anatomical plate showed similar results in terms of the pre- and postoperative HKA angle, MPTA, and tibial slope. The TomoFix anatomical group showed a significantly greater plate angle ($39.2° \pm 8.1°$ vs. $31.7° \pm 7.0°$, $p < 0.001$) and less screw angles, indicating that the TomoFix anatomical plates allowed a more posterior plate position than the conventional plate. The plate-to-cortex distance was significantly less in the TomoFix anatomical group than in the TomoFix conventional group ($p < 0.001$). *Conclusion*: The TomoFix anatomical plate showed a more posteromedial plating position, better proximal screw direction to the lateral hinge, and improved post-correction tibial contour compared to the TomoFix conventional plate.

Keywords: high tibial osteotomy; TomoFix; plate position; anatomical conformity

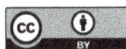

1. Introduction

High tibial osteotomy is a well-established surgical procedure for the management of medial unicompartmental arthritis of the knee joint [1–4]. A lateral closed-wedge high tibial osteotomy has potential disadvantages, including difficulty in intraoperatively controlling the amount of correction and concerns of neurologic deficits [5,6]. Due to these disadvantages, open-wedge high tibial osteotomy (OWHTO) is becoming popular [7].

The mechanical stability of the osteotomy site is a major issue following OWHTO. Correction loss and non-union of the osteotomy site have been observed after surgery [8–10]. However, with the introduction of the TomoFix plate (Synthes GmbH, Oberdorf, Switzerland), which is characterized by a T-shaped, long, rigid-angle stable implant, the incidence of non-union following OWHTO has declined significantly [8,9].

Plate position and proximal screw angles are important for fixation stability in OWHTO [11]. Posteromedial plating provides better fixation stability than anteromedial plating [11,12]. The proximal screw in the direction of the lateral hinge rather than the posterior tibial cortex is associated with increased stability and less neurovascular injury [12]. Anatomical contouring to the post-correction medial tibial geometry is also important for decreasing the distance between the plate and cortex [13,14]. The TomoFix anatomical plate was developed to improve plate position, proximal screw direction, and post-correction tibial contouring (Figure 1).

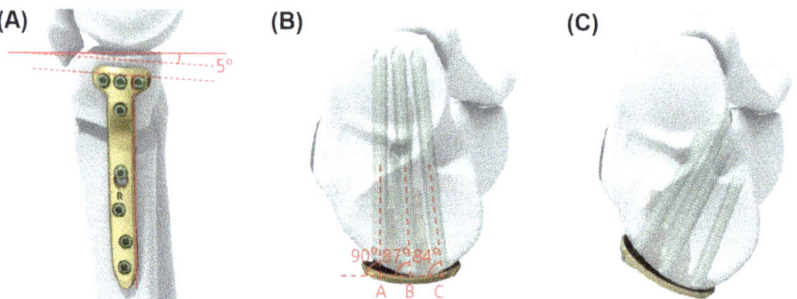

Figure 1. (**A**) Schematic diagram of the new plate lateral view. While the previous plate was a 90° T-shaped plate with no left and right distinction, the TomoFix anatomical plate has a 5° posterior slope, allowing the plate to be positioned relatively backward. As a result, the new plate system (**B**) enables parallel screw fixation than the previous plate (**C**).

Therefore, the purpose of the current study is to compare postoperative configurations between the new modified plate and the conventional plate (the TomoFix Anatomical plate versus the TomoFix conventional plate). It was hypothesized that the new modified plate would provide a better anatomical fitness than the conventional plate.

2. Materials and Methods

This study enrolled patients with primary medial osteoarthritis who underwent primary OWHTO between March 2015 and February 2021. The included subjects were patients aged <65 years who had osteoarthritis with persistent pain despite conservative management for more than three months. Patients were excluded if they had severe osteoarthritis of the patellofemoral joint or lateral compartment, ligament laxity, rheumatoid arthritis, or flexion contracture > 15°, and required an angle of correction > 20°. A total of 116 cases (112 patients) were enrolled in the current study. Among them, 63 patients underwent surgery using the conventional TomoFix plate and 53 using the TomoFix Anatomical plate. For patients who underwent surgery between March 2015 and July 2018, OWHTO was performed using the TomoFix conventional plate, after which surgery was performed using the TomoFix anatomical plate. Both plates were made of titanium. The patient demographics and preoperative data are summarized in Table 1. This study was approved by the Ethics Committee of our institution (SMC2021-05-051 at 26 May 2021), and written informed consent was obtained from all patients.

Table 1. Demographic and preoperative data.

Number of Cases, n	116
Sex, M:F	35:81
Age, year	56.9 ± 7.0 (43–77)
BMI, kg/m^2	27.5 ± 3.4 (20.4–38.0)
Direction, R:L	50:66
Preoperative HKA angle, °	8.6 ± 3.0 (5–20.1)
Preoperative MPTA, °	84.6 ± 2.0 (79.5–89.3)
Preoperative tibial slope, °	10.1 ± 3.7 (1.7–20.7)

BMI, body mass index; HKA, hip-knee-ankle; MPTA, medial proximal tibial angle.

2.1. Surgical Technique

All surgeries were performed by the senior author. The correction angle was measured using Miniaci's method [15,16]. The alignment of the lower limb was adjusted by passing the point located at 62.5% of the tibial plateau width when measured from the edge of the proximal tibial medial plateau [17]. Biplanar osteotomy was performed in all knees. After skin incision, a guide wire was inserted with visual assistance by an image intensifier. The oblique part of the osteotomy was performed with a saw for a distance of up to 1 cm from the lateral cortex. The osteotomy of the vertical part was performed at the posterior aspect of the tibial tubercle, thus not violating the bony portion to which the patellar tendon was attached, leaving most of the tendon attached to the distal tibial fragment. The anterior gap of the osteotomy sited behind the tibial tuberosity was intended to be approximately 1/2 to 2/3 of the posterior opening gap at the posteromedial corner of the proximal tibia to maintain tibial slope. Target alignment was achieved under intraoperative fluoroscopy, and the osteotomy was stabilized using the TomoFix conventional plate or the TomoFix anatomical plate. A cortical screw was used on the most proximal hole of the distal holes (the so-called #1 hole), if the bone-to-plate distance was more than 5 mm, to avoid fixative failure [18]. An allogenic bone graft (Junyoung Medical, Seoul, South Korea) was inserted into the osteotomy gap to minimize postoperative loss of correction.

The patients were started on isometric quadriceps, active ankle, and straight leg-raising exercises on the day after surgery. Knee motion exercises were initiated on the second postoperative day. Patients were restricted toe toe-touch weight bearing for the first 2 postoperative weeks, followed by partial weight bearing for next 4–6 weeks. Full weight-bearing was permitted by 6–8 weeks.

2.2. Radiographic Evaluation

Plain radiographs were obtained before surgery and three months postoperatively. The radiographs included whole leg standing radiographs (patella facing forward and full knee extension) and lateral views with 30° flexion. The change in limb alignment from before to after surgery was determined by measuring the hip–knee–ankle (HKA) angle on full-length standing radiographs, using a picture archiving and communication system (Centricity; General Electric, Chicago, IL, USA) [19,20]. The HKA angle was measured by the angle subtended by a line drawn from the center of the femoral head to the center of the knee and a line drawn from the center of the knee to the center of the talus. The medial proximal tibial angle (MPTA) was measured as the angle between the proximal anatomical axis of the tibia and the tangent along the articular surface of the tibial plateau on full-length standing radiographs [21]. The angle of the tibial slope was defined using the proximal tibial anatomical axis method [19]. The MPTA and tibial slope were also compared before and after surgery and between both plate systems.

Computed tomography (CT) scans (MDCT; Brilliance 64, Phillips, Cleveland, OH, USA) were performed on the fifth postoperative day. The proximal plate position was evaluated by the proximal plate angle on the axial CT images [14]. The proximal plate angle was defined as the angle between the posterior cortex line and the line connecting the front and back of the plate proximal area (Figure 2A). The most proximal screw (A screw, B screw, and C screw, each from front to back, respectively, Figure 2B) angles were also measured on axial CT images. Each screw angle was defined as the angle between the posterior cortex and the line drawn along the screw. The plate-to-cortex (just below the osteotomy site) distance at #1 hole was measured, and the usage of cortical screw on #1 hole was counted to evaluate the post-correction tibial contouring of the plate (Figure 3).

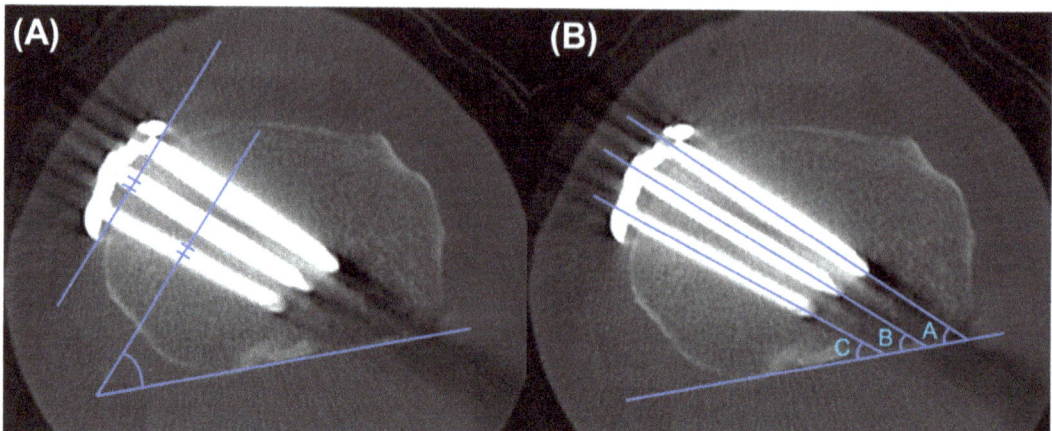

Figure 2. Measurement of the plate angle and screw angles on the CT axial scan. (**A**) The plate angle was defined as the angle between the anteroposterior line connecting the proximal part of the plate and the posterior tibial condylar line. (**B**) The A, B, and C screw angle was defined as the angle between the line drawn along the screw and the posterior tibial condylar line. (A, B, and C screws from anterior to posterior, respectively).

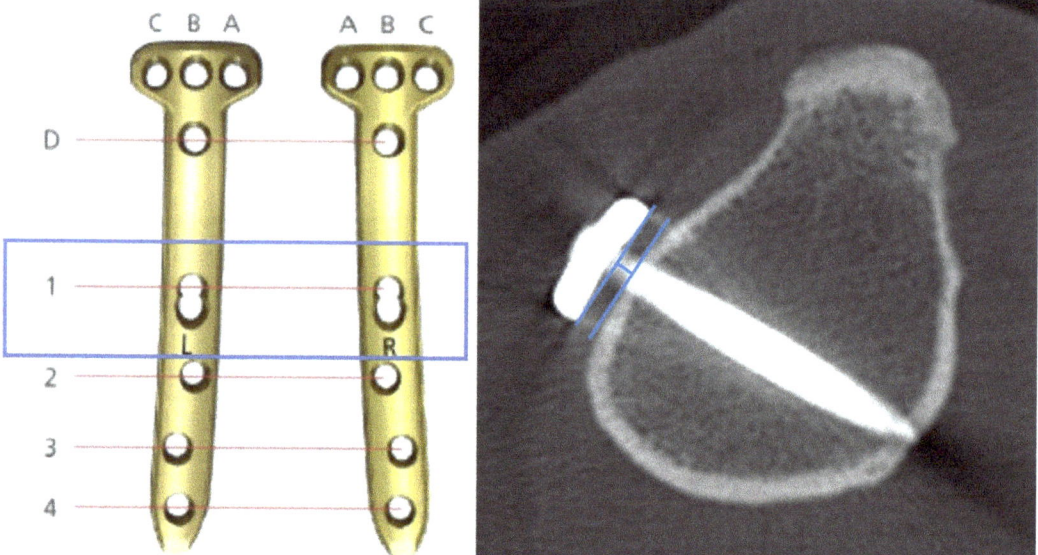

Figure 3. Measurement of the plate-to-cortex distance at #1 hole. It was defined as the distance between the inner surface of the plate and the outer surface of the tibial cortex at #1 hole.

All measurements were performed by two orthopedic surgeons with significant experience in OWHTO, but who were not associated with the subject of this study to assess interobserver reliability, and were repeated six weeks later to assess intra-observer reliability.

2.3. Statistical Analysis

The *Shapiro–Wilk* test was used to investigate the normality of distribution. The *Student's t*-test was used for continuous variables, whereas the *chi-squared* test was used for categorical variables to compare the demographic data and radiographic data. Statistical significance was set at $p < 0.05$. All data were analyzed using SPSS software (version 22, IBM Corp, Armonk, NY, USA). To have a 90% probability of detecting a 1 mm difference in the plate-to-cortex distance, we needed to enroll 72 patients, assuming an overall standard deviation in 2 mm and a 2-tailed alpha-level of 5%.

3. Results

All inter- and intra-observer intraclass correlation coefficients showed good agreement for all radiographic measurement reliabilities (>0.80).

Compared to the TomoFix conventional group, the TomoFix anatomical group showed similar results in terms of sex distribution, mean age, body mass index, and preoperative and postoperative simple radiographic measurements (Table 2).

Table 2. Comparison of the demographic and simple radiographic data between the TomoFix conventional plate and the TomoFix anatomical plate groups.

	TomoFix Conventional	TomoFix Anatomical	p-Value
Number of cases, n	63	53	
Sex, M:F	17:46	18:35	0.415
Age, year	56.0 ± 7.4	57.8 ± 6.5	0.171
BMI, kg/m^2	27.4 ± 3.3	27.7 ± 3.5	0.681
Direction, R:L	28:35	22:31	0.851
Preoperative HKA angle, °	8.3 ± 2.7	9.0 ± 3.3	0.156
Preoperative MPTA, °	84.8 ± 2.2	84.3 ± 1.9	0.26
Preoperative tibial slope, °	10.4 ± 3.7	9.7 ± 3.6	0.308
Opening width, mm	10.6 ± 2.6	11.2 ± 1.7	0.169
Postoperative HKA angle, °	−3.1 ± 2.5	−2.5 ± 2.3	0.135
Postoperative MPTA, °	92.8 ± 2.5	92.5 ± 2.5	0.469
Postoperative tibial slope, °	11.8 ± 4.2	11.4 ± 3.8	0.549

BMI, body mass index; HKA, hip–knee–ankle; MPTA, medial proximal tibial angle.

With respect to CT scan measurements, the TomoFix anatomical group showed a greater plate angle than the TomoFix conventional group (39.2° ± 8.1° vs. 31.7° ± 7.0°, $p < 0.001$, Table 3). This result indicates that the TomoFix anatomical plates allowed a more posterior plate position than the conventional plate. Moreover, all screw angles were significantly lower in the TomoFix anatomical group. These results were also caused by positioning the plate more posteriorly than in the TomoFix conventional group.

Table 3. Comparison of the fixative device position on CT scan between the two groups.

	TomoFix Conventional	TomoFix Anatomical	p-Value
Plate angle, °	31.7 ± 7.0	39.2 ± 8.1	0.001
A screw angle, °	61.4 ± 6.6	51.8 ± 7.4	<0.001
B screw angle, °	57.8 ± 7.3	49.6 ± 7.7	<0.001
C screw angle, °	54.2 ± 7.4	46.6 ± 7.4	<0.001
Using cortical screw on #1 hole	16 cases (25.4%)	8 cases (15.1%)	0.128
Plate-to-cortex distance (all cases), mm	3.2 ± 1.7	1.7 ± 1.3	<0.001
Plate-to-cortex distance (only using locking screw), mm	3.9 ± 1.1	1.9 ± 1.2	<0.001

In the TomoFix conventional group, a cortical screw on #1 hole (the most proximal hole of distal 4 holes) was used in 16 cases (25.4%). However, cortical screws were used in eight cases (15.1%) in the TomoFix anatomical group. The anatomical plate group used fewer cortical screws on #1 hole, but the difference was not statistically significant ($p = 0.18$). The plate-to-cortex distance was significantly shorter in the TomoFix anatomical group than in the TomoFix conventional group regardless of the use of a cortical screw on the #1 hole. ($p < 0.001$).

4. Discussion

The principal finding of the current study was that the TomoFix anatomical plate represented a more posteromedial plating position, proximal screw toward the lateral hinge rather than posterior cortex, and improved post-correction tibial contour compared to the TomoFix conventional plate.

Numerous studies have demonstrated that posteromedial plating provides better fixative stability than anteromedial plating in OWHTO [11,12,22]. Takeuchi et al. [11]. compared the stress on the TomoFix plate between the anteromedial and medial plating positions. They reported that the medial plate position provided significantly less stress on the plate than the anteromedial plate position. Moreover, previous studies reported that the anterior plate position was associated with an increased posterior tibial slope, which might lead to anterior cruciate ligament damage after OWHTO [23,24]. The TomoFix conventional plate was a 90° T-shaped plate with no left and right distinction, while the TomoFix anatomical plate had a 5° posterior slope, allowing the plate to be positioned relatively backward. In the current study, the patients using the TomoFix anatomical plate showed a significantly posterior position compared to those using the conventional plate among single-surgeon cases. These results are consistent with the intent of the TomoFix anatomical plate design.

It is well known that an increased plate–bone distance might reduce the fixative stability when using a locking compression plate and screws. Ahmad et al. [18]. demonstrated that, 5 mm from the bone, the locking plate exhibited increased plastic deformation during cyclical compression and required lower loads to induce mechanical failure when compared to a lesser distance between the bone and plate. Therefore, post-correction anatomical contouring is important for reducing the plate–bone distance in OWHTO. The plate-fitting technique using cortical lag screws was widely performed [25]. However, it might induce a change in the opening gap or lateral hinge fracture [26]. In the current study, in the patients with the TomoFix anatomical plate, fewer cortical screws were used on #1 hole (15.1% vs. 25.4%, $p = 0.128$). Moreover, the plate-to-cortex distances were significantly shorter in the TomoFix anatomical group regardless of the use of a cortical screw. These results demonstrated that the TomoFix anatomical plate showed better anatomical contouring to the post-correction tibia.

OWHTO is a promising surgery for medial compartmental knee joint osteoarthritis. However, adverse events were reported following OWHTO in 37% to 55% of cases [25,27,28]. Sidhu et al. [29] demonstrated that a low rate of serious complications (6.5%) requiring unplanned additional surgery was noted after OWHTO using a TomoFix locking plate. However, 52% of the knees required elective hardware removal due to soft tissue irritation. The TomoFix anatomical plate is expected to have a lower hardware removal rate as it has a more posterior position and is more suitable for the post-correction anatomical structure of the tibia.

This study has some limitations. First, although the TomoFix anatomical plate provided a better configuration than the previous version plate system, the superiority of the actual mechanical stability was not proven. An investigation including a mechanical test is needed to identify the association between fixative configuration and mechanical stability in the future. Second, the current study did not include clinical outcomes, including patient-reported outcome measurements, union rate, union period, and correction loss rate. Therefore, this study was not able to identify the effects of plate design changes on clinical outcomes. Third, the two groups had OWHTO performed at different times (TomoFix conventional plate was used between March 2015 and July 2018, TomoFix anatomical plate was used between August 2018 to February 2021), which may have affected the outcome. However, this study was based on data from a single surgeon, which would have had little effect on the results.

5. Conclusions

The TomoFix anatomical plate showed a more posteromedial plating position, proximal screw direction toward the lateral hinge rather than posterior cortex, and improved post-correction tibial contour compared to the TomoFix conventional plate.

Author Contributions: Conceptualization, S.-S.L. and D.-H.L.; methodology, S.-S.L. and D.-H.L.; validation, S.-S.L. and J.P.; formal analysis, S.-S.L. and J.P.; investigation, J.P.; data curation, S.-S.L. and J.P.; writing—original draft preparation, S.-S.L. and D.-H.L.; writing—review and editing, S.-S.L. and D.-H.L.; visualization, S.-S.L. and J.P.; supervision, D.-H.L.; project administration, D.-H.L. All authors have read and agreed to the published version of the manuscript.

Funding: This research received no external funding.

Institutional Review Board Statement: The protocol used to evaluate radiographic findings and intraoperative navigation data was approved by our institution's investigational review board. (SMC2021-05-051 at May 26 2021).

Informed Consent Statement: Informed consent was obtained from all individual participants included in the study.

Data Availability Statement: Not applicable.

Conflicts of Interest: The authors declare that they have no conflict of interest.

References

1. Amendola, A.; Bonasia, D.E. Results of high tibial osteotomy: Review of the literature. *Int. Orthop.* **2010**, *34*, 155–160. [CrossRef]
2. Na, Y.G.; Lee, B.K.; Choi, J.U.; Lee, B.H.; Sim, J.A. Change of joint-line convergence angle should be considered for accurate alignment correction in high tibial osteotomy. *Knee Surg. Relat. Res.* **2021**, *33*, 4. [CrossRef]
3. Lorbergs, A.L.; Birmingham, T.B.; Primeau, C.A.; Atkinson, H.F.; Marriott, K.A.; Giffin, J.R. Improved Methods to Measure Outcomes After High Tibial Osteotomy. *Clin. Sports Med.* **2019**, *38*, 317–329. [CrossRef] [PubMed]
4. Song, I.S.; Kwon, J. Analysis of changes in tibial torsion angle on open-wedge high tibial osteotomy depending on the osteotomy level. *Knee Surg. Relat. Res.* **2022**, *34*, 17. [CrossRef] [PubMed]
5. Coventry, M.B. Upper tibial osteotomy. *Clin. Orthop. Relat. Res.* **1984**, *182*, 46–52. [CrossRef]
6. Staubli, A.E.; De Simoni, C.; Babst, R.; Lobenhoffer, P. TomoFix: A new LCP-concept for open wedge osteotomy of the medial proximal tibia—Early results in 92 cases. *Injury* **2003**, *34* (Suppl. S2), B55–B62. [CrossRef]
7. Kim, H.J.; Shin, J.Y.; Lee, H.J.; Park, K.H.; Jung, C.H.; Kyung, H.S. Can medial stability be preserved after open wedge high tibial osteotomy? *Knee Surg. Relat. Res.* **2020**, *32*, 51. [CrossRef]
8. Kyung, H.S.; Lee, B.J.; Kim, J.W.; Yoon, S.D. Biplanar Open Wedge High Tibial Osteotomy in the Medial Compartment Osteoarthritis of the Knee Joint: Comparison between the Aescula and TomoFix Plate. *Clin. Orthop. Surg.* **2015**, *7*, 185–190. [CrossRef]
9. Staubli, A.E.; Jacob, H.A. Evolution of open-wedge high-tibial osteotomy: Experience with a special angular stable device for internal fixation without interposition material. *Int. Orthop.* **2010**, *34*, 167–172. [CrossRef]
10. Kang, B.Y.; Lee, D.K.; Kim, H.S.; Wang, J.H. How to achieve an optimal alignment in medial opening wedge high tibial osteotomy? *Knee Surg. Relat. Res.* **2022**, *34*, 3. [CrossRef]
11. Takeuchi, R.; Woon-Hwa, J.; Ishikawa, H.; Yamaguchi, Y.; Osawa, K.; Akamatsu, Y.; Kuroda, K. Primary stability of different plate positions and the role of bone substitute in open wedge high tibial osteotomy. *Knee* **2017**, *24*, 1299–1306. [CrossRef]
12. Wang, J.H.; Bae, J.H.; Lim, H.C.; Shon, W.Y.; Kim, C.W.; Cho, J.W. Medial open wedge high tibial osteotomy: The effect of the cortical hinge on posterior tibial slope. *Am. J. Sports Med.* **2009**, *37*, 2411–2418. [CrossRef]
13. Yoo, O.S.; Lee, Y.S.; Lee, M.C.; Elazab, A.; Choi, D.G.; Jang, Y.W. Evaluation of the screw position and angle using a post-contoured plate in the open wedge high tibial osteotomy according to the correction degree and surgical technique. *Clin. Biomech.* **2016**, *35*, 111–115. [CrossRef]
14. Lee, E.S.; Kim, T.W.; Jo, I.H.; Lee, Y.S. Comparative analysis of fixation configurations and their effect on outcome after medial open-wedge high tibial osteotomy. *J. Orthop. Sci.* **2020**, *25*, 627–634. [CrossRef] [PubMed]
15. Moore, J.; Mychaltchouk, L.; Lavoie, F. Applicability of a modified angular correction measurement method for open-wedge high tibial osteotomy. *Knee Surg. Sports Traumatol. Arthrosc.* **2017**, *25*, 846–852. [CrossRef]
16. Matsushita, T.; Watanabe, S.; Araki, D.; Nagai, K.; Hoshino, Y.; Kanzaki, N.; Matsumoto, T.; Niikura, T.; Kuroda, R. Differences in preoperative planning for high-tibial osteotomy between the standing and supine positions. *Knee Surg. Relat. Res.* **2021**, *33*, 8. [CrossRef]
17. Sabzevari, S.; Ebrahimpour, A.; Roudi, M.K.; Kachooei, A.R. High Tibial Osteotomy: A Systematic Review and Current Concept. *Arch. Bone Jt. Surg.* **2016**, *4*, 204–212.

18. Ahmad, M.; Nanda, R.; Bajwa, A.S.; Candal-Couto, J.; Green, S.; Hui, A.C. Biomechanical testing of the locking compression plate: When does the distance between bone and implant significantly reduce construct stability? *Injury* **2007**, *38*, 358–364. [CrossRef]
19. Lee, S.S.; Nha, K.W.; Lee, D.H. Posterior cortical breakage leads to posterior tibial slope change in lateral hinge fracture following opening wedge high tibial osteotomy. *Knee Surg. Sports Traumatol. Arthrosc.* **2019**, *27*, 698–706. [CrossRef]
20. Batra, S.; Malhotra, R. Medial Ball and Socket Total Knee Arthroplasty in Indian Population: 5-Year Clinical Results. *Clin. Orthop. Surg.* **2022**, *14*, 90–95. [CrossRef]
21. Kubota, M.; Ohno, R.; Sato, T.; Yamaguchi, J.; Kaneko, H.; Kaneko, K.; Ishijima, M. The medial proximal tibial angle accurately corrects the limb alignment in open-wedge high tibial osteotomy. *Knee Surg. Sports Traumatol. Arthrosc.* **2019**, *27*, 2410–2416. [CrossRef]
22. Martinez de Albornoz, P.; Leyes, M.; Forriol, F.; Del Buono, A.; Maffulli, N. Opening wedge high tibial osteotomy: Plate position and biomechanics of the medial tibial plateau. *Knee Surg. Sports Traumatol. Arthrosc.* **2014**, *22*, 2641–2647. [CrossRef]
23. Noyes, F.R.; Mayfield, W.; Barber-Westin, S.D.; Albright, J.C.; Heckmann, T.P. Opening wedge high tibial osteotomy: An operative technique and rehabilitation program to decrease complications and promote early union and function. *Am. J. Sports Med.* **2006**, *34*, 1262–1273. [CrossRef] [PubMed]
24. Black, M.S.; d'Entremont, A.G.; McCormack, R.G.; Hansen, G.; Carr, D.; Wilson, D.R. The effect of wedge and tibial slope angles on knee contact pressure and kinematics following medial opening-wedge high tibial osteotomy. *Clin. Biomech.* **2018**, *51*, 17–25. [CrossRef] [PubMed]
25. Valkering, K.P.; van den Bekerom, M.P.; Kappelhoff, F.M.; Albers, G.H. Complications after tomofix medial opening wedge high tibial osteotomy. *J. Knee Surg.* **2009**, *22*, 218–225. [CrossRef]
26. Weng, P.W.; Chen, C.H.; Luo, C.A.; Sun, J.S.; Tsuang, Y.H.; Cheng, C.K.; Lin, S.C. The effects of tibia profile, distraction angle, and knee load on wedge instability and hinge fracture: A finite element study. *Med. Eng. Phys.* **2017**, *42*, 48–54. [CrossRef]
27. Miller, B.S.; Dorsey, W.O.; Bryant, C.R.; Austin, J.C. The effect of lateral cortex disruption and repair on the stability of the medial opening wedge high tibial osteotomy. *Am. J. Sports Med.* **2005**, *33*, 1552–1557. [CrossRef]
28. Nelissen, E.M.; van Langelaan, E.J.; Nelissen, R.G. Stability of medial opening wedge high tibial osteotomy: A failure analysis. *Int. Orthop.* **2010**, *34*, 217–223. [CrossRef]
29. Sidhu, R.; Moatshe, G.; Firth, A.; Litchfield, R.; Getgood, A. Low rates of serious complications but high rates of hardware removal after high tibial osteotomy with Tomofix locking plate. *Knee Surg. Sports Traumatol. Arthrosc.* **2020**, *29*, 3361–3367. [CrossRef] [PubMed]

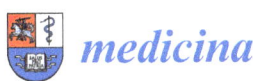

Article

Central Sensitization Is Associated with Inferior Patient-Reported Outcomes and Increased Osteotomy Site Pain in Patients Undergoing Medial Opening-Wedge High Tibial Osteotomy

Jae-Jung Kim [1], In-Jun Koh [2], Man-Soo Kim [1], Keun-Young Choi [2], Ki-Ho Kang [1] and Yong In [1,*]

[1] Department of Orthopaedic Surgery, Seoul St. Mary's Hospital, College of Medicine, The Catholic University of Korea, 222, Banpo-daero, Seocho-gu, Seoul 06591, Republic of Korea
[2] Department of Orthopaedic Surgery, EunPyeong St. Mary's Hospital, College of Medicine, The Catholic University of Korea, 1021, Tongil Ro, Eunpyeong-gu, Seoul 03312, Republic of Korea
* Correspondence: iy1000@catholic.ac.kr

Abstract: *Background and Objectives*: Studies have shown that centrally sensitized patients have worse clinical outcomes following total knee arthroplasty (TKA) than non-centrally sensitized patients. It is unclear whether central sensitization (CS) affects patient-reported outcomes (PROs) and/or level of osteotomy site pain in patients undergoing medial opening-wedge high tibial osteotomy (MOWHTO). The purpose of this study was to determine whether CS is associated with PROs and osteotomy site pain following MOWHTO. *Materials and Methods*: A retrospective evaluation was conducted on 140 patients with varus knee osteoarthritis (OA) who were treated with MOWHTO and monitored for two years. Before surgery, the Central Sensitization Inventory (CSI) was used to assess CS status, and a CSI of 40 or higher was considered indicative of CS. The Western Ontario and McMaster Universities Osteoarthritis Index (WOMAC) and pain visual analogue scale (VAS) were used to assess PROs. The minimal clinically important difference (MCID) for the WOMAC was set as 4.2 for the pain subscore, 1.9 for the stiffness subscore, 10.1 for the function subscore, and 16.1 for the total based on the results of a previous study. The WOMAC score, pain VAS score of the osteotomy site, and the achievement rates of WOMAC MCID were compared between the CS and non-CS groups. *Results*: Thirty-seven patients were assigned to the CS group, whereas 84 were assigned to the non-CS group. Before surgery, the CS group showed a higher WOMAC score than the non-CS group (58.7 vs. 49.4, $p < 0.05$). While there was a statistically significant improvement in WOMAC subscores (pain, stiffness, function, and total) for both groups at two years after surgery (all $p < 0.05$), the CS group had a higher WOMAC score than the non-CS group (37.1 vs. 21.8, $p < 0.05$). The CS group showed significantly inferior results in pre- and postoperative changes of WOMAC subscores (pain, function, and total) relative to the non-CS group (all $p < 0.05$). In addition, pain at the osteotomy site was more severe in the CS group than in the non-CS group at two years after surgery (4.8 vs. 2.2, $p < 0.05$). Patients with CS had worse MCID achievement rates across the board for WOMAC pain, function, and total scores (all $p < 0.05$) compared to the non-CS group. *Conclusions*: Centrally sensitized patients following MOWHTO had worse PROs and more severe osteotomy site pain compared to non-centrally sensitized patients. Furthermore, the WOMAC MCID achievement rate of patients with CS was lower than that of patients without CS. Therefore, appropriate preoperative counseling and perioperative pain management are necessary for patients with CS undergoing MOWHTO. *Level of Evidence*: Level III, case-control study.

Keywords: medial opening-wedge high tibial osteotomy; central sensitization; patient-reported outcomes; osteotomy site pain; minimal clinically important difference

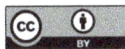

1. Introduction

Medial compartment osteoarthritis (OA) with varus deformity [1,2] is the most common indication for medial opening-wedge high tibial osteotomy (MOWHTO). Chondral lesions in the medial compartment [3], osteonecrosis of the medial femoral condyle [4], and varus thrust instability [3] are all reasons to consider MOWHTO if they are accompanied by varus deformity. By moving the mechanical axis to the lateral compartment, it is possible to reduce load on the medial compartment and postpone the progression of knee OA [5,6].

While total knee arthroplasty (TKA) is effective in eliminating pain by cutting off the source at the joint periphery, about 20–40% of patients are dissatisfied with the results and complain of persistent pain [7]. Due to these results, research into the mechanisms of central pain has increased [8]. Studies have shown that centrally sensitized patients had worse clinical outcomes and pain following TKA than non-centrally sensitized patients [9–11]. Central sensitization (CS) is considered an etiology of persistent pain and dissatisfaction following TKA [9–12]. Hyperalgesia and allodynia are hallmarks of CS, which is caused by dysfunction in the central nervous system [10,11]. However, there is a lack of studies on patient-reported outcomes (PROs) in CS patients following MOWHTO. In addition, unlike TKA, in which the painful lesion is surgically removed, MOWHTO is performed on the bone around the lesion. Currently, no studies have examined the PROs and degree of osteotomy site pain after MOWHTO according to the presence or absence of CS.

PROs have gained traction in recent years, and patient-reported outcome measures (PROMs) are widely used to assess the success of orthopedic procedures [13]. One of the most common and reliable PROMs used following knee surgery is the Western Ontario and McMaster Universities Arthritis Index (WOMAC) [14,15]. The pain visual analogue scale (VAS) score is also extensively used for evaluating outcomes following orthopedic surgery [16]. Understanding the minimal clinically important difference (MCID) and factors that may be used to forecast whether the MCID will be exceeded might have a major bearing on the definition of surgical outcomes and on the development of patient-centered decision-making aids [17,18]. Due to its emphasis on clinical relevance over statistical significance, it is recommended to use the MCID in PROMs [18,19].

It is currently unclear whether CS affects PROs and/or osteotomy site pain in patients undergoing MOWHTO. Therefore, the purpose of this study was to determine whether CS is associated with PROs and osteotomy site pain following MOWHTO. We predicted that centrally sensitized patients would have worse PROs and increased osteotomy site pain than those who were not centrally sensitized.

2. Materials and Methods

As part of a retrospective record review research, we included 140 patients who received MOWHTO between May 2015 and April 2019 at a single hospital. The criteria for inclusion were age < 70 years and isolated medial compartment OA with varus deformity. Patients with lateral compartment and patellofemoral OA, osteonecrosis, inflammatory or traumatic OA, missing data, and/or loss to follow-up within two years were excluded from the study to reduce the potential impact of preoperative variables on MOWHTO outcomes. The final study contained 121 patients, after excluding 19 for various reasons (Figure 1). Informed consent was acquired from all patients, and the study was approved by the Institutional Review Board of Seoul St. Mary's Hospital (KC22RASI0419 and 15 June 2022).

Surgical procedure

A tourniquet was placed in the proximal femur and maintained during surgery with a pressure of 300 mmHg. Arthroscopy was performed prior to osteotomy in all cases. If the meniscus tear was present including medial meniscal root tear, partial meniscectomy was performed. Multiple drilling was also performed for cartilage defects. A 7 cm long skin incision was made in the middle between the tibial tuberosity and the posteromedial border of the tibia, beginning 1 cm below the knee joint. Same skin incision was used in all patients. The Dugdale method [20] was used to determine the correction angle, and the Fujisawa point [21] was chosen as the surgical target. The Dugdale method requires the use of two lines to calculate the correction angle. Two lines are drawn: one from the center of the femoral head to 62.5% of the tibial width and the other from the center of the tibiotalar joint to the same percentage of the tibial width. The angle between these two lines is known as the correction angle [22]. Biplanar osteotomy was used in the surgical operation. A locking plating system (TomoFix®, DePuy Synthes, Oberdorf, Switzerland) was used to secure the osteotomy site. No bone grafts or artificial materials were used to fill the opening gap space.

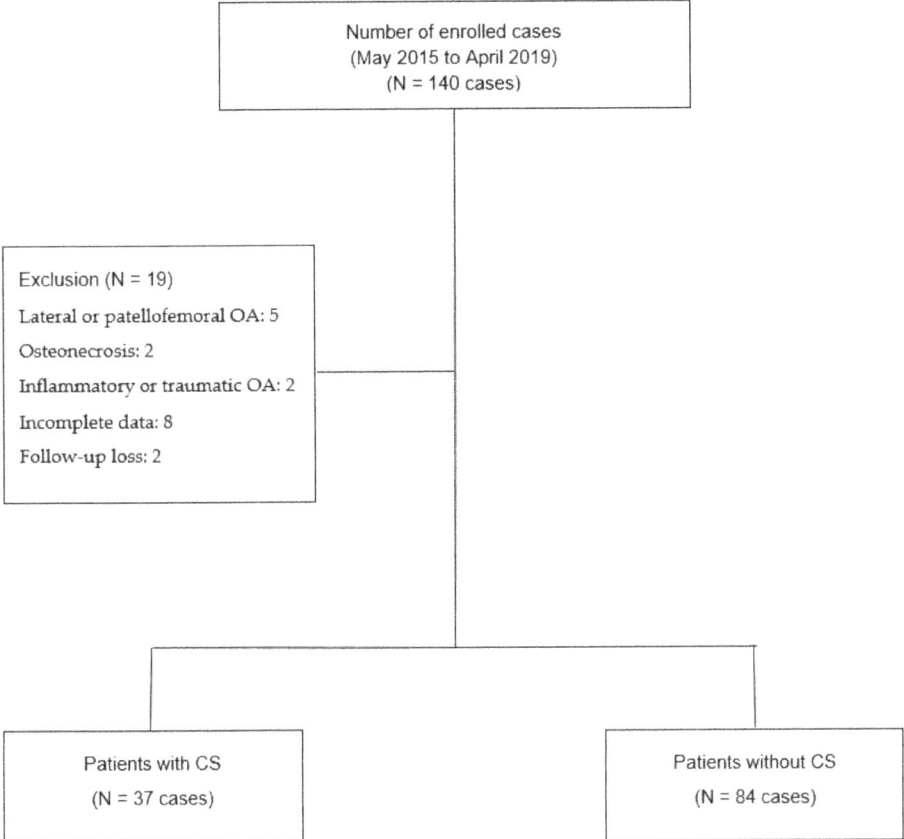

Figure 1. Patient flowchart.

Postoperative rehabilitation

Following surgical procedures, all patients participated in the same rehabilitation regimen. To improve knee flexion range, exercise on a continuous passive motion machine was started on postoperative day one at 60 degrees and progressed by 5 degrees daily up to 130 degrees of flexion. Within four weeks, patients were allowed to walk with crutches, and after six weeks, they were permitted full weight bearing.

Clinical assessment and Radiographic evaluation

The Central Sensitization Inventory (CSI) was used to assess the status of CS, and patients were given the questionnaire the day before the surgery [23]. The CSI is a valid and reliable self-report assessment of central sensitivity [23,24]. The purpose of this 25-item survey is to evaluate both emotional state and pain perception in the course of daily living. Each survey uses a Likert scale ranging from 0 to 4 to collect data. Based on the findings of prior research, a CSI of 40 or higher is considered indicative of CS, and a CSI score less than 40 indicates non-CS [24]. In this study, 37 patients were assigned to the CS group, whereas 84 were assigned to the non-CS group (Figure 1).

Preoperatively and at two years postoperatively, the WOMAC scores were used to assess knee PROs [25]. The 24-item disease-specific questionnaire (WOMAC) is a popular tool for assessing patient progress following knee surgery. It is comprised of three subscores evaluating pain (five items), stiffness (two items), and function (17 items). Each of the items has five possible responses, with scores ranging from 0 to 4. Scores range from 0 to 96, with 20 points assigned to pain, 8 points to stiffness, and 68 points to function. A lower score indicates a more favorable clinical result. In addition, pain VAS scores were used to assess pain at the osteotomy site at two years after surgery. The MCID for the WOMAC was set as 4.2 for the pain subscore, 1.9 for the stiffness subscore, 10.1 for the function subscore, and 16.1 for the total score based on the results of a previous study [26] that refers to the smallest improvement that a patient might perceive as beneficial. The achievement rates of WOMAC MCID were also measured. Between the CS and non-CS groups, the WOMAC scores, pain VAS scores of the osteotomy site, and the achievement rates of WOMAC MCID were compared.

Age, sex, operation side, body mass index (BMI), American Society of Anesthesiologists (ASA) score, comorbidities (diabetes and hypertension), alcohol intake, smoking, and preoperative OA severity were also recorded. The Kellgren and Lawrence (K-L) grade was used to quantify the severity of OA [27]. Hip–knee–ankle (HKA) angle and weight-bearing line (WBL) ratio were assessed as radiological variables preoperatively and after 2 years postoperatively. HKA angle is a measure of lower limb alignment, defined as the angle between the mechanical axes of the femur and the tibia. The WBL ratio was estimated by measuring from the medial border of the proximal tibia to the spot where the WBL meets the proximal tibia and dividing that number by the total width of the tibia. HKA angle and WBL ratio were measured on weight-bearing bilateral standing long-leg radiographs. In addition, correction angles were collected for surgical factors.

Preoperative and postoperative HKA angle and WBL ratio were analyzed twice by two orthopedic surgeons. They were orthopedic surgeons with more than five years of experience. Each analyzer was blinded to the results of the other and to all patient information. The average of the two analyzers' results was used. Using the intraclass correlation coefficient (ICC), intraobserver and interobserver reliability were evaluated to determine the reliability of the measurement. In this study, both intraobserver and interobserver ICC values were greater than 0.8.

Statistical Analysis

The mean and standard deviation are presented as descriptive statistics for all continuous variables, and frequency statistics are supplied for all noncontinuous variables. We compared preoperative PROMs, two-year postoperative PROMs, and osteotomy site pain between the CS and non-CS groups using Student's t-test. The rate of WOMAC MCID achievement was compared between the two groups using the chi-square test. A post hoc power analysis was conducted to evaluate whether our findings had sufficient statistical power. SPSS was used conduct statistical analyses (version 21.0; IBM). A p-value less than 0.05 was considered statistically significant.

3. Results

The 121 patients included 37 (30.5%) patients with CS and 84 (69.4%) patients without CS. The mean follow-up period was 2.0 ± 0.1 years. Table 1 shows the demographic data comparing patients with and without CS.

Before surgery, the CS group showed a significantly higher mean WOMAC score than the non-CS group ($p < 0.05$, Table 2). While there was a statistically significant improvement in WOMAC subscores (pain, stiffness, function, and total) for both groups (all $p < 0.05$), the CS group had a significantly lower two-year postoperative score and lower WOMAC subscores (pain, function, and total) than in the non-CS group (all $p < 0.05$, Table 2). In addition, pain VAS at the osteotomy site was more severe in the CS group at two years after surgery ($p < 0.05$, Table 2). With an alpha value of 0.05, a post hoc power analysis revealed greater than 90% power to detect a difference in postoperative two-year WOMAC (pain, function, and total) and postoperative two-year osteotomy site pain VAS.

Table 1. Patient characteristics.

Variables	CS Group (n = 37)	Non-CS Group (n = 84)	p Value
Age (years)	57.6 ± 5.8	55.9 ± 6.1	0.170
Sex			0.064
Male	1 (2.7%)	12 (14.3%)	
Female	36 (97.3%)	72 (85.7%)	
Operation side			0.891
Right	18 (48.6%)	42 (50.0%)	
Left	19 (51.4%)	42 (50.0%)	
Body mass index (kg/m^2)	26.1 ± 4.1	26.2 ± 3.1	0.817
CSI score	45.3 ± 6.7	21.2 ± 8.6	0.000
K-L grade			0.415
2	11 (29.7%)	17 (20.2%)	
3	25 (67.5%)	61 (72.6%)	
4	1 (2.7%)	6 (7.1%)	
Preoperative HKA angle, deg	6.9 ± 2.9	7.2 ± 2.8	0.529
Preoperative WBL ratio, %	19.3 ± 11.9	16.8 ± 11.3	0.267
Postoperative two-year HKA angle, deg	−1.4 ± 2.0	−0.9 ± 2.5	0.277
Postoperative two-year WBL ratio, %	55.1 ± 10.9	53.5 ± 9.8	0.447
Surgical correction angle	10.5 ± 2.7	11.2 ± 2.7	0.243
ASA score			0.275
1	15 (40.5%)	23 (27.3%)	
2	22 (59.4%)	59 (70.2%)	
3	0 (0.0%)	2 (2.3%)	
Diabetes	5 (13.5%)	7 (8.3%)	0.510
Hypertension	12 (32.4%)	24 (28.6%)	0.669
Alcohol consumption	6 (16.2%)	16 (19.0%)	0.710
Smoking	5 (13.5%)	8 (9.5%)	0.534

Data are provided as mean ± SD or n (%). CS, central sensitization; CSI, Central Sensitization Inventory; K–L, Kellgren–Lawrence; ASA, American Society of Anesthesiologists.

Table 2. Preoperative and two-year postoperative WOMAC scores and two-year postoperative osteotomy site pain.

Variables	CS Group (n = 37)	Non-CS Group (n = 84)	p Value
Preoperative WOMAC			
Pain	11.8 ± 3.0	9.3 ± 3.3	0.000
Stiffness	5.0 ± 1.7	4.4 ± 2.2	0.198
Function	41.8 ± 9.3	35.6 ± 11.7	0.003
Total	58.7 ± 12.5	49.4 ± 16.1	0.001
Postoperative two-year WOMAC			
Pain	7.8 ± 2.2	3.9 ± 3.5	0.000
Stiffness	2.7 ± 1.1	2.2 ± 1.6	0.067
Function	26.5 ± 4.8	15.6 ± 11.3	0.000
Total	37.1 ± 6.2	21.8 ± 14.6	0.000
Change WOMAC			
Pain	3.9 ± 2.1	5.3 ± 3.0	0.016
Stiffness	2.3 ± 1.6	2.2 ± 2.1	0.897
Function	15.3 ± 8.7	19.9 ± 14.3	0.031
Total	21.5 ± 9.7	27.5 ± 17.6	0.019
Postoperative two-year osteotomy site pain VAS	4.8 ± 1.8	2.2 ± 2.1	0.000

Data are provided as mean ± SD or n (%). WOMAC, Western Ontario and McMaster Universities arthritis index score; VAS, visual analogue scale.

MCID achievement was examined using the results of a previous study [26]. Patients with CS had worse MCID achievement rates across the board for WOMAC pain, function, and total scores (all $p < 0.05$) compared with the non-CS group (Table 3).

Table 3. MCID achievement.

Variables	CS Group (n = 37)	Non-CS Group (n = 84)	p Value
MCID achievement			
Pain	23 (62.2%)	67 (79.8%)	0.041
Stiffness	19 (51.4%)	44 (52.4%)	0.917
Function	21 (56.8%)	64 (76.2%)	0.031
Total	21 (56.8%)	64 (76.2%)	0.031

Data are provided as mean ± SD or n (%). MCID, minimal clinically important difference.

During the follow-up, there were no major complications requiring additional surgery. Minor complications occurred in four knees. Three patients had superficial wound infections that were treated with intravenous antibiotics. Routine DVT evaluation was not performed. However, one symptomatic patient was confirmed as DVT under CT venography and was treated with oral anticoagulants. No neurovascular injury, pulmonary embolism, or delayed union case was observed during the follow-up period.

4. Discussion

The most important finding of this study was that patients with CS showed inferior outcomes in terms of PROs and greater osteotomy site pain compared to those without CS despite significant improvement in WOMAC subscores.

It has been established that CS is a major contributor to persistent pain following TKA [9–12]. It is believed that severe chronic pain is induced by reduced activation of the descending antinociceptive pathway, perhaps as a result of inactivation by norepinephrine/serotonin [10,11]. Unlike neurogenic or inflammatory pain, central pain is defined as dysfunctional [28,29]. The Central Sensitization Inventory (CSI) is frequently used to evaluate CS [23,24]; in addition, a whole-body pain diagram or quantitative sensory testing (QST) can be used for assessment [30–33]. In our study, the CSI was used for diagnosis of CS.

There have been many studies that focused on CS in relation to the spine and joints, especially in the field of TKA. It has been reported that CS patients showed inferior PROs to non-CS patients in the short term (three months to two years) after TKA [9–11].

Although MOWHTO is a surgical procedure that also involves bone cutting, there has been no research on the relationships between clinical outcomes and CS. As such, this study investigated the relationships between CS and clinical outcomes following MOWHTO.

Even though the PROs of the CS group showed significant improvement after surgery, scores for the preoperative, postoperative, and amount of change in WOMAC in patients with CS were worse than those for patients without CS. Two years after surgery, pain at the osteotomy site of patients with CS was more severe than in non-CS patients. Therefore, surgery outcome, including osteotomy site pain, may be inferior for CS patients who undergo MOWHTO.

Most recently, the MCID (minimum gain judged clinically important vs. statistically significant) has been given more weight [34,35]. Due to the lower improvement in WOMAC scores of patients with CS compared to those without CS, obtaining a minimally acceptable improvement in clinical outcomes is more difficult. In our study, the WOMAC scores of CS patients improved statistically significantly after surgery, but the WOMAC MCID achievement rate of the CS group was only 56.8%. This means that it is difficult to expect clinical improvement in nearly half of patients when performing MOWHTO in the CS group, possibly explaining why CS patients who undergo MOWHTO report lower levels of satisfaction.

Although there was no statistically significant difference in sex between the two groups, the proportion of females in the CS group tended to be higher than in the non-CS group ($p = 0.064$). Women have been shown in several studies to be more sensitive to centrally mediated pain than males [36–38]. This is due to their decreased modulation of conditioned pain [36], increased referred pain following intramuscular experimental pain [37], and increased temporal summation to thermal pain [38]. However, there has been a lack of studies that clearly examine sex differences in pain sensitivity in patients with knee OA, which may be attributable to the confounding factor of disease.

The reason for the differences in PROs and osteotomy site pain between patients with and without CS is not well understood. It is considered that individuals with and without CS have different clinical results after surgery [9–11]. Even before surgery, patients with CS had worse pain and function than patients without CS. Despite the clinical improvement following surgery for both groups, patients with CS might experience more pain in response to the same stimulus (hyperalgesia) and could interpret normal stimulation as painful (allodynia) [9,10]. As a result, it is recommended that patients with CS be given different perioperative pain control when assessing the PROs and osteotomy site pain in patients undergoing MOWHTO. With an incidence of 30.5% of patients with CS in our study, active pain control regimens should be incorporated focusing on preemptive, multimodal pain management in patients with CS undergoing MOWHTO. Studies exist that have demonstrated the efficacy of duloxetine in TKA patients [11,39,40]. Additionally, a recent study suggested that perioperative duloxetine could reduce pain after HTO [41]. Although we think duloxetine can help control pain in MOWHTO patients, further randomized study is warranted. A better understanding of differences in PROs and osteotomy site pain between patients with and without CS for MOWHTO would lead to better overall patient perioperative pain management.

There were limitations in this study. First, as seen in previous research with Koreans who have been diagnosed with OA, patients in this study were all Korean, with females as the majority of patients, which limits the application of the study to other environments [42,43]. In Korea, women have been shown to account for 80–90% of cases of degenerative arthritis and TKA [44,45], indicating an acceptable degree of bias in our study. Second, as a retrospective analysis, there is a chance of selection bias, even though CSI and WOMAC scores were prospectively assessed in all patients. Additional prospective studies are required to verify these findings. Third, due to the nature of the study, only 37 patients were included in the CS group, even though 121 patients who had MOWHTO were studied to compare the PROs and osteotomy site pain according to CS [46,47]. However, our preoperative prevalence of CS was consistent with other studies that found central sensitization in 20–40% of patients before surgery [46–49], which was 30.5% in our study. Fourth, there is a variety of questionnaires that can be used to evaluate the degree of CS [23,24,30–33], which means that study results may vary depending on which questionnaire is used. Unfortunately, there is no agreed-upon approach for assessing CS, and it is unclear whether previous evaluations were validated for use in knee OA patients undergoing MOWHTO. In this study, CS was evaluated using the CSI, which should be considered before applying our results to other studies. Finally, to determine the degree of WOMAC score improvement, we depended on the previously reported MCID of 16.1 points [26]. It has been reported that there are several variables related to MCID, and these differences are clinically significant [34,35]. Despite these limitations, the findings in this study are consistent with those of previous studies, indicating some degree of generalizability [11,46,47]. Therefore, this study contributes important knowledge on CS and its impact on PROs following MOWHTO.

5. Conclusions

The PROs and severity of osteotomy site pain of patients with CS following MOWHTO were worse than those of patients without CS. Moreover, the MCID achievement rate of patients with CS was lower than that of patients without CS. Therefore, appropriate preoperative counseling and perioperative pain management should be considered for patients with CS undergoing MOWHTO.

Author Contributions: Conceptualization, J.-J.K. and Y.I.; methodology, J.-J.K., I.-J.K., M.-S.K. and Y.I.; software, J.-J.K., K.-Y.C. and K.-H.K.; validation, J.-J.K., I.-J.K., M.-S.K. and Y.I.; formal analysis, J.-J.K., K.-Y.C. and K.-H.K.; investigation, J.-J.K., I.-J.K. and M.-S.K.; resources, J.-J.K., K.-Y.C. and K.-H.K.; data curation, K.-Y.C. and K.-H.K.; writing—original draft preparation, J.-J.K.; writing—review and editing, J.-J.K., I.-J.K., M.-S.K., K.-Y.C., K.-H.K. and Y.I.; visualization, K.-Y.C. and K.-H.K.; supervision, I.-J.K., M.-S.K. and Y.I.; project administration, J.-J.K. and Y.I. All authors have read and agreed to the published version of the manuscript.

Funding: This research received no external funding.

Institutional Review Board Statement: The study was conducted in accordance with the Declaration of Helsinki and approved by the Institutional Review Board of Seoul St. Mary's Hospital (KC22RASI0419, 15 June 2022).

Informed Consent Statement: Informed consent was obtained from all subjects involved in the study.

Data Availability Statement: The data published in this research are available on request from the first author (J.-J.K).

Conflicts of Interest: The authors declare no conflict of interest.

References

1. Ogawa, H.; Matsumoto, K.; Ogawa, T.; Takeuchi, K.; Akiyama, H. Preoperative varus laxity correlates with overcorrection in medial opening wedge high tibial osteotomy. *Arch. Orthop. Trauma. Surg.* **2016**, *136*, 1337–1342. [CrossRef] [PubMed]
2. Song, S.J.; Bae, D.K. Computer-Assisted Navigation in High Tibial Osteotomy. *Clin. Orthop. Surg.* **2016**, *8*, 349–357. [CrossRef] [PubMed]
3. Sabzevari, S.; Ebrahimpour, A.; Roudi, M.K.; Kachooei, A.R. High Tibial Osteotomy: A Systematic Review and Current Concept. *Arch. Bone Jt. Surg.* **2016**, *4*, 204–212. [PubMed]
4. Goshima, K.; Sawaguchi, T.; Shigemoto, K.; Iwai, S.; Fujita, K.; Yamamuro, Y. Open-wedge high tibial osteotomy for spontaneous osteonecrosis of the medial tibial plateau shows excellent clinical outcomes. *J. Exp. Orthop.* **2020**, *7*, 14. [CrossRef] [PubMed]
5. Lee, S.C.; Jung, K.A.; Nam, C.H.; Jung, S.H.; Hwang, S.H. The Short-term Follow-up Results of Open Wedge High Tibial Osteotomy with Using an Aescula Open Wedge Plate and an Allogenic Bone Graft: The Minimum 1-Year Follow-up Results. *Clin. Orthop. Surg.* **2010**, *2*, 47–54. [CrossRef]
6. Sterett, W.I.; Steadman, J.R.; Huang, M.J.; Matheny, L.M.; Briggs, K.K. Chondral Resurfacing and High Tibial Osteotomy in the Varus Knee: Survivorship Analysis. *Am. J. Sport. Med.* **2010**, *38*, 1420–1424. [CrossRef]
7. Scott, C.E.; Howie, C.R.; MacDonald, D.; Biant, L.C. Predicting dissatisfaction following total knee replacement: A prospective study of 1217 patients. *J. Bone Jt. Surg.* **2010**, *92*, 1253–1258. [CrossRef]
8. Petersen, K.K.; Graven-Nielsen, T.; Simonsen, O.; Laursen, M.B.; Arendt-Nielsen, L. Preoperative pain mechanisms assessed by cuff algometry are associated with chronic postoperative pain relief after total knee replacement. *Pain* **2016**, *157*, 1400–1406. [CrossRef]
9. Kim, M.S.; Koh, I.J.; Lee, S.Y.; In, Y. Central sensitization is a risk factor for wound complications after primary total knee arthroplasty. *Knee Surg. Sport. Traumatol. Arthrosc.* **2018**, *26*, 3419–3428. [CrossRef]
10. Kim, S.H.; Yoon, K.B.; Yoon, D.M.; Yoo, J.H.; Ahn, K.R. Influence of Centrally Mediated Symptoms on Postoperative Pain in Osteoarthritis Patients Undergoing Total Knee Arthroplasty: A Prospective Observational Evaluation. *Pain Pract.* **2015**, *15*, E46–E53. [CrossRef]
11. Koh, I.J.; Kim, M.S.; Sohn, S.; Song, K.Y.; Choi, N.Y.; In, Y. Duloxetine reduces pain and improves quality of recovery following total knee arthroplasty in centrally sensitized patients: A prospective, randomized controlled study. *J. Bone Jt. Surg. Am.* **2019**, *101*, 64–73. [CrossRef]
12. Kurien, T.; Arendt-Nielsen, L.; Petersen, K.K.; Graven-Nielsen, T.; Scammell, B.E. Preoperative Neuropathic Pain-like Symptoms and Central Pain Mechanisms in Knee Osteoarthritis Predicts Poor Outcome 6 Months After Total Knee Replacement Surgery. *J. Pain* **2018**, *19*, 1329–1341. [CrossRef]
13. Gagnier, J.J. Patient reported outcomes in orthopaedics. *J. Orthop. Res.* **2017**, *35*, 2098–2108. [CrossRef]
14. McConnell, S.; Kolopack, P.; Davis, A. The Western Ontario and McMaster Universities Osteoarthritis Index (WOMAC): A review of its utility and measurement properties. *Arthritis Rheum.* **2001**, *45*, 453–461. [CrossRef]
15. Webb, M.; Dewan, V.; Elson, D. Functional results following high tibial osteotomy: A review of the literature. *Eur. J. Orthop. Surg. Traumatol.* **2018**, *28*, 555–563. [CrossRef]
16. Wei, W.; Shen, J. Effectiveness of double-plane high tibial osteotomy in treatment of medial compartment osteoarthritis. *Chin. J. Reparative Reconstr. Surg.* **2018**, *32*, 1406–1410.

17. Ccedilelik, D.; Çoban, Ö.; Kılıçoğlu, Ö. Minimal clinically important difference of commonly used hip-, knee-, foot-, and ankle-specific questionnaires: A systematic review. *J. Clin. Epidemiol.* **2019**, *113*, 44–57. [CrossRef]
18. Maredupaka, S.; Meshram, P.; Chatte, M.; Kim, W.H.; Kim, T.K. Minimal clinically important difference of commonly used patient-reported outcome measures in total knee arthroplasty: Review of terminologies, methods and proposed values. *Knee Surg. Relat. Res.* **2020**, *32*, 19. [CrossRef]
19. Copay, A.G.; Subach, B.R.; Glassman, S.D.; Polly, D.W., Jr.; Schuler, T.C. Understanding the minimum clinically important difference: A review of concepts and methods. *Spine J.* **2007**, *7*, 541–546. [CrossRef]
20. Lee, D.C.; Byun, S.J. High tibial osteotomy. *Knee Surg. Relat. Res.* **2012**, *24*, 61–69. [CrossRef]
21. Fujisawa, Y.; Masuhara, K.; Shiomi, S. The Effect of High Tibial Osteotomy on Osteoarthritis of the Knee: An arthroscopic study of 54 knee joints. *Orthop. Clin. North Am.* **1979**, *10*, 585–608. [CrossRef] [PubMed]
22. Kim, M.S.; Son, J.M.; Koh, I.J.; Bahk, J.H.; In, Y. Intraoperative adjustment of alignment under valgus stress reduces outliers in patients undergoing medial opening-wedge high tibial osteotomy. *Arch. Orthop. Trauma Surg.* **2017**, *137*, 1035–1045. [CrossRef] [PubMed]
23. Mayer, T.G.; Neblett, R.; Cohen, H.; Howard, K.J.; Choi, Y.H.; Williams, M.J.; Perez, Y.; Gatchel, R.J. The Development and Psychometric Validation of the Central Sensitization Inventory. *Pain Pract.* **2012**, *12*, 276–285. [CrossRef] [PubMed]
24. Neblett, R.; Cohen, H.; Choi, Y.; Hartzell, M.M.; Williams, M.; Mayer, T.G.; Gatchel, R.J. The Central Sensitization Inventory (CSI): Establishing Clinically Significant Values for Identifying Central Sensitivity Syndromes in an Outpatient Chronic Pain Sample. *J. Pain* **2013**, *14*, 438–445. [CrossRef] [PubMed]
25. Bellamy, N.; Buchanan, W.W.; Goldsmith, C.H.; Campbell, J.; Stitt, L.W. Validation study of WOMAC: A health status instrument for measuring clinically important patient relevant outcomes to antirheumatic drug therapy in patients with osteoarthritis of the hip or knee. *J. Rheumatol.* **1988**, *15*, 1833–1840.
26. Kim, M.S.; Koh, I.J.; Choi, K.Y.; Sung, Y.G.; Park, D.C.; Lee, H.J.; In, Y. The Minimal Clinically Important Difference (MCID) for the WOMAC and Factors Related to Achievement of the MCID after Medial Opening Wedge High Tibial Osteotomy for Knee Osteoarthritis. *Am. J. Sports Med.* **2021**, *49*, 2406–2415. [CrossRef]
27. Kohn, M.D.; Sassoon, A.A.; Fernando, N.D. Classifications in Brief: Kellgren-Lawrence Classification of Osteoarthritis. *Clin. Orthop. Relat. Res.* **2016**, *474*, 1886–1893. [CrossRef]
28. Song, S.J.; Kim, K.I.; Bae, D.K.; Park, C.H. Mid-term lifetime survivals of octogenarians following primary and revision total knee arthroplasties were satisfactory: A retrospective single center study in contemporary period. *Knee Surg. Relat. Res.* **2020**, *32*, 50. [CrossRef]
29. Takamura, D.; Iwata, K.; Sueyoshi, T.; Yasuda, T.; Moriyama, H. Relationship between early physical activity after total knee arthroplasty and postoperative physical function: Are these related? *Knee Surg. Relat. Res.* **2021**, *33*, 35. [CrossRef]
30. Lape, E.C.; Selzer, F.; Collins, J.E.; Losina, E.; Katz, J.N. Stability of Measures of Pain Catastrophizing and Widespread Pain Following Total Knee Replacement. *Arthritis Care Res.* **2020**, *72*, 1096–1103. [CrossRef]
31. Dave, A.; Selzer, F.; Losina, E.; Usiskin, I.; Collins, J.; Lee, Y.; Band, P.; Dalury, D.; Iorio, R.; Kindsfater, K.; et al. The association of pre-operative body pain diagram scores with pain outcomes following total knee arthroplasty. *Osteoarthr. Cartil.* **2016**, *25*, 667–675. [CrossRef]
32. Wylde, V.; Palmer, S.; Learmonth, I.; Dieppe, P. The association between pre-operative pain sensitisation and chronic pain after knee replacement: An exploratory study. *Osteoarthr. Cartil.* **2013**, *21*, 1253–1256. [CrossRef]
33. Wylde, V.; Sayers, A.; Lenguerrand, E.; Gooberman-Hill, R.; Pyke, M.; Beswick, A.D.; Dieppe, P.; Blom, A.W. Preoperative widespread pain sensitization and chronic pain after hip and knee replacement: A cohort analysis. *Pain* **2015**, *156*, 47–54. [CrossRef]
34. Angst, F.; Aeschlimann, A.; Angst, J. The minimal clinically important difference raised the significance of outcome effects above the statistical level, with methodological implications for future studies. *J. Clin. Epidemiol.* **2017**, *82*, 128–136. [CrossRef]
35. Clement, N.D.; MacDonald, D.; Simpson, A.H.R.W. The minimal clinically important difference in the Oxford knee score and Short Form 12 score after total knee arthroplasty. *Knee Surg. Sport. Traumatol. Arthrosc.* **2013**, *22*, 1933–1939. [CrossRef]
36. Arendt-Nielsen, L.; Sluka, K.A.; Nie, H.L. Experimental muscle pain impairs descending inhibition. *Pain* **2008**, *140*, 465–471. [CrossRef]
37. Law, L.A.F.; Sluka, K.; McMullen, T.; Lee, J.; Arendt-Nielsen, L.; Graven-Nielsen, T. Acidic buffer induced muscle pain evokes referred pain and mechanical hyperalgesia in humans. *Pain* **2008**, *140*, 254–264. [CrossRef]
38. Fillingim, R.B.; Maixner, W.; Kincaid, S.; Silva, S. Sex differences in temporal summation but not sensory-discriminative processing of thermal pain. *Pain* **1998**, *75*, 121–127. [CrossRef]
39. Kim, M.S.; Koh, I.J.; Choi, K.Y.; Yang, S.C.; In, Y. Efficacy of duloxetine compared with opioid for postoperative pain control following total knee arthroplasty. *PLoS ONE* **2021**, *16*, e0253641. [CrossRef]
40. Kim, M.; Koh, I.; Sung, Y.; Park, D.; Na, J.; In, Y. Preemptive Duloxetine Relieves Postoperative Pain and Lowers Wound Temperature in Centrally Sensitized Patients Undergoing Total Knee Arthroplasty: A Randomized, Double-Blind, Placebo-Controlled Trial. *J. Clin. Med.* **2021**, *10*, 2809. [CrossRef]
41. Otsuki, S.; Okamoto, Y.; Ikeda, K.; Wakama, H.; Okayoshi, T.; Neo, M. Perioperative duloxetine administration reduces pain after high tibial osteotomy and non-steroidal anti-inflammatory administration: A prospective, controlled study. *Knee* **2022**, *38*, 42–49. [CrossRef] [PubMed]

42. Song, S.J.; Kang, S.G.; Park, C.H.; Bae, D.K. Comparison of Clinical Results and Risk of Patellar Injury between Attune and PFC Sigma Knee Systems. *Knee Surg. Relat. Res.* **2018**, *30*, 334–340. [CrossRef] [PubMed]
43. Yoo, J.-H.; Kim, J.-G.; Chung, K.; Lee, S.H.; Oh, H.-C.; Park, S.-H.; Seok, S.-O. Vascular Calcification in Patients Undergoing Total Knee Arthroplasty: Frequency and Effects on the Surgery. *Clin. Orthop. Surg.* **2020**, *12*, 171–177. [CrossRef] [PubMed]
44. Koh, I.J.; Kim, T.K.; Chang, C.B.; Cho, H.J.; In, Y. Trends in Use of Total Knee Arthroplasty in Korea from 2001 to 2010. *Clin. Orthop. Relat. Res.* **2013**, *471*, 1441–1450. [CrossRef] [PubMed]
45. Koh, I.J.; Cho, W.-S.; Choi, N.Y.; Kim, T.K. Causes, Risk Factors, and Trends in Failures After TKA in Korea Over the Past 5 Years: A Multicenter Study. *Clin. Orthop. Relat. Res.* **2014**, *472*, 316–326. [CrossRef]
46. Kim, M.S.; Koh, I.J.; Choi, K.Y.; Seo, J.Y.; In, Y. Minimal Clinically Important Differences for Patient-Reported Outcomes After TKA Depend on Central Sensitization. *J. Bone Jt. Surg.* **2021**, *103*, 1374–1382. [CrossRef]
47. Kim, M.S.; Koh, I.J.; Choi, K.Y.; Ju, G.I.; In, Y. Centrally sensitized patients undergoing total knee arthroplasty have higher expectations than do non-centrally sensitized patients. *Knee Surg. Sport. Traumatol. Arthrosc.* **2021**, *30*, 1257–1265. [CrossRef]
48. Hochman, J.; Gagliese, L.; Davis, A.; Hawker, G. Neuropathic pain symptoms in a community knee OA cohort. *Osteoarthr. Cartil.* **2011**, *19*, 647–654. [CrossRef]
49. Ohtori, S.; Orita, S.; Yamashita, M.; Ishikawa, T.; Ito, T.; Shigemura, T.; Nishiyama, H.; Konno, S.; Ohta, H.; Takaso, M.; et al. Existence of a Neuropathic Pain Component in Patients with Osteoarthritis of the Knee. *Yonsei Med. J.* **2012**, *53*, 801–805. [CrossRef]

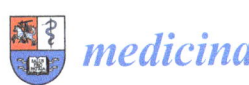

Article

Automated Detection of Surgical Implants on Plain Knee Radiographs Using a Deep Learning Algorithm

Back Kim [1,†], Do Weon Lee [2,†], Sanggyu Lee [3], Sunho Ko [4], Changwung Jo [5], Jaeseok Park [1], Byung Sun Choi [4], Aaron John Krych [6], Ayoosh Pareek [6], Hyuk-Soo Han [1,4] and Du Hyun Ro [1,4,7,*]

1. College of Medicine, Seoul National University, Seoul 03080, Republic of Korea
2. Department of Orthopedic Surgery, Korean Armed Forces Yangju Hospital, Yangju-si 11429, Republic of Korea
3. Department of Computer Science and Engineering, Seoul National University, Seoul 08826, Republic of Korea
4. Department of Orthopedic Surgery, Seoul National University Hospital, Seoul 03080, Republic of Korea
5. Seoul National University Hospital, Seoul 03080, Republic of Korea
6. Department of Orthopedic Surgery, Mayo Clinic, Rochester, MN 55902, USA
7. CONNECTEVE Co., Ltd., Seoul 03080, Republic of Korea
* Correspondence: duhyunro@gmail.com; Tel.: +82-2-2072-4060
† These authors contributed equally to this paper.

Abstract: *Background and Objectives*: The number of patients who undergo multiple operations on a knee is increasing. The objective of this study was to develop a deep learning algorithm that could detect 17 different surgical implants on plain knee radiographs. *Materials and Methods*: An internal dataset consisted of 5206 plain knee antero-posterior X-rays from a single, tertiary institute for model development. An external set contained 238 X-rays from another tertiary institute. A total of 17 different types of implants including total knee arthroplasty, unicompartmental knee arthroplasty, plate, and screw were labeled. The internal dataset was approximately split into a train set, a validation set, and an internal test set at a ratio of 7:1:2. You Only look Once (YOLO) was selected as the detection network. Model performances with the validation set, internal test set, and external test set were compared. *Results*: Total accuracy, total sensitivity, total specificity value of the validation set, internal test set, and external test set were (0.978, 0.768, 0.999), (0.953, 0.810, 0.990), and (0.956, 0.493, 0.975), respectively. Means ± standard deviations (SDs) of diagonal components of confusion matrix for these three subsets were 0.858 ± 0.242, 0.852 ± 0.182, and 0.576 ± 0.312, respectively. True positive rate of total knee arthroplasty, the most dominant class of the dataset, was higher than 0.99 with internal subsets and 0.96 with an external test set. *Conclusion*: Implant identification on plain knee radiographs could be automated using a deep learning technique. The detection algorithm dealt with overlapping cases while maintaining high accuracy on total knee arthroplasty. This could be applied in future research that analyzes X-ray images with deep learning, which would help prompt decision-making in clinics.

Keywords: automated detection; detection algorithm; deep learning

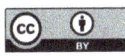

1. Introduction

As knee operations are increasing in number, the number of patients who undergo multiple knee surgeries is increasing [1,2]. Surgical history must be identified to check whether there is an existing implant and what type of implant it is [3]. However, some patients undergo surgeries at multiple institutions, which hinders obtaining accurate surgical history [4]. According to a 2012 survey on American Association of Hip and Knee Surgeons (AAHKS) members, 10% of implants before operations and 2% of implants during surgery could not be identified [5]. Moreover, the median time taken for implant identification by surgeons was 20 min [5].

Automated identification using artificial intelligence (AI) is an efficient way to overcome this situation. Machine learning (ML) methods have been demonstrated to be fast and accurate in processing medical images such as X-ray, MRI, and pathology slides [6,7]. Among diverse ML approaches, deep learning (DL) especially stands out because it can find distinctive features in given data without direct human supervision, unlike classic ML models [8]. DL model could significantly reduce time and cost spent in identifying implants by examining X-ray images directly and automatically. Tiwari et al. [9] and Patel et al. [10] have directly compared DL models with human experts in examining X-ray images and proven that DL models are better in both speed and accuracy.

Ren et al. [11] have reviewed studies on identification of orthopedic implants using AI. Their systematic review covered several different anatomic sites such as hip, knee, and shoulder. It is reasonable because basic concepts are similar regardless of anatomical locations. Among the 11 studies they included, those conducted by Yi et al. [12] and Karnuta et al. [13] dealt with knee X-rays.

Yi et al. [12] were the first who tried to identify implants on knee plain radiographs using AI. They developed three different DL models: (1) a model that judges whether there is total knee arthroplasty (TKA) on the image, (2) a model that classifies TKA and unicompartmental knee arthroplasty (UKA), and (3) a model that distinguishes between two TKA models. They utilized 237 to 274 images, which varied by each model. All three models with binary classifications achieved a perfect AUC of 1.0.

Karnuta et al. [13] have expanded the task into multi-class classification. Their DL system classified nine different implant models with AUC of 0.99. They also increased the size of the dataset into 682 images.

Contrary to these previous studies [12,13], this study employed a detection network because there were 'overlapping' cases in the dataset. A majority of previous studies focused on classifying companies and models within the scope of TKA, whereas this study aimed to figure out the type and location of every implant on an X-ray image. For example, some images might include TKA and three screws simultaneously. Such images could be easily identified with detection networks.

Covering a variety of implants other than TKA is important because TKA is not the only surgical intervention that a patient may have undergone. For instance, if a patient received high tibial osteotomy (HTO), a plate and screws would appear on the X-ray, but there would be no TKA. Another example is anterior cruciate ligament (ACL) reconstruction. Usually, only screws would appear in this case. Most of the previous studies could not deal with these surgeries because their models classified TKA only. Thus, the main purpose of this study was to develop a DL model to identify 17 different types of objects and determine their locations in the form of bounding boxes.

2. Materials and Methods

This study was approved by the Institutional Review Board (No. H-1801-061-915). The overall process of this study, from organizing dataset to evaluating the trained DL model, is summarized in Figure 1.

2.1. Dataset and Pre-Processing

The internal dataset consisted of 5206 X-rays taken at a single, tertiary hospital from 4435 patients. The external test contained 238 X-rays from another tertiary institution. X-rays from each hospital were retrospectively collected from 2009-01-01 to 2019-12-31.

All images were knee anteroposterior (AP) view images. These images were first converted from Digital Imaging and Communications in Medicine (DICOM) format to Portable Network Graphics (PNG) format. They were subsequently converted into Joint Photographic Expert Group (JPG) format. JPG quality was 70 for internal data and 95 for external data.

The external dataset consisted of 71 images including both legs (29.8%), 73 images including only the left leg (30.7%), and 94 images including only the right leg (39.5%). Those images were flipped horizontally and concatenated with the original ones. If the original image contained the right leg, the flipped one was put left to it. If the original one included the left leg, the flipped one was placed right to it.

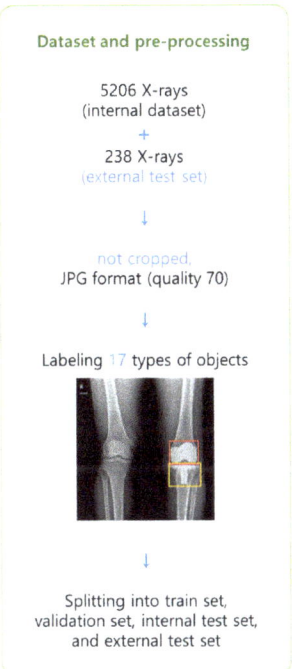 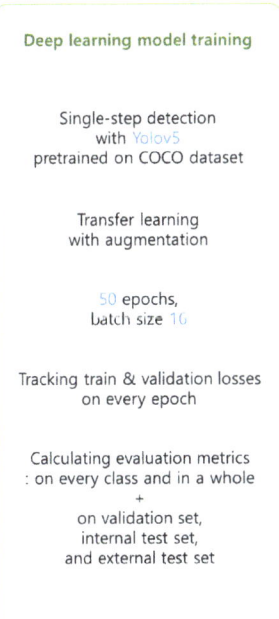 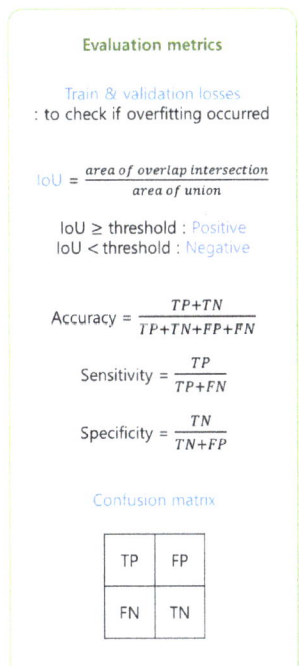

Figure 1. A schematic process of the deep learning system development in this study. (TP = true positive, TN = true negative, FP = false positive, FN = false negative, mAP = mean average precision).

A total of 17 different types of objects were labeled: TKA_femur, TKA_tibia, UKA, staple, wire, screw, plate, IM nail, washer, smooth pin, metal button, bone cement, tumor prosthesis, ruler, External fixator, Patellofemoral arthroplasty, and TKA_stem (TKA = total knee arthroplasty, UKA = unicompartmental knee arthroplasty, IM nail = intramedullary nail). The type and location of each object were labeled so that both classification and detection were possible. Table 1 shows the number of images and instances that belong to each class in internal and external datasets.

Table 1. The number of images and instances by class in internal and external dataset.

Class	The Internal Dataset		The External Dataset	
	Number of Images	Number of Object Instances	Number of Images	Number of Object Instances
TKA_femur	3913	6107	46	85
TKA_tibia	3911	6101	41	76
UKA	154	173	21	41
staple	189	310	23	55
wire	89	126	26	68
screw	1035	3348	113	1184
plate	283	371	65	151
IM nail	83	89	40	79
washer	200	245	19	42
smooth pin	62	170	7	12
metal button	155	204	29	99

Table 1. *Cont.*

Class	The Internal Dataset		The External Dataset	
	Number of Images	Number of Object Instances	Number of Images	Number of Object Instances
bone cement	11	11	11	20
tumor prosthesis	12	12	20	37
ruler	237	237	16	31
External fixator	6	10	1	4
Patellofemoral arthroplasty	10	13	22	31
TKA_stem	310	521	10	25

TKA, total knee arthroplasty; UKA, unicompartmental knee arthroplasty; IM, intramedullary.

The internal dataset was split into train set, validation set, and internal test set. The split ratio was train: validation: test = (about) 7:1:2. Multiple X-rays from a single patient were assigned to the same subset. In addition, the class imbalance was adjusted by applying a ratio of 7:1:2 in a per-class manner. Except for this principle, the splitting process was done in a random manner. Finally, 3701, 517, and 1042 images were assigned to the train set, validation set, and internal test set, respectively. The external dataset was solely used as the external test set. These 238 images were neither used in the training nor in the validation of DL process.

2.2. Deep Learning Model Training

You only look once (YOLO) was utilized as the DL algorithm. The detection approach before YOLO was divided into two steps. For example, R-CNN could "first generate potential bounding boxes in an image and then run a classifier on these proposed boxes" [14]. Using YOLO, the detection process became a single-step, "straight from image pixels to bounding box coordinates and class probabilities" [14]. In other words, it can judge the type and location of an object simultaneously. YOLO is fast and light because of this feature. Yolov5, the latest version of YOLO, was employed in this research. Yolov5 offers multiple options such as size and complexity, whose basic approaches are identical. Yolov5s has the most simple and lightest architecture among them. Thus, it was selected in this study.

The programming language and the deep learning framework used for model training were Python 3.8.5 and PyTorch, respectively. Graphics processing unit (GPU) NVIDIA GeForce RTX 3090 was utilized for fast training. Transfer learning was conducted. That is, Yolov5s trained with Common Objects in Context (COCO) dataset was fine-tuned to adjust to our dataset. COCO is a large-scale dataset frequently used in detection and segmentation tasks like ImageNet in classification tasks. It consists of 330K images with 1.5 million object instances labeled into 80 object categories [15]. Detection models pretrained with COCO is expected to perform well even on novel tasks because it has already learned how to find meaningful features on various kinds of objects (e.g., finding contours or rectangles). The model was trained and validated in 50 epochs. The batch size was 16. Online imagespace and colorspace augmentations were applied to the train set [16]. Three random images were presented with the original image each time when an image was loaded for training [17].

2.3. Evaluation Metrics

Train losses and validation losses of each epoch were examined to verify that no overfitting occurred. In that case, the model 'memorizes the answers' of the training set instead of recognizing genuine features of each image. This phenomenon can be sensed by tracking validation loss because an overfitted model cannot perform well on novel data. Thus, validation loss increases with each epoch in the overfitted model.

Accuracy, sensitivity, specificity, and confusion matrix were used to evaluate the model's performance. These metrics were each measured with the validation set, internal test set, and external test set separately. Accuracy, sensitivity, and specificity of each class were first calculated. The total score was defined as their weighted average, whose weight was the number of instances that belonged to each class. Accuracy was defined as (TP+TN)/(TP+TN+FP+FN). Sensitivity was defined as TP/(TP+FN) and specificity was defined as TN/(TN+FP). The confusion matrix is a figure that shows TP, TN, FP, and FN rates of each class. TP, TN, FP, and FN mean true positive, true negative, false positive, and false negative, respectively. The metrics of each class could be figured out by treating the task like a binary classification problem. For instance, the sensitivity value of TKA_stem was figured out by defining TKA_stem as 'True' and all other classes as 'False'. The judgment of true and false is intuitive in classification. For example, if the ground truth is '0' and the model prediction is '0', it is true. If the model prediction is '1', it is false. However, in the case of detection, the location of the bounding box was also taken into consideration.

Intersection over union (IoU) was used as a criterion for detection. IoU was defined as (area of overlap intersection)/(area of union). It was determined by overlap intersection and union between two boxes: ground truth and prediction. IoU became higher when the two boxes overlapped more, i.e., the area of intersection of the two boxes was larger while the area of symmetric difference was smaller. It is because the area of union is the sum of the area of intersection and symmetric difference. The threshold of minimum IoU can be selected by users. In this study, a threshold of 0.5 was used for accuracy, sensitivity, and specificity, while a threshold of 0.45 was for confusion matrices. It means that if the threshold is 0.7, predictions with IoU lower than 0.7 are false predictions.

3. Results

Figure 2 shows no overfitting in the training process. There was no abnormal increase in validation loss during the task.

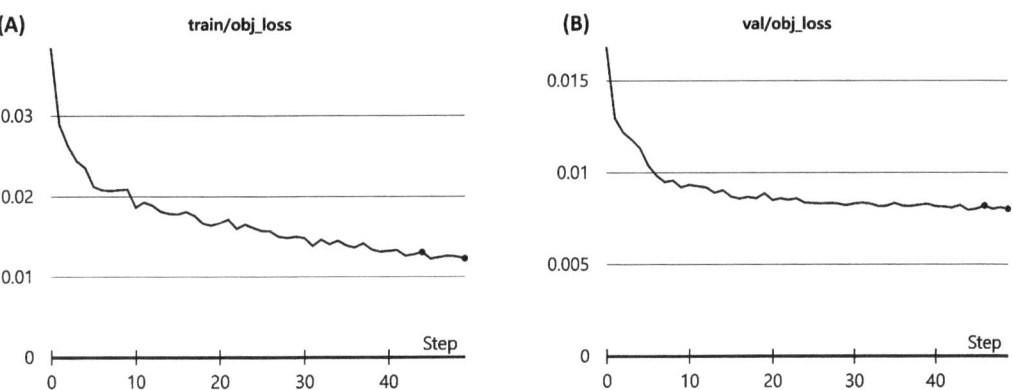

Figure 2. Train (**A**) & validation (**B**) losses of the Yolov5s model in the study. As the number of epochs increases, train losses always decrease. Validation losses decrease if the model is robust on new data. If the model is overfitted to the train set, validation losses would increase.

Tables 2–4 present accuracy, sensitivity, and specificity tested with the validation set, internal test set, and external test set, respectively. Total accuracy, total sensitivity, total specificity value of each subset were (0.978, 0.768, 0.999), (0.953, 0.810, 0.990), and (0.956, 0.493, 0.975), respectively.

Table 2. Evaluation metrics on the validation set.

	Accuracy	Sensitivity	Specificity
TKA_femur	0.999	0.998	1
TKA_tibia	1	1	1
UKA	1	1	1
staple	0.991	0.6	0.999
wire	0.999	0.75	1
screw	0.952	0.737	0.996
plate	0.997	0.806	1
IM nail	0.998	0.818	0.999
washer	0.994	0.654	0.999
smooth pin	0.997	0.733	0.999
metal button	0.999	1	0.999
bone cement	1	1	1
tumor prosthesis	1	1	1
ruler	0.999	0.952	0.999
External fixator	0.999	0	1
Patellofemoral arthroplasty	0.703	0.002	1
TKA_stem	0.999	1	0.999
Total	**0.978**	**0.768**	**0.999**

TKA, total knee arthroplasty; UKA, unicompartmental knee arthroplasty; IM, intramedullary.

Table 3. Evaluation metrics on the internal test set.

	Accuracy	Sensitivity	Specificity
TKA_femur	0.998	0.998	0.998
TKA_tibia	0.994	0.997	0.985
UKA	0.999	1	0.999
staple	0.979	0.754	0.987
wire	0.995	0.818	0.998
screw	0.888	0.868	0.901
plate	0.99	0.92	0.993
IM nail	0.994	0.647	0.997
washer	0.987	0.864	0.99
smooth pin	0.984	0.5	0.994
metal button	0.995	0.971	0.996
bone cement	0.999	1	0.999
tumor prosthesis	0.999	1	0.999
ruler	0.999	0.979	0.999
External fixator	0.999	0.5	1
Patellofemoral arthroplasty	0.402	0.002	0.999
TKA_stem	0.993	0.948	0.996
Total	**0.953**	**0.810**	**0.990**

TKA, total knee arthroplasty; UKA, unicompartmental knee arthroplasty; IM, intramedullary.

Table 4. Evaluation metrics on the external test set.

	Accuracy	Sensitivity	Specificity
TKA_femur	0.988	1	0.987
TKA_tibia	0.981	0.987	0.981
UKA	1	1	1
staple	0.944	0.527	0.958
wire	0.975	0.588	0.99
screw	0.67	0.644	0.725
plate	0.982	0.848	0.995
IM nail	0.979	0.658	0.994

Table 4. Cont.

	Accuracy	Sensitivity	Specificity
washer	0.974	0.238	0.992
smooth pin	0.993	0	1
metal button	0.966	0.505	0.994
bone cement	0.989	0.35	0.997
tumor prosthesis	0.979	0.243	0.995
ruler	0.979	0.161	0.994
External fixator	0.998	0	1
Patellofemoral arthroplasty	0.878	0.118	0.999
TKA_stem	0.972	0.52	0.979
Total	**0.956**	**0.493**	**0.975**

TKA, total knee arthroplasty; UKA, unicompartmental knee arthroplasty; IM, intramedullary.

As for the internal validation set, the accuracy ranged from 0.703 to 1. Accuracy values for TKA_tibia, UKA, bone cement, and tumor prosthesis were 1. The value for Patellofemoral arthroplasty was 0.703. Sensitivity values for TKA_tibia, UKA, metal button, bone cement, tumor prosthesis, and TKA_stem were 1. Specificity values for TKA_femur, TKA_tibia, UKA, wire, plate, bone cement, tumor prosthesis, External fixator, and Patellofemoral arthroplasty were also 1.

As for the internal test set, the accuracy ranged from 0.402 to 0.999. Accuracy values for UKA, bone cement, tumor prosthesis, ruler, and External fixator were 0.999. This value for Patellofemoral arthroplasty was 0.402. Sensitivity values for UKA, bone cement, and tumor prosthesis were 1. The specificity value for External fixator was also 1.

As for the external test set, the accuracy ranged from 0.670 to 0.998. The accuracy value for External fixator was 0.998. This value for screw was 0.670. Sensitivity values for TKA_femur and UKA were 1. Specificity values for UKA, smooth pin, and External fixator were also 1.

Confusion matrices of the validation set, internal test set, and external test set are displayed in Figure 3. Means ± SDs of diagonal components of the validation set, internal test set, and external test set in the confusion matrices were 0.858 ± 0.242, 0.852 ± 0.182, and 0.576 ± 0.312, respectively.

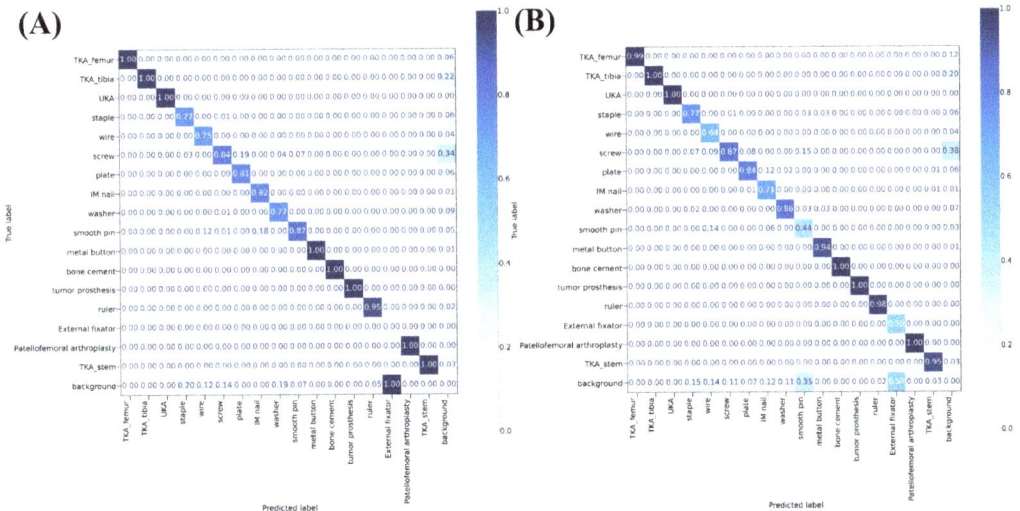

Figure 3. Cont.

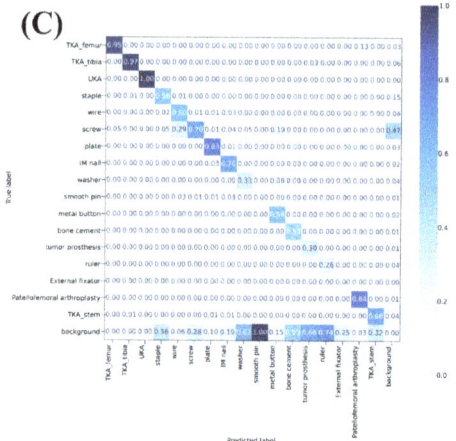

Figure 3. Confusion matrices on validation set (**A**), internal test set (**B**), and external test set (**C**). Among 18 labels on each axis, only 'background' is not an object class. If the 'True label' is background and the 'Predicted label' belongs to one of the object classes, it means that the model made a false positive judgment on the presence of an implant. If the 'Predicted label' is background and the 'True label' belongs to one of the object classes, it means that the model made a false negative judgment on the presence of an implant.

4. Discussion

The most dominant orthopedic implant of our dataset was TKA. This is because the number of arthritis patients is increasing due to the aging population. In addition, TKA has been acknowledged as a highly effective treatment, especially for senior patients. Nevertheless, there are other types of implants for other diseases. The number of these cases was not negligible. Thus, the authors tried to define as diverse classes as possible to cover a wide range of knee implants.

Table 5 compares the approach and the result of this research with previous studies. Among previous studies that automatically identified implants on X-rays, seven studies that dealt with knee radiographs were included. In comparison, our study dealt with large amount of dataset with comparable accuracy to other DL models while adapting a different kind of approach (detection method) to identify multiple different kinds of implants.

Table 5. Comparison with previous studies.

Author	Year	Total Dataset Size	External Test Set	Radiograph Location	Mode of Judgement	Accuracy
Yi et al. [12]	2020	511	No	knee	classification	Not reported (AUC = 1.00)
Karnuta et al. [13]	2021	682	No	knee	classification	99%
Belete et al. [18]	2021	588	No	knee	classification	100%
Sharma et al. [19]	2021	1240	Yes	knee	classification	96%
Tiwari et al. [9]	2022	521	No	knee	classification	96%
Patel et al. [10]	2021	1547	No	knee and hip	segmentation and classification	99%
Klemt et al. [20]	2020	11204	No	knee and hip	classification	Not reported (AUC = 0.97)
Kim et al. (This study)	2022	5444	Yes	knee	detection	96%

AUC = Area Under the Curve.

Belete et al. [18] have developed a DL model with eight different classes, and they considered calculating the probability with the softmax function in the evaluation process.

Sharma et al. [19] have classified six implant types using 1078 images and compared four different networks with an external test set that consists of 162 images. Tiwari et al. [9] have classified six implant types using 521 images, and they have shown the superiority of ML models over human experts regarding the average accuracy. Patel et al. [10] have used both knee and hip radiographs, identifying 12 implant types using 427 knee and 922 hip unilateral images. Klemt et al. [20] have also classified both knee and hip arthroplasties, identifying 14 TKA designs and 24 total hip arthroplasty (THA) designs using a total of 11,204 knee X-rays.

Gurung et al. [21] have reviewed nine studies using AI for the identification of orthopedic implants. They also analyzed three articles that focused on predicting the risk of implant surgery failure. Ren et al. [11] and Gurung et al. [21] both pointed out that most of the existing studies didn't use external datasets, which means they only used radiographs from one institution. Our model was tested on a balanced external test set to resolve this problem.

Among studies that only handled locations other than the knee, such as the hip and shoulder, the one conducted by Kang et al. [22] was notable because they automatically cropped images with YOLOv3, a detection network. The final prediction was done with a simple CNN classification network. The research by Urban et al. [23] was also noticeable because they compared the performances of DL networks with other ML classifiers (e.g., Gradient Boosting).

The current study employed YOLO, a detection network, unlike majority of previous studies that utilized classification networks such as ResNet. These previous studies have focused on identifying different companies or models of arthroplasty implants like TKA because different models of arthroplasties are usually incompatible. In contrast, this study aims to identify implants that can appear simultaneously in the same image. In other words, images that include each type of object are not disjoint in our dataset. For example, both UKA and screw can appear in some images. Therefore, when applying classification networks, this task becomes not only a multi-class classification, but also a multi-label classification. To handle this problem, either the dataset or model algorithm should be transformed. That was why this study employed detection approach instead. Unlike classification, detection networks can inherently handle overlapping cases. The model output includes every object in an image. For example, the model can detect eight smooth pins and two wires in an image and figure out their locations.

As to the pre-processing of images, conversion into low-quality JPGs can reduce not only computational resources required for DL training and inference, but also model training and predicting time. Another way to save time and resources is by cropping images to only include the region of interest (ROI), i.e., the area around the knee joint. However, cropped dataset limits types and locations of implants that can be detected. For example, detection of TKA_stem and differentiation between IM_nail and TKA_stem becomes easier with the dataset that is uncropped. Thus, the whole image was used in this study.

In terms of defining object classes, the reason why TKA was split into TKA_femur and TKA_tibia and why there were classes that were not surgical implants (i.e., ruler and external fixator) was related to the performance of the detection model. TKA was split into TKA_femur and TKA_tibia because unless it was separated, bounding boxes became too large and the performance of the detection model would decline. The reason why there were 'ruler' and 'external fixator' classes was because unless they were assigned to some classes, the detection model could mistake them for some other implants like screws or staples.

As for model evaluation, the metrics were measured with three subsets for comparison. Test sets were more novel than the validation set to the model. The external test set was from different institution. Thus, how the model would respond in a new situation can be predicted by comparing its performances with these three subsets. Moreover, the reason why the 'weighted' average of accuracy, sensitivity, and specificity was calculated was because it could help deal with the class imbalance problem by reflecting the number of instances. Despite covering diverse cases, the proportion of TKA instances was high, which was more than half of the entire dataset.

Confusion matrices in Figure 3 showed that the model was more than 99% accurate on TKA in the case of internal subsets. This score was almost the same as the binary TKA classifier described by Yi et al. [12]. TP rate of TKA on external subset was also high, which was about 0.96. The fact TKA was the most dominant class might explain this result. However, this result might also be due to fact that TKA implant is relatively big and easy to identify owing to its distinct shape. UKA shares these characteristics with TKA. Its TP rates were 1.00 in all subsets. Interestingly, TP rates of screw, the second most dominant class after TKA, were less than 0.9 in all three subsets. It might be because the model confused screws with other small implants like staples.

External fixator was not detected successfully because the number of their instances was too small. In the case of tumor prosthesis whose number of instances was also small, the model showed perfect TP rates with internal subsets, but a poor TP rate of 0.3 with the external dataset. It means the model is not robust enough for detecting tumor prosthesis. Notably, the score on patellofemoral arthroplasty was fine, although its number of instances was similar to that of tumor prosthesis. The fact that its shape and location are very distinct from other implants might explain this outcome.

The metrics in Tables 2–4 display similar tendencies with the confusion matrices. Performances for TKA and UKA were high in all three subsets. The model could successfully identify the presence of TKA and UKA. Overall scores with the external dataset show that the robustness of the model needs to be improved. However, the evenness of the external test set should be considered, which can be verified through the number of images by class such as those shown in Table 1.

This research would be helpful not only in clinical fields including medical centers performing orthopedic surgeries, but also in future DL studies. Inclusion or exclusion criteria for DL research on X-rays may contain whether a patient has undergone knee surgeries. Automated identification of implants would help us quickly screen images for implants.

This study has several limitations. First, there was a class imbalance problem in the internal dataset. The proportion of TKA instances was very high, which was more than half of the entire dataset. It can make an objective evaluation of the DL models difficult. This problem could be partly resolved by using a relatively balanced external dataset. Second, the sensitivity of the model for certain kinds of implants such as staples was low. Since this was the first study, to our knowledge, that dealt with these low profile implants, further study is needed to improve the sensitivity of the model. Third, default hyperparameters were used for model training. The model performance could become better if hyperparameter tuning was applied.

5. Conclusions

In conclusion, this study explored automation of implant identification process on plain knee radiographs using DL techniques. True positive rates of TKA, the most dominant class, for the validation set, internal test set, and external test set were 1.00, 0.99, and 0.95, respectively. The total accuracy value of the internal test set was 0.953, meaning that the model classified other classes with a fine performance as well. Unlike the models presented in previous studies, the one in this study can identify various cases other than TKA in clinical fields by detecting multiple implants that can be overlapped. Approaches of this study can also be applied in future research that analyzes X-ray images with DL techniques.

Author Contributions: Conceptualization, D.H.R. and B.K.; methodology, B.K.; software, S.K.; validation, S.L., J.P. and D.W.L.; formal analysis, B.K.; investigation, J.P.; resources, S.K., A.J.K., A.P. and H.-S.H.; data curation, S.L.; writing—original draft preparation, B.K.; writing—review and editing, D.W.L. and B.S.C.; visualization, C.J.; supervision, D.H.R.; project administration, D.H.R. All authors have read and agreed to the published version of the manuscript.

Funding: This research received no external funding.

Institutional Review Board Statement: The study was conducted in accordance with the Declaration of Helsinki, and approved by the Institutional Review Board of Seoul National University Hospital. (No. H-1801-061-915, 16 September 2022).

Informed Consent Statement: Patient consent was waived due to anonymity of the data used in the study. It was approved by the Institutional Review Board of Seoul National University Hospital.

Data Availability Statement: The data presented in this study are available on request from the corresponding author. The data are not publicly available due to privacy.

Conflicts of Interest: The authors declare no conflict of interest.

References

1. Postler, A.; Lützner, C.; Beyer, F.; Tille, E.; Lützner, J. Analysis of total knee arthroplasty revision causes. *BMC Musculoskelet. Disord.* **2018**, *19*, 55. [CrossRef] [PubMed]
2. Sun, X.; Wang, J.; Su, Z. A meta-analysis of total knee arthroplasty following high tibial osteotomy versus primary total knee arthroplasty. *Arch. Orthop. Trauma Surg.* **2020**, *140*, 527–535. [CrossRef]
3. Baré, J.; MacDonald, S.J.; Bourne, R.B. Preoperative evaluations in revision total knee arthroplasty. *Clin. Orthop. Relat. Res.* **2006**, *446*, 40–44.
4. Dy, C.J.; Bozic, K.J.; Padgett, D.E.; Pan, T.J.; Marx, R.G.; Lyman, S. Is changing hospitals for revision total joint arthroplasty associated with more complications? *Clin. Orthop. Relat. Res.* **2014**, *472*, 2006–2015. [CrossRef]
5. Wilson, N.A.; Jehn, M.; York, S.; Davis, C.M., III. Revision total hip and knee arthroplasty implant identification: Implications for use of unique device identification 2012 AAHKS member survey results. *J. Arthroplast.* **2014**, *29*, 251–255. [CrossRef] [PubMed]
6. De Bruijne, M. Machine learning approaches in medical image analysis: From detection to diagnosis. *Med. Image Anal.* **2016**, *33*, 94–97. [CrossRef] [PubMed]
7. Madabhushi, A.; Lee, G. Image analysis and machine learning in digital pathology: Challenges and opportunities. *Med. Image Anal.* **2016**, *33*, 170–175. [CrossRef] [PubMed]
8. Shen, D.; Wu, G.; Suk, H.I. Deep learning in medical image analysis. *Annu. Rev. Biomed. Eng.* **2017**, *19*, 221–248. [CrossRef] [PubMed]
9. Tiwari, A.; Yadav, A.K.; Bagaria, V. Application of deep learning algorithm in automated identification of knee arthroplasty implants from plain radiographs using transfer learning models: Are algorithms better than humans? *J. Orthop.* **2022**, *32*, 139–145. [CrossRef] [PubMed]
10. Patel, R.; Thong, E.H.; Batta, V.; Bharath, A.A.; Francis, D.; Howard, J. Automated identification of orthopedic implants on radiographs using deep learning. *Radiol. Artif. Intell.* **2021**, *3*, e200183. [CrossRef] [PubMed]
11. Ren, M.; Yi, P.H. Artificial intelligence in orthopedic implant model classification: A systematic review. *Skelet. Radiol.* **2021**, *51*, 407–416. [CrossRef] [PubMed]
12. Paul, H.Y.; Wei, J.; Kim, T.K.; Sair, H.I.; Hui, F.K.; Hager, G.D.; Fritz, J.; Oni, J.K. Automated detection & classification of knee arthroplasty using deep learning. *Knee* **2020**, *27*, 535–542.
13. Karnuta, J.M.; Haeberle, H.S.; Luu, B.C.; Roth, A.L.; Molloy, B.M.; Nystrom, L.M.; Piuzzi, N.S.; Schaffer, J.L.; Chen, A.F.; Iorio, R.; et al. Artificial intelligence to identify arthroplasty implants from radiographs of the knee. *J. Arthroplast.* **2021**, *36*, 935–940. [CrossRef] [PubMed]
14. Redmon, J.; Divvala, S.; Girshick, R.; Farhadi, A. You only look once: Unified, real-time object detection. In Proceedings of the IEEE Conference on Computer Vision and Pattern Recognition, Las Vegas, NV, USA, 27–30 June 2016; pp. 779–788.
15. COCO—Common Objects in Context. Available online: https://cocodataset.org/#home (accessed on 18 May 2020).
16. YOLOv5 Documentation. Augmentation—YOLOv5 Documentation. Available online: https://docs.ultralytics.com/FAQ/augmentation/ (accessed on 18 May 2020).
17. YOLOv5. yolov5/datasets.py. Available online: https://github.com/ultralytics/yolov5/blob/90b7895d652c3bd3d361b2d6e9aee900fd67f5f7/utils/datasets.py#L678-L732 (accessed on 18 May 2020).
18. Belete, S.C.; Batta, V.; Kunz, H. Automated classification of total knee replacement prosthesis on plain film radiograph using a deep convolutional neural network. *Inform. Med. Unlocked* **2021**, *25*, 100669. [CrossRef]
19. Sharma, S.; Batta, V.; Chidambaranathan, M.; Mathialagan, P.; Mani, G.; Kiruthika, M.; Datta, B.; Kamineni, S.; Reddy, G.; Masilamani, S.; et al. Knee Implant Identification by Fine-Tuning Deep Learning Models. *Indian J. Orthop.* **2021**, *55*, 1295–1305. [CrossRef] [PubMed]
20. Klemt, C.; Uzosike, A.C.; Cohen-Levy, W.B.; Harvey, M.J.; Subih, M.A.; Kwon, Y.-M. The Ability of Deep Learning Models to Identify Total Hip and Knee Arthroplasty Implant Design From Plain Radiographs. *J. Am. Acad. Orthop. Surg.* **2020**, *30*, 409–415. [CrossRef] [PubMed]
21. Gurung, B.; Liu, P.; Harris, P.D.R.; Sagi, A.; Field, R.E.; Sochart, D.H.; Tucker, K.; Asopa, V. Artificial intelligence for image analysis in total hip and total knee arthroplasty: A scoping review. *Bone Jt. J.* **2022**, *104*, 929–937. [CrossRef] [PubMed]

22. Kang, Y.J.; Yoo, J.I.; Cha, Y.H.; Park, C.H.; Kim, J.T. Machine learning–based identification of hip arthroplasty designs. *J. Orthop. Transl.* **2020**, *21*, 13–17. [CrossRef] [PubMed]
23. Urban, G.; Porhemmat, S.; Stark, M.; Feeley, B.; Okada, K.; Baldi, P. Classifying shoulder implants in X-ray images using deep learning. *Comput. Struct. Biotechnol. J.* **2020**, *18*, 967–972. [CrossRef] [PubMed]

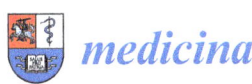

Article

Dual-Energy CT-Based Bone Mineral Density Has Practical Value for Osteoporosis Screening around the Knee

Keun Young Choi [1,2,†], Sheen-Woo Lee [3,†], Yong In [2,4], Man Soo Kim [2,4], Yong Deok Kim [1,2], Seung-yeol Lee [1,2], Jin-Woo Lee [1,2] and In Jun Koh [1,2,*]

1. Joint Replacement Center, Eunpyeong St. Mary's Hospital, Seoul 03312, Korea
2. Department of Orthopaedic Surgery, College of Medicine, The Catholic University of Korea, Seoul 06591, Korea
3. Department of Radiology, Eunpyeong St. Mary's Hospital, Seoul 03312, Korea
4. Department of Orthopaedic Surgery, Seoul St. Mary's Hospital, Seoul 06591, Korea
* Correspondence: esmh.jrcenter@gmail.com; Tel.: +82-2-2030-2655; Fax: +82-2-2030-4629
† These authors contributed equally to this work.

Abstract: *Introduction*: Adequate bone quality is essential for long term biologic fixation of cementless total knee arthroplasty (TKA). Recently, vertebral bone quality evaluation using dual-energy computed tomography (DECT) has been introduced. However, the DECT bone mineral density (BMD) in peripheral skeleton has not been correlated with Hounsfield units (HU) or central dual-energy X-ray absorptiometry (DXA), and the accuracy remains unclear. *Materials and methods*: Medical records of 117 patients who underwent TKA were reviewed. DXA was completed within three months before surgery. DECT was performed with third-generation dual source CT in dual-energy mode. Correlations between DXA, DECT BMD and HU for central and periarticular regions were analyzed. Receiver operating characteristic (ROC) curves were plotted and area under the curve (AUC), optimal threshold, and sensitivity and specificity of each region of interest (ROI) were calculated. *Results*: Central DXA BMD was correlated with DECT BMD and HU in ROIs both centrally and around the knee (all $p < 0.01$). The diagnostic accuracy of DECT BMD was higher than that of DECT HU and was also higher when the T-score for second lumbar vertebra (L2), rather than for the femur neck, was used as the reference standard (all AUC values: L2 > femur neck; DECT BMD > DECT HU, respectively). Using the DXA T-score at L2 as the reference standard, the optimal DECT BMD cut-off values for osteoporosis were 89.2 mg/cm^3 in the distal femur and 78.3 mg/cm^3 in the proximal tibia. *Conclusion*: Opportunistic volumetric BMD assessment using DECT is accurate and relatively simple, and does not require extra equipment. DECT BMD and HU are useful for osteoporosis screening before cementless TKA.

Keywords: dual-energy CT; Hounsfield unit; bone mineral density; volumetric phantomless BMD; opportunistic CT

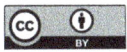

1. Introduction

The number of younger and more active patients treated with total knee arthroplasty (TKA) continues to increase rapidly [1–5], but TKA in younger patients has exhibited a lower 10-year survivorship with higher demand for revision [6–9]. Thus, long-term and biologic fixation after TKA has been revisited, and interest in cementless TKA, which theoretically enables physiologic fixation, has increased [10,11]. The earlier cementless TKA prostheses had unacceptably high failure rates and poor clinical outcomes [12,13], but major advances in design and materials in recent years have greatly improved the newer generation of cementless prostheses [14–16]. Stereo imaging analysis has shown that the new cementless prosthesis is superior to traditional press fit design and cemented prostheses in reducing micromotion, and it is anticipated that the risk of aseptic loosening will be greatly reduced [17].

Preoperative bone quality and bone mineral density (BMD) around the knee joint are strongly associated with adequate bone ingrowth and initial prosthesis stability after cementless TKA [16,18,19]. However, there is no gold standard method as yet to evaluate BMD around the knee joint. Previous study has shown that BMD around the knee can be estimated by CT attenuation in Hounsfield units (HU), which are a measure of the standardized linear attenuation coefficient of CT [20]. However, the HU-based BMD is limited due to distortion by changes in marrow composition, and diagnostic value around the knee joint remains unclear [20–23]. Dual-energy CT (DECT), which acquires CT attenuation data at two different energy levels, can generate images of soft tissue or bone marrow by decomposing different tissue characteristics [24]. It has recently been proposed as a tool to screen for osteoporosis with greater diagnostic accuracy than traditional quantitative CT (QCT) [22,25]. However, the DECT BMD for peripheral bone assessment has not been studied yet.

Therefore, the purposes of this study were (1) to assess the strength of correlation between central dual-energy X-ray absorptiometry (DXA) BMD, DECT BMD and HU at the lumbar spine, femur neck, distal femur, and proximal tibia; and (2) to calculate the diagnostic accuracy of DECT BMD and HU for bone quality assessment around the knee joint when the T-score of central DXA is used as the reference standard. We hypothesized that the volumetric BMD and HU from DECT would be well correlated with DXA BMD. We also hypothesized that the diagnostic accuracy of DECT BMD and HU in bone quality assessment around the knee joint would be high.

2. Material and Methods

A total of 125 patients who underwent TKA between November 2021 and January 2022 and had both preoperative third-generation dual-source DECT and DXA within three months before surgery were considered for study inclusion. The study was approved by the Institutional Review Board of our institute (PC22RISI0049) and it was exempted from informed consent because it is a retrospective medical and radiological record review. Patients with metal prosthesis, fracture or infection in central (spine or hip) or peripheral (distal femur or proximal tibia) regions were excluded (Figure 1). DXA at the lumbar spine and left pelvic area had been taken within 3 months before TKA (Figure 2A), and had identified osteoporosis in 11% of L2 vertebral bodies and in 14.5% of femur necks (Table 1). Lower extremity CT was performed for the purpose of preoperative planning for TKA with a measured resection technique. All CT studies were performed on a third-generation dual-source CT system in dual-energy mode (SOMATOM Force; Siemens Healthineers, Erlangen, Germany), with tube A at 90 kVp and 180 mAs and tube B at Sn150 kVp [0.64-mm tin filter] and 180 mAs. Image series were collected in a craniocaudal direction with the patient in a supine position without administration of a contrast agent. Three image sets, 90 kVp, Sn150 kVp, and weighted average (ratio 0.5:0.5), were acquired in each CT examination to resemble the contrast properties of single-energy bone CT images. The images were reconstructed with a dual-energy bone kernel (B69f), transferred to the image archiving system (SyngoVia, Siemens Healthineers, Erlangen, Germany), and then transferred to a personal computer carrying the analysis software for postprocessing.

Phantomless volumetric BMD assessment of L2 and the left femur neck with DECT requires manual delineation of trabecular volumes of interest (VOI) in the L2 vertebra and the left pelvis, which was carried out by one of the authors with dedicated software (Examine, Siemens Healthcare, Erlangen, Germany). Regions of interest (ROIs) defined to best include trabecular bone and exclude any cortical bone were also drawn manually on the images loaded into the software (Figure 2B). The software then performed calculations according to a dedicated algorithm and the resulting output included the volumetric BMD values.

For DECT HU analysis, one of the authors, working at a conventional PACS workstation, manually defined polygonal ROIs on standard bone reconstructions in sagittal or axial image series (Figure 2C). The ROIs were positioned in the anterior trabecular bone space of the L2 vertebral body, as proposed by several studies [26–28]. Thereby, the reader was instructed to avoid attenuation heterogeneity by placing the ROIs in areas of spinal hemangiomas or other causes of attenuation heterogeneity. All HU values were obtained as averages of three serial polygonal ROIs.

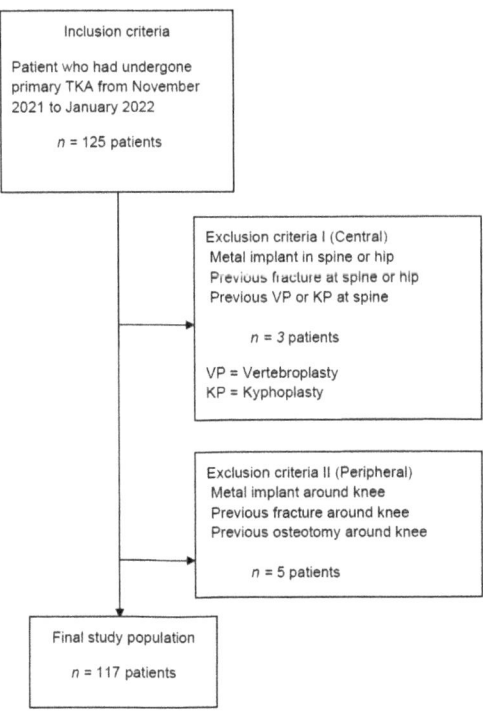

Figure 1. Standards for Reporting of Diagnostic Accuracy Studies (STARD) flow chart of patient inclusion.

Table 1. Patient demographics and preoperative characteristics.

Demographic Data	n = 117	
Age *	70.6 ± 6.5 (54~88)	
Sex (male: female) [†]	15 (13): 102 (87)	
Height (cm) *	153.7 ± 7.2 (140~178)	
Weight (kg) *	63.0 ± 10.6 (44~89)	
BMI (kg/m^2) *	26.6 ± 3.4 (21.0~35.2)	
Diagnosis of Osteoporosis (%) [†]	L2	Femur neck
Normal	44 (38)	31 (26.5)
Osteopenia	60 (51)	69 (59)
Osteoporosis	13 (11)	17 (14.5)
DXA	L2	Femur neck
BMD *	0.859 ± 0.166 (0.556~1.468)	0.640 ± 0.097 (0.451~0.945)
T-score *	−1.055 ± 1.419 (−3.7~3.3)	−1.532 ± 0.899 (−3.3~1.3)

[†] Data are presented as numbers (percentage) of patients. * Data are presented as the means ± standard deviations (range). DXA, dual x-ray absorptiometry; BMD, bone mineral density.

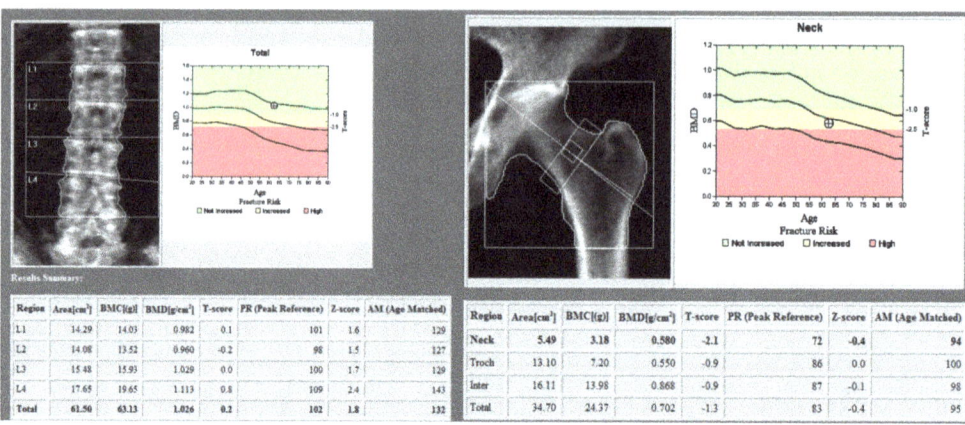

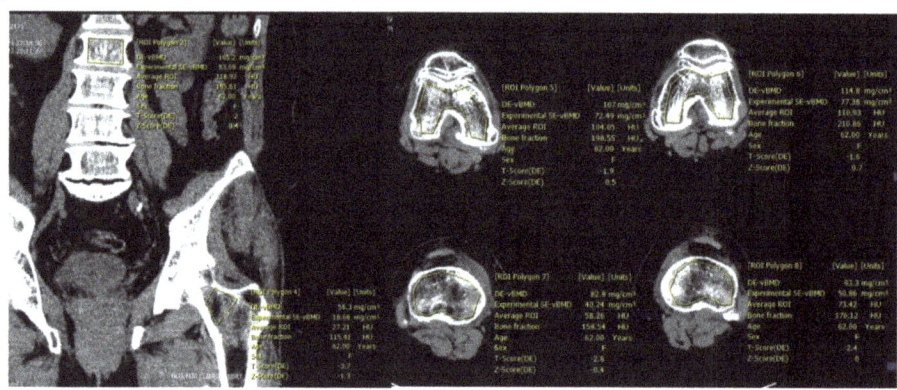

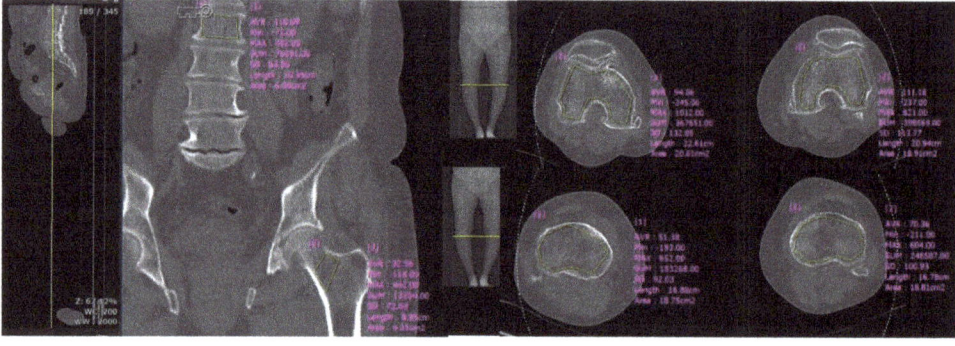

Figure 2. (**A**) Assessment of dual x-ray absorptiometry (DXA) in the lumbar spine and femur neck; (**B**) Manual definition of the region of interest (ROI) and assessment of bone mineral density (BMD) derived from dual-energy computed tomography (DECT) in the distal femur and proximal tibia using dedicated DECT postprocessing software; (**C**) Manual definition of the region of interest (ROI) and assessment of Hounsfield unit (HU) derived from dual-energy computed tomography (DECT) in the distal femur and proximal tibia using dedicated DECT postprocessing software.

Correlation between DXA BMD or T-scores for L2 or the left femur neck and DECT BMD or HU of L2, left femur neck, distal femur, and proximal tibia was analyzed and receiver-operating characteristic (ROC) curves were plotted to evaluate diagnostic accuracy. In addition, the area under the curve (AUC), optimal threshold, and sensitivity and specificity of DECT BMD and HU for distal femur and proximal tibia were determined by using the DXA T-scores for L2 and femur neck as the reference standards.

The values assessed by the researchers were obtained as the average of two evaluators. Each researcher assessed every radiological variable two times with the interval at least two weeks. Intra- and inter-observer reliability for each measurement were expressed as intraclass correlation coefficients (ICCs).

Statistical Analysis

All computations were performed with Statistical Package for Social Sciences (SPSS) version 21 (IBM Corp., Armonk, NY, USA), with significance set at $p < 0.05$. Variables are presented as mean ± standard deviation. The correlation between DXA BMD and DECT BMD or HU was analyzed by using the Pearson product moment correlation. ROC curve analysis and calculation of the AUC were performed to evaluate optimal cut-off values for distinguishing osteoporosis from normal BMD. Osteoporosis [$T < -2.5$], osteopenia [$-1.0 \leq T \leq -2.5$], and normal BMD [$T > -1.0$] were classified according to the DXA T-score. Sensitivity, specificity, positive and negative predictive values (PPV and NPV), and accuracy were computed from these cut-off values.

3. Results

Of a total of 125 patients, three patients with a history of metal implants in spine or hip, tumor or previous fracture at spine or hip, previous vertebroplasty or kyphoplasty at spine, or previous infection at spine or hip were excluded. Five patients with metal implant, previous fracture, or history of previous osteotomy around a knee were excluded. Thus, a total of 117 patients were finally included and their medical and radiographic data were reviewed (Figure 1). The mean age was 70.6 years and the mean body mass index (BMI) was 26.6 kg/m^2 (Table 1).

DXA BMD of L2 and femur neck were strongly correlated with DECT BMD and HU at their own region (all $r > 0.5$, all $p < 0.01$). In addition, the DXA BMD of L2 and the femur neck were significantly correlated with DECT BMD and HU in the other ROIs, surpassing moderate degree (all $r > 0.3$), except for the DXA BMD of the femur neck and HU of the proximal tibia ($r = 0.286$) (all $p < 0.01$) (Table 2). In addition, the correlation value (r) was higher for L2 than for the femur neck for all ROIs except for their own region.

The DECT BMD showed a stratified result from normal bone quality for osteoporosis measured by the DXA T-score in every ROI (Figure 3A–D). When the DXA T-score at L2 was used as the reference standard, the optimal cut-off values of DECT BMD for diagnosing osteoporosis were calculated as 89.2 mg/cm^3 in the distal femur and as 78.3 mg/cm^3 in the proximal tibia. In terms of DECT HU, the optimal cut-off values were 104.5 in the distal femur and 66.5 in the proximal tibia. When the DXA T-score at the left femur neck was used as the reference standard, the optimal DECT BMD cut-off values for diagnosing osteoporosis were 96.9 mg/cm^3 in the distal femur and 80.9 mg/cm^3 in the proximal tibia and the optimal cut-off values of DECT HU were 117.4 in the distal femur and 66.8 in the proximal tibia (Table 3). In addition, all AUC values of L2 surpassed femur neck and AUC values of DECT BMD surpassed DECT HU, respectively (Table 3). Thus, the diagnostic accuracy of both DECT BMD and HU was better when the DXA T-score for L2, rather than the femur neck, was used as the reference standard (Figure 4A,B).

Table 2. Correlation analysis between DECT BMD or HU and central DXA BMD or T-score.

		DXA							
		L2				Femur Neck			
		BMD (g/cm²)		T-Score		BMD (g/cm²)		T-Score	
		Pearson r	p Value	Pearson r	p Value	Pearson r	p Value	Pearson r	p Value
DECT HU	L2	0.529	<0.01	0.524	<0.01	0.417	<0.01	0.408	<0.01
	Femur neck	0.351	<0.01	0.352	<0.01	0.593	<0.01	0.578	<0.01
	Distal femur	0.458	<0.01	0.450	<0.01	0.307	<0.01	0.286	<0.01
	Proximal tibia	0.342	<0.01	0.342	<0.01	0.286	<0.01	0.267	0.015
DECT BMD (g/cm³)	L2	0.585	<0.01	0.585	<0.01	0.476	<0.01	0.479	<0.01
	Femur neck	0.379	<0.01	0.384	<0.01	0.546	<0.01	0.550	<0.01
	Distal femur	0.458	<0.01	0.446	<0.01	0.454	<0.01	0.444	<0.01
	Proximal tibia	0.466	<0.01	0.479	<0.01	0.382	<0.01	0.381	<0.01

Pearson correlation analysis demonstrated significant correlation of dual-energy computed tomography (DECT) bone mineral density (BMD) and Hounsfield unit (HU) values with DXA (dual x-ray absorptiometry)-based BMD and T-score values.

Table 3. Diagnostic accuracy of DECT BMD and HU for osteoporosis diagnosis in distal femur and proximal tibia using DXA as the reference standard.

		L2 DXA as Standard of Reference				95% CI		Femur Neck DXA as Standard of Reference				95% CI	
		AUC	Cut-Off	Sensitivity	Specificity	Min	Max	AUC	Cut-Off	Sensitivity	Specificity	Min	Max
Distal femur	DECT BMD	0.872	89.2	82%	92%	0.809	0.936	0.714	96.9	70%	71%	0.616	0.813
	DECT HU	0.796	104.5	78%	77%	0.673	0.919	0.643	117.4	67%	65%	0.503	0.783
Proximal tibia	DECT BMD	0.935	78.3	85%	85%	0.871	0.999	0.738	80.9	76%	71%	0.609	0.866
	DECT HU	0.800	66.5	75%	77%	0.706	0.894	0.697	66.8	75%	71%	0.560	0.823

AUC: area under the curve. CI: confidence intervals. BMD: bone mineral density. HU: Hounsfield unit. DXA: dual-energy X-ray absorptiometry. Min: Minimum. Max: Maximum. L2: second lumbar spine.

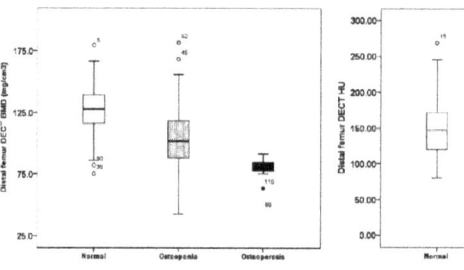

A

Figure 3. Cont.

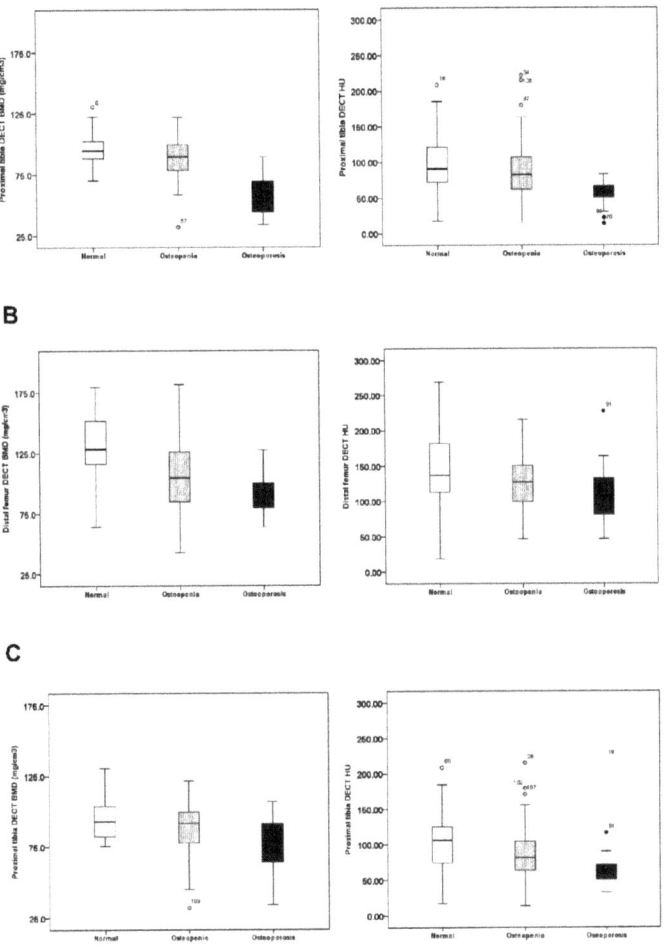

Figure 3. (**A**) Box plots of volumetric bone mineral density (BMD) and Hounsfield unit (HU) values in the distal femur derived from dual-energy computed tomography (DECT). The plots show the distribution of values that were categorized as normal BMD, osteopenia, and osteoporosis according to the dual x-ray absorptiometry (DXA)-derived T-score in the lumbar spine, which served as the reference standard; (**B**) Box plots of volumetric bone mineral density (BMD) and Hounsfield unit (HU) values in the proximal tibia derived from dual-energy computed tomography (DECT). The plots show the distribution of values that were categorized as normal BMD, osteopenia, and osteoporosis according to the dual x-ray absorptiometry (DXA)-derived T-score in the lumbar spine, which served as the reference standard; (**C**) Box plots of volumetric bone mineral density (BMD) and Hounsfield unit (HU) values in the distal femur derived from dual-energy computed tomography (DECT). The plots show the distribution of values that were categorized as normal BMD, osteopenia, and osteoporosis according to the dual x-ray absorptiometry (DXA)-derived T-score in the femur neck, which served as the reference standard; (**D**) Box plots of volumetric bone mineral density (BMD) and Hounsfield unit (HU) values in the proximal tibia derived from dual-energy computed tomography (DECT). The plots show the distribution of values that were categorized as normal BMD, osteopenia, and osteoporosis according to the dual x-ray absorptiometry (DXA)-derived T-score in the femur neck, which served as the reference standard.

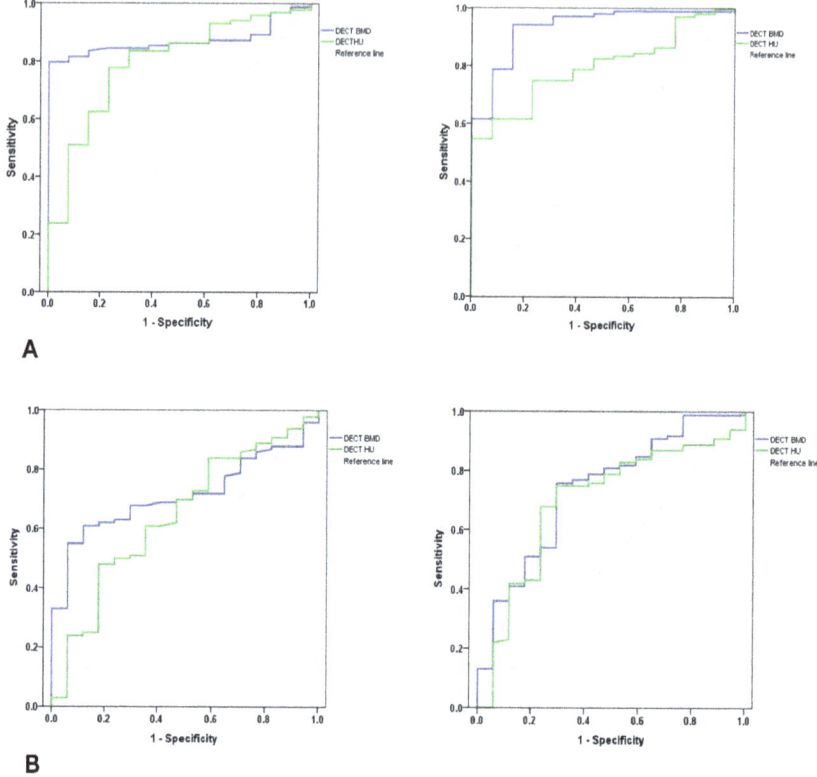

Figure 4. (**A**) Representative receiver operating characteristic (ROC) curves of phantomless volumetric bone mineral density (BMD) (blue line) values and Hounsfield unit (HU) measurements (green line) derived from dual-energy computed tomography (DECT) for the detection of osteoporosis using the dual x-ray absorptiometry (DXA) derived T-score of the lumbar spine as the reference standard. (Left: values in distal femur; Right: values in proximal tibia); (**B**) Representative receiver operating characteristic (ROC) curves of phantomless volumetric bone mineral density (BMD) (blue line) values and Hounsfield unit (HU) measurements (green line) derived from dual-energy computed tomography (DECT) for the detection of osteoporosis using the dual x-ray absorptiometry (DXA) derived T-score of the femur neck as the reference standard. (Left: values in distal femur; Right: values in proximal tibia).

Intra- and inter-observer reliability for all radiographic measurements was considered acceptable, ranging from 0.81 to 0.99 and 0.81 to 0.96, respectively.

4. Discussion

Aseptic loosening is a major cause of failure after TKA in young and active patients, and the need for optimal biological fixation of cementless prostheses is growing [1,6–9,29,30]. Preoperative poor bone quality is associated with a higher rate of micromotion and migration in cementless prostheses. Meanwhile, there is no gold standard method for evaluating bone quality in peripheral regions [19,31]. We investigated the diagnostic accuracy of DECT BMD and HU for osteoporosis around the knee and compared the DECT values with the central DXA. In addition, we calculated the optimal cut-off values of DECT BMD and HU for diagnosing osteoporosis around the knee.

We found that BMD of central DXA was significantly correlated with DECT BMD and HU in both central and peripheral ROIs. The DXA BMD and T-scores for L2 and the femur neck were strongly correlated with DECT BMD and HU in their own region (all correlation coefficients > 0.5). In addition, the DXA BMD of L2 and the femur neck were moderately correlated with DECT BMD and HU in all other ROIs, except for a weak correlation of the DXA BMD at the femur neck with DECT HU at the proximal tibia. Our results concur with previous studies reporting the correlation between DXA BMD and radiologic values obtained from opportunistic CT scans [20,26,27]. However, while a substantial number of studies have found correlations between central DXA BMD and DECT BMD or HU [20–22,26,27], it is difficult to compare those studies with ours because all of the previous studies were confined to ROIs other than the knee joint. According to our study, DECT BMD and HU were more strongly correlated with DXA BMD at L2 than at the femur neck. In addition, there was stronger correlation between DECT BMD than DECT HU with DXA BMD. These results concur with a previous study reporting a stronger correlation between DXA BMD and DECT BMD than DECT HU [21]. Our study results demonstrate that DECT can yield more accurate and precise volumetric BMD than HU, permitting opportunistic BMD measurements in routine CT scans without the need for calibration phantoms. Our results indicate that DECT for the routine preoperative evaluation of lower extremity axial alignment can also be a useful method of evaluating preoperative bone quality in patients who are about to undergo cementless TKA.

The result of this study, using DXA T-score as the reference standard, also supports the hypothesis that DECT BMD and HU can provide reliable diagnostic accuracy in assessing bone quality around the knee joint. DECT BMD provided the highest diagnostic accuracy with DXA BMD at L2 as the reference standard (all AUC values: L2 > femur neck; DECT BMD > DECT HU, respectively) (Table 3). Moreover, the reference of L2 provided more precise diagnostic value in the tibia than in the femur. This result concurs with previous studies finding that phantomless volumetric DECT BMD offered significantly more accurate BMD assessment and superior diagnostic accuracy for osteoporosis than DECT HU [21]. Our results suggest that DECT BMD has the potential to be a gold standard method for evaluation of BMD around the knee joint. However, because this finding is based on the central DXA T-score as the reference standard, further biomechanical research regarding the correlation between DECT BMD or HU and the true bone strength around the knee is required.

Interestingly, BMD evaluation using DECT may have additional benefits and possibilities compared to DXA. Although DXA has been regarded as a gold standard preferred by the International Society for Clinical Densitometry (ISCD), it has certain limitations in clinical application, and variations in body composition can lead to up to 20% error [32]. DXA cannot be used in patients with scoliosis or calcifications from chronic disease, metal implants in both hips or at multiple levels of the spine, or cement in a vertebral body. In addition, DXA is based in two dimensions, meaning it cannot distinguish cancellous bone from cortical bone quality. On the other hand, the three-dimensional DECT analysis can discriminate cancellous bone, which may comprise most of the bone-prosthesis interface between cementless TKA and cortical bone. There are already studies reporting a higher rate of successful fusion and lower rates of adjacent spine fracture following spine surgery in patients with higher HU [33–36]. Moreover, there also are studies reporting no significant difference between HU measurements on sagittal and axial CT images [27]. These previous studies may further support the possibility of utilizing DECT BMD and HU as a tool for evaluation of preoperative bone quality around the knee in patients undergoing TKA. This study assessing BMD around the knee joint proposes a novel method in evaluating bone quality around peripheral regions. Moreover, there is a possibility to expand this method to other peripheral joints. If surgeons can get information about a patient's bone quality around the knee or other peripheral joints from a preoperative CT scan, they may be able to screen for the suitability of a cementless implant and modify their technique or type of implant according to the findings. Routine preoperative DECT may be helpful for detecting unexpected poor bone quality that could provoke early prosthesis failure.

This study had several limitations. First, it was confined to an Asian population, and most of the patients undergoing TKA who were included in this study are women

(102/117, 87%), and it may be difficult to generalize our results to other ethnicities. It is not yet clear why the majority of patients with arthritis in Korea are females [37]. Second, the study was confined to middle-aged and older patients (70.6 ± 6.5, 54 to 88) because only patients who underwent TKA were included. Third, although there was significant correlation between DXA BMD and DECT BMD, the clinical meaning of DECT BMD values remains unclear. As a way to overcome this limitation, further study examining the direct correlation between DECT BMD values and the properties of actual bone is required. Fourth, there are concerns of increased radiation exposure by utilizing DECT. However, DECT has been reported not to increase radiation exposure compared with single energy CT [38]. In addition, preoperative lower extremity CT is already part of the routine preoperative planning protocol for TKA by measured resection technique. Thus, the opportunistic measurement of BMD around the knee using DECT does not seem to increase radiation exposure compared with standard clinical practice. Fifth, because of the small study population, it is possible that the study was underpowered and subject to type-II error with respect to detecting all relevant outcomes. Sixth, analysis on factors possibly affecting BMD is not done in this study. Further study focused on the possible factors is required to expand the clinical relevance and would provide more valuable information. Finally, there is a possibility of limited reproducibility because of discrepancies in HU and BMD values among institutions with different CT scanners, DXA devices, and software [20]. Nonetheless, it is still possible to use DECT BMD as a tool to evaluate BMD around the knee, and despite these limitations, our study appears to provide valuable information on the practical use of DECT for osteoporosis screening around the knee in patients scheduled for cementless TKA.

5. Conclusions

Volumetric BMD assessment using DECT is accurate, relatively simple, and does not require further equipment. DECT BMD and HU are useful tools for osteoporosis screening before cementless TKA in clinical practice. Further research focused on the correspondence between the actual bone quality of the distal femur and proximal tibia and DECT BMD and HU is required to expand the clinical relevance.

Author Contributions: Data curation, I.J.K. and S.-W.L.; Software, S.-W.L.; Investigation, K.Y.C., Y.I., M.S.K., Y.D.K., S.-y.L. and J.-W.L.; Supervision, I.J.K.; Visualization, K.Y.C.; Writing—original draft, K.Y.C.; Writing—review and editing, K.Y.C., S.-W.L. and I.J.K. All authors have read and agreed to the published version of the manuscript.

Funding: This research was supported by a grant funded by The Catholic University of Korea, Eunpyeong St. Mary's Hospital, Research Institute of Medical Science in program year 2022. (EPSMH-C-2022-01).

Institutional Review Board Statement: The study was conducted according to the guidelines of the Declaration of Helsinki and approved by the Institutional Review Board of Eunpyeong St. Mary's Hospital (PC22RISI0049, 2018-05-04).

Informed Consent Statement: Patient consent was waived because this study is a retrospective medical and radiologic record review.

Data Availability Statement: Data collected for this study, including individual patient data, will not be made available.

Acknowledgments: We thank Seongyong Pak, Siemens Healthcare, for technical consultation.

Conflicts of Interest: The authors declare no conflict of interest.

References

1. Shah, S.H.; Schwartz, B.E.; Schwartz, A.R.; Goldberg, B.A.; Chmell, S.J. Total Knee Arthroplasty in the Younger Patient. *J. Knee Surg.* **2017**, *30*, 555–559. [PubMed]
2. Roof, M.A.; Kreinces, J.B.; Schwarzkopf, R.; Rozell, J.C.; Aggarwal, V.K. Are there avoidable causes of early revision total knee arthroplasty? *Knee Surg. Relat. Res.* **2022**, *34*, 29. [CrossRef] [PubMed]

3. Lee, S.H.; Kim, D.H.; Lee, Y.S. Is there an optimal age for total knee arthroplasty? A systematic review. *Knee Surg. Relat. Res.* **2020**, *32*, 60. [CrossRef] [PubMed]
4. Kulshrestha, V.; Sood, M.; Kumar, S.; Sood, N.; Kumar, P.; Padhi, P.P. Does Risk Mitigation Reduce 90-Day Complications in Patients Undergoing Total Knee Arthroplasty? A Cohort Study. *Clin. Orthop. Surg.* **2022**, *14*, 56–68. [CrossRef] [PubMed]
5. Kulshrestha, V.; Sood, M.; Kanade, S.; Kumar, S.; Datta, B.; Mittal, G. Early Outcomes of Medial Pivot Total Knee Arthroplasty Compared to Posterior-Stabilized Design: A Randomized Controlled Trial. *Clin. Orthop. Surg.* **2020**, *12*, 178–186. [CrossRef] [PubMed]
6. Rand, J.A.; Trousdale, R.T.; Ilstrup, D.M.; Harmsen, W.S. Factors affecting the durability of primary total knee prostheses. *J. Bone Jt. Surgery. Am. Vol.* **2003**, *85*, 259–265. [CrossRef] [PubMed]
7. Annette, W.D.; Robertsson, O.; Lidgren, L. Surgery for knee osteoarthritis in younger patients. *Acta Orthop.* **2010**, *81*, 161–164.
8. Parvizi, J.; Nunley, R.M.; Berend, K.R.; Lombardi, A.V., Jr.; Ruh, E.L.; Clohisy, J.C.; Hamilton, W.G.; Della Valle, C.J.; Barrack, R.L. High level of residual symptoms in young patients after total knee arthroplasty. *Clin. Orthop. Relat. Res.* **2014**, *472*, 133–137. [CrossRef] [PubMed]
9. Bisschop, R.; Brouwer, R.W.; Van Raay, J.J. Total knee arthroplasty in younger patients: A 13-year follow-up study. *Orthopedics* **2010**, *33*, 876. [CrossRef] [PubMed]
10. Kamath, A.F.; Siddiqi, A.; Malkani, A.L.; Krebs, V.E. Cementless Fixation in Primary Total Knee Arthroplasty: Historical Perspective to Contemporary Application. *J. Am. Acad. Orthop. Surg.* **2021**, *29*, e363–e379. [CrossRef]
11. Grau, L.C.; Ong, A.C.; Restrepo, S.; Griffiths, S.Z.; Hozack, W.J.; Smith, E.B. Survivorship, Clinical and Radiographic Outcomes of a Novel Cementless Metal-Backed Patella Design. *J. Arthroplast.* **2021**, *36*, S221–s226. [CrossRef] [PubMed]
12. Berger, R.A.; Lyon, J.H.; Jacobs, J.J.; Barden, R.M.; Berkson, E.M.; Sheinkop, M.B.; Rosenberg, A.G.; Galante, J.O. Problems with cementless total knee arthroplasty at 11 years followup. *Clin. Orthop. Relat. Res.* **2001**, *392*, 196–207. [CrossRef] [PubMed]
13. Robertsson, O.; Bizjajeva, S.; Fenstad, A.M.; Furnes, O.; Lidgren, L.; Mehnert, F.; Odgaard, A.; Pedersen, A.B.; Havelin, L.I. Knee arthroplasty in Denmark, Norway and Sweden. A pilot study from the Nordic Arthroplasty Register Association. *Acta Orthop.* **2010**, *81*, 82–89. [CrossRef] [PubMed]
14. Søballe, K.; Hansen, E.S.; Brockstedt-Rasmussen, H.; Bünger, C. Hydroxyapatite coating converts fibrous tissue to bone around loaded implants. *J. Bone Jt. Surgery. Br. Vol.* **1993**, *75*, 270–278. [CrossRef] [PubMed]
15. Chen, C.; Shi, Y.; Wu, Z.; Gao, Z.; Chen, Y.; Guo, C.; Bao, X. Long-term effects of cemented and cementless fixations of total knee arthroplasty: A meta-analysis and systematic review of randomized controlled trials. *J. Orthop. Surg. Res.* **2021**, *16*, 590. [CrossRef] [PubMed]
16. Bobyn, J.D.; Stackpool, G.J.; Hacking, S.A.; Tanzer, M.; Krygier, J.J. Characteristics of bone ingrowth and interface mechanics of a new porous tantalum biomaterial. *J. Bone Jt. Surgery. Br. Vol.* **1999**, *81*, 907–914. [CrossRef]
17. Nakama, G.Y.; Peccin, M.S.; Almeida, G.J.; Lira Neto Ode, A.; Queiroz, A.A.; Navarro, R.D. Cemented, cementless or hybrid fixation options in total knee arthroplasty for osteoarthritis and other non-traumatic diseases. *Cochrane Database Syst. Rev.* **2012**, *10*, Cd006193. [CrossRef] [PubMed]
18. Petersen, M.M.; Nielsen, P.T.; Lebech, A.; Toksvig-Larsen, S.; Lund, B. Preoperative bone mineral density of the proximal tibia and migration of the tibial component after uncemented total knee arthroplasty. *J. Arthroplast.* **1999**, *14*, 77–81. [CrossRef]
19. Andersen, M.R.; Winther, N.S.; Lind, T.; Schrøder, H.M.; Flivik, G.; Petersen, M.M. Low Preoperative BMD Is Related to High Migration of Tibia Components in Uncemented TKA-92 Patients in a Combined DEXA and RSA Study With 2-Year Follow-Up. *J. Arthroplast.* **2017**, *32*, 2141–2146. [CrossRef] [PubMed]
20. Gausden, E.B.; Nwachukwu, B.U.; Schreiber, J.J.; Lorich, D.G.; Lane, J.M. Opportunistic Use of CT Imaging for Osteoporosis Screening and Bone Density Assessment: A Qualitative Systematic Review. *J. Bone Jt. Surgery. Am. Vol.* **2017**, *99*, 1580–1590. [CrossRef] [PubMed]
21. Booz, C.; Noeske, J.; Albrecht, M.H.; Lenga, L.; Martin, S.S.; Yel, I.; Huizinga, N.A.; Vogl, T.J.; Wichmann, J.L. Diagnostic accuracy of quantitative dual-energy CT-based bone mineral density assessment in comparison to Hounsfield unit measurements using dual x-ray absorptiometry as standard of reference. *Eur. J. Radiol.* **2020**, *132*, 109321. [CrossRef] [PubMed]
22. Koch, V.; Hokamp, N.G.; Albrecht, M.H.; Gruenewald, L.D.; Yel, I.; Borggrefe, J.; Wesarg, S.; Eichler, K.; Burck, I.; Gruber-Rouh, T.; et al. Accuracy and precision of volumetric bone mineral density assessment using dual-source dual-energy versus quantitative CT: A phantom study. *Eur. Radiol. Exp.* **2021**, *5*, 43. [CrossRef] [PubMed]
23. Mazess, R.B. Errors in measuring trabecular bone by computed tomography due to marrow and bone composition. *Calcif. Tissue Int.* **1983**, *35*, 148–152. [CrossRef] [PubMed]
24. Rajiah, P.; Sundaram, M.; Subhas, N. Dual-Energy CT in Musculoskeletal Imaging: What Is the Role Beyond Gout? *AJR Am. J. Roentgenol.* **2019**, *213*, 493–505. [CrossRef]
25. Gruenewald, L.D.; Koch, V.; Martin, S.S.; Yel, I.; Eichler, K.; Gruber-Rouh, T.; Lenga, L.; Wichmann, J.L.; Alizadeh, L.S.; Albrecht, M.H.; et al. Diagnostic accuracy of quantitative dual-energy CT-based volumetric bone mineral density assessment for the prediction of osteoporosis-associated fractures. *Eur. Radiol.* **2022**, *32*, 3076–3084. [CrossRef] [PubMed]
26. Pickhardt, P.J.; Pooler, B.D.; Lauder, T.; del Rio, A.M.; Bruce, R.J.; Binkley, N. Opportunistic screening for osteoporosis using abdominal computed tomography scans obtained for other indications. *Ann. Intern. Med.* **2013**, *158*, 588–595. [CrossRef]

27. Lee, S.J.; Binkley, N.; Lubner, M.G.; Bruce, R.J.; Ziemlewicz, T.J.; Pickhardt, P.J. Opportunistic screening for osteoporosis using the sagittal reconstruction from routine abdominal CT for combined assessment of vertebral fractures and density. *Osteoporos. Int. J. Establ. Result Coop. Between Eur. Found. Osteoporos. Natl. Osteoporos. Found. USA* **2016**, *27*, 1131–1136. [CrossRef]
28. Garner, H.W.; Paturzo, M.M.; Gaudier, G.; Pickhardt, P.J.; Wessell, D.E. Variation in Attenuation in L1 Trabecular Bone at Different Tube Voltages: Caution Is Warranted When Screening for Osteoporosis With the Use of Opportunistic CT. *AJR Am. J. Roentgenol.* **2017**, *208*, 165–170. [CrossRef]
29. Julin, J.; Jämsen, E.; Puolakka, T.; Konttinen, Y.T.; Moilanen, T. Younger age increases the risk of early prosthesis failure following primary total knee replacement for osteoarthritis. A follow-up study of 32,019 total knee replacements in the Finnish Arthroplasty Register. *Acta Orthop.* **2010**, *81*, 413–419. [CrossRef] [PubMed]
30. Harwin, S.F.; Elmallah, R.K.; Jauregui, J.J.; Cherian, J.J.; Mont, M.A. Outcomes of a Newer-Generation Cementless Total Knee Arthroplasty Design. *Orthopedics* **2015**, *38*, 620–624. [CrossRef]
31. Kanis, D.R.; Ratner, M.A.; Marks, T.J.J.C.R. Design and construction of molecular assemblies with large second-order optical nonlinearities. *Quantum Chem. Asp.* **1994**, *94*, 195–242.
32. Yu, E.W.; Thomas, B.J.; Brown, J.K.; Finkelstein, J.S. Simulated increases in body fat and errors in bone mineral density measurements by DXA and QCT. *J. Bone Miner. Res. Off. J. Am. Soc. Bone Miner. Res.* **2012**, *27*, 119–124. [CrossRef]
33. Kim, D.H.; Shanti, N.; Tantorski, M.E.; Shaw, J.D.; Li, L.; Martha, J.F.; Thomas, A.J.; Parazin, S.J.; Rencus, T.C.; Kwon, B. Association between degenerative spondylolisthesis and spinous process fracture after interspinous process spacer surgery. *Spine J. Off. J. N. Am. Spine Soc.* **2012**, *12*, 466–472. [CrossRef]
34. Schreiber, J.J.; Hughes, A.P.; Taher, F.; Girardi, F.P. An association can be found between hounsfield units and success of lumbar spine fusion. *HSS J. Musculoskelet. J. Hosp. Spec. Surg.* **2014**, *10*, 25–29. [CrossRef] [PubMed]
35. Meredith, D.S.; Schreiber, J.J.; Taher, F.; Cammisa, F.P., Jr.; Girardi, F.P. Lower preoperative Hounsfield unit measurements are associated with adjacent segment fracture after spinal fusion. *Spine* **2013**, *38*, 415–418. [CrossRef] [PubMed]
36. Nguyen, H.S.; Shabani, S.; Patel, M.; Maiman, D. Posterolateral lumbar fusion: Relationship between computed tomography Hounsfield units and symptomatic pseudoarthrosis. *Surg. Neurol. Int.* **2015**, *6*, S611–S614. [CrossRef] [PubMed]
37. Koh, I.J.; Kim, T.K.; Chang, C.B.; Cho, H.J.; In, Y. Trends in use of total knee arthroplasty in Korea from 2001 to 2010. *Clin. Orthop. Relat. Res.* **2013**, *471*, 1441–1450. [CrossRef] [PubMed]
38. Lenga, L.; Leithner, D.; Peterke, J.L.; Albrecht, M.H.; Gudauskas, T.; D'Angelo, T.; Booz, C.; Hammerstingl, R.; Vogl, T.J.; Martin, S.S.; et al. Comparison of Radiation Dose and Image Quality of Contrast-Enhanced Dual-Source CT of the Chest: Single-Versus Dual-Energy and Second-Versus Third-Generation Technology. *AJR Am. J. Roentgenol.* **2019**, *212*, 741–747. [CrossRef]

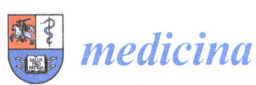

Article

Guided-Motion Bicruciate-Stabilized Total Knee Arthroplasty Reproduces Native Medial Collateral Ligament Strain

Dai-Soon Kwak [1], Yong Deok Kim [2,3], Nicole Cho [4], Ho-Jung Cho [1], Jaeryong Ko [2,3], Minji Kim [5], Jae Hyuk Choi [5], Dohyung Lim [5] and In Jun Koh [2,3,*]

1. Catholic Institute for Applied Anatomy, Department of Anatomy, College of Medicine, The Catholic University of Korea, Seoul 06591, Republic of Korea
2. Joint Replacement Center, Eunpyeong St. Mary's Hospital, Seoul 03312, Republic of Korea
3. Department of Orthopaedic Surgery, College of Medicine, The Catholic University of Korea, Seoul 06591, Republic of Korea
4. Boston College, Morrissey College of Arts and Sciences, Chestnut Hill, MA 02467, USA
5. Department of Mechanical Engineering, Sejong University, Seoul 05006, Republic of Korea
* Correspondence: esmh.jrcenter@gmail.com; Tel.: +82-2-2030-2655; Fax: +82-2-2030-4629

Abstract: *Background and Objectives*: Guided-motion bicruciate-stabilized (BCS) total knee arthroplasty (TKA) includes a dual cam-post mechanism with an asymmetric bearing geometry that promotes normal knee kinematics and enhances anterior-posterior stability. However, it is unclear whether the improved biomechanics after guided-motion BCS TKA reproduce soft tissue strain similar to the strain generated by native knees. The purpose of this cadaveric study was to compare medial collateral ligament (MCL) strain between native and guided-motion BCS TKA knees using a video extensometer. *Materials and Methods*: Eight cadaver knees were mounted onto a customized knee squatting simulator to measure MCL strain during flexion in both native and guided-motion BCS TKA knees (Journey II-BCS; Smith & Nephew, Memphis, TN, USA). MCL strain was measured using a video extensometer (Mercury® RT RealTime tracking system, Sobriety s.r.o, Kuřim, Czech Republic). MCL strain level and strain distribution during knee flexion were compared between the native and guided-motion BCS TKA conditions. *Results*: The mean and peak MCL strain were similar between native and guided-motion BCS TKA knees at all flexion angles ($p > 0.1$). MCL strain distribution was similar between native and BCS TKA knees at 8 of 9 regions of interest (ROIs), while higher MCL strain was observed after BCS TKA than in the native knee at 1 ROI in the mid portion of the MCL at early flexion angles ($p < 0.05$ at $\leq 30°$ of flexion). *Conclusions*: Guided-motion BCS TKA restored the amount and distribution of MCL strain to the values observed on native knees.

Keywords: knee; medial collateral ligament; strain; video extensometer; total knee arthroplasty

Citation: Kwak, D.-S.; Kim, Y.D.; Cho, N.; Cho, H.-J.; Ko, J.; Kim, M.; Choi, J.H.; Lim, D.; Koh, I.J. Guided-Motion Bicruciate-Stabilized Total Knee Arthroplasty Reproduces Native Medial Collateral Ligament Strain. *Medicina* **2022**, *58*, 1751. https://doi.org/10.3390/medicina58121751

Academic Editor: Jose Antonio de Paz

Received: 25 October 2022
Accepted: 26 November 2022
Published: 29 November 2022

Publisher's Note: MDPI stays neutral with regard to jurisdictional claims in published maps and institutional affiliations.

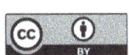

Copyright: © 2022 by the authors. Licensee MDPI, Basel, Switzerland. This article is an open access article distributed under the terms and conditions of the Creative Commons Attribution (CC BY) license (https://creativecommons.org/licenses/by/4.0/).

1. Introduction

Despite advancements in total knee arthroplasty (TKA), many patients have residual symptoms or unsatisfactory outcomes after TKA [1–6]. Recently, guided-motion bicruciate-stabilized (BCS) TKA, which involves asymmetric bearing geometry and dual substitution for the anterior cruciate ligament (ACL) and posterior cruciate ligament, has been introduced [7–9]. Guided-motion BCS TKA has an asymmetric femoral component, a polyethylene insert with 3° of tibial varus, a medially concave and laterally convex shape, and a dual cam-post mechanism (Figure 1). The goal of guided-motion BCS TKA is to facilitate guided motion that is closest to normal knee kinematics. A growing body of evidence supports that guided-motion BCS TKA can mimic native knee kinematics, improve recovery and activity, and provide more natural knee sensations compared to conventional TKA [5,6,8–11]. However, the biomechanical mechanisms that underlie these improved results remain unclear.

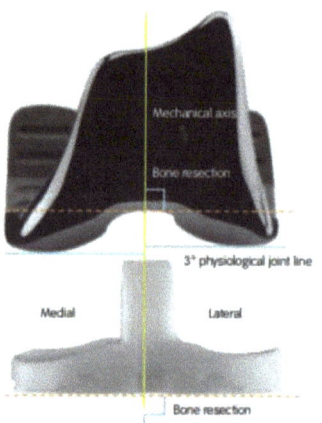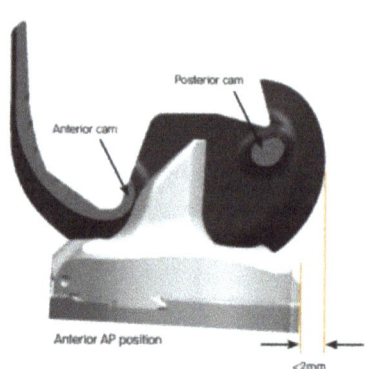

Figure 1. The JOURNEYTM II Bi-cruciate Stabilized Total Knee System (Smith & Nephew, Memphis, TN, USA) has an asymmetric femoral component, a polyethylene insert replicating 3° of the tibial varus, a medially concave and laterally convex shape, and a dual cam-post mechanism.

As the medial collateral ligament (MCL) plays critical roles in primary restraint against mechanical stresses and neurosensory feedback, changes in MCL tension after TKA affect postoperative kinematics and outcomes. Therefore, restoration of appropriate MCL strain is essential for optimal performance after TKA. Despite the significant influence of the ACL on restoring native knee kinematics, most TKA designs sacrifice the ACL without providing a substitute for its function. In the conventional ACL-deficient TKA design, the MCL and remaining capsular structures provide restraint against anterior tibial translation. Previous studies have reported that MCL strain, compared to native knees, worsened after conventional ACL-deficient TKA [12–18]. Theoretically, BCS TKA may restore post-TKA MCL strain to levels observed in native knees by enhancing anterior-posterior stability. However, no previous studies have investigated the changes in MCL strain after BCS TKA, and it is unclear whether BCS TKA restores native strain of the MCL.

The purpose of this study was to compare MCL strain between native knees and guided-motion BCS TKA knees using a video extensometer, a highly accurate tool for measuring surface strain in human cadavers [19,20]. We hypothesized that guided-motion BCS TKA would restore the strain level and distribution of the MCL to the values observed in native healthy knees.

2. Materials and Methods

Eight fresh-frozen knees from eight men with a mean age of 79 years (range: 49–96 years) were used. The specimens were macroscopically intact and did not exhibit any gross pathology. The specimens were frozen at −20 °C until the evening before dissection, when they were thawed at room temperature. The lower extremity specimens were prepared by disarticulating the hip joint; high-resolution photographs were obtained to measure the preoperative hip-knee-ankle axis. The hip-knee-ankle axis showed a varus angle of $1.3 \pm 3.2°$ (range: varus 4° to valgus 6°). The skin and subcutaneous tissue were dissected without damage to the extensor mechanism, retinaculum, knee capsule, or periarticular soft tissues. The quadriceps femoris was separated into the vastus medialis, rectus femoris/vastus intermedius, and vastus lateralis. The hamstring muscles were separated into the biceps femoris and semimembranosus/semitendinosus. The separated muscle branches were sutured using wire to connect the muscles and allow transmission of force. The femur was cut 30 cm proximal to the joint line; the tibia was cut 25 cm distal to the joint line. The ends of the femur and tibia were anatomically positioned and a cylindrical resin mold (Z-Grip, Evercoat, OH, USA) was created to mount the knee squatting simulator. Each specimen was securely mounted in its original axial alignment on a customized knee squatting simulator system (RNX & Corentec, Seoul, Republic of Korea) based on the original Oxford rig (Figure 2) [21]. This system, which is an opened loop control system with a motor type actuator with 7.5°/sec angular velocity, produced continuous flexion-extension motion while permitting physiological muscle loading and 6° of freedom positioning. The multi-plane loading of the quadriceps and hamstring muscles was used to simulate physiological loading of the knee joint (vastus medialis 51 N, rectus femoris/ vastus intermedius 87 N, and vastus lateralis 77 N, biceps femoris 31 N, semimembranosus/ semitendinosus 54 N). The total loading was 300 N [17]. These loading parameters were based on the ratios of the physiological cross-sectional area of the muscles as described in a previous anatomical study [22]. The muscles were loaded in a multiplanar fashion as described in previous studies [23,24].

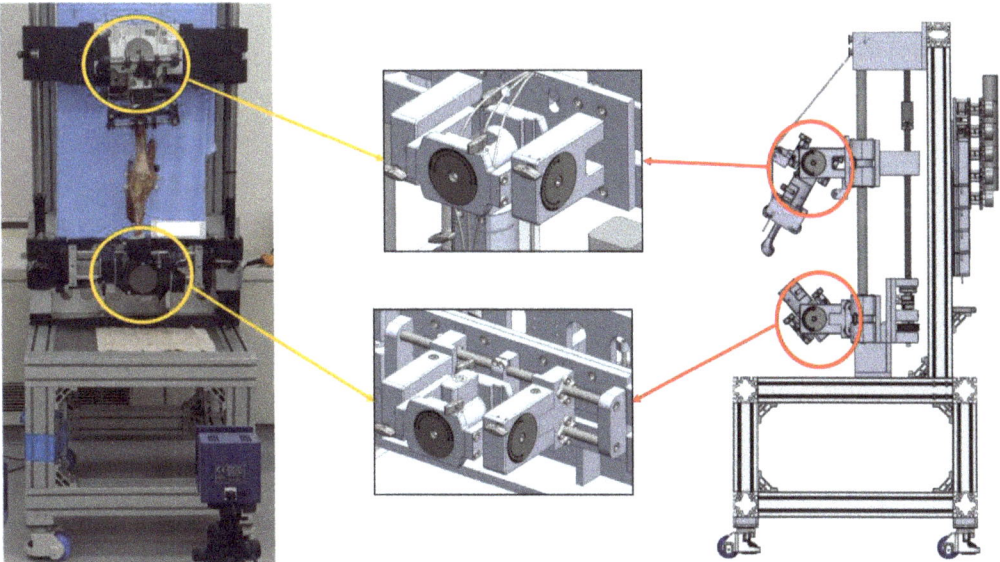

Figure 2. Schematic drawing of knee squatting simulator with six degrees-of-freedom.

A single experienced surgeon (one of authors) performed the arthroplasties using the JOURNEY™ II Bi-cruciate Stabilized Total Knee System (Smith & Nephew, Memphis, TN, USA). A subvastus approach was used to expose the knee joint, whereas the patellae were left un-resurfaced. TKA was performed using the conventional measured resection technique. The distal femur was resected using individualized intramedullary instrumentation based on the difference between the mechanical and anatomical axes of the specimen. The trans-epicondylar axis served as a reference to determine the extent of external rotation of the femoral component. Coronal and sagittal resection of the proximal tibia was performed using extramedullary instrumentation at a cutting angle of 90° to the tibial axis. Finally, flexion gaps at 0 and 90° were measured using a tensor device (B Braun-Aesculap, Tuttlingen, Germany) with a 200-N distraction force [25].

The superficial MCL was identified as previously described, then stained with multiple random speckles prior to measurement of MCL strain [18,26]. Real-time changes in MCL strain during flexion were analyzed using a non-contact video extensometer that consisted of a high-resolution digital camera (ISG, MONET 3D, Sobriety s.r.o, Czech Republic) and real-time image processing software (ISG, Mercury RT x64 2.7, Sobriety s.r.o). The camera was installed 1 m from the specimen to produce a field of view of 485 (w) × 383 mm and resolution of 1.87 μm. Illumination was minimized by performing the tests in darkness under two 36-watt light-emitting diode lights (Figure 3). MCL strain was measured at knee flexion angles of 0–120°, at intervals of 15°. Repeatability was checked in real-time to raise reliability. Each measurement was performed in three flexion-extension cycles and all of graphs following each of the three cycles were plotted at the same time. The patterns of all three cycles were compared and repeatability was analyzed. After repeatability was confirmed, data from the 3rd cycle were used for statistical analyses in all specimens. The native and post-TKA MCL strains were compared in terms of quantity and distribution. The mean MCL strain was determined by measuring the strain over the entire MCL and the peak MCL strain at one-fourth of the entire MCL area. The distribution of MCL strain was evaluated by measuring MCL strain at 9 regions of interest (ROIs), drawn by dividing the ligament vertically (front to back) into equal anterior (A), middle (M), and posterior (P) regions, and horizontally (top to bottom) into equal regions numbered 1–3. MCL strain was measured in all specimens before and after arthroplasty.

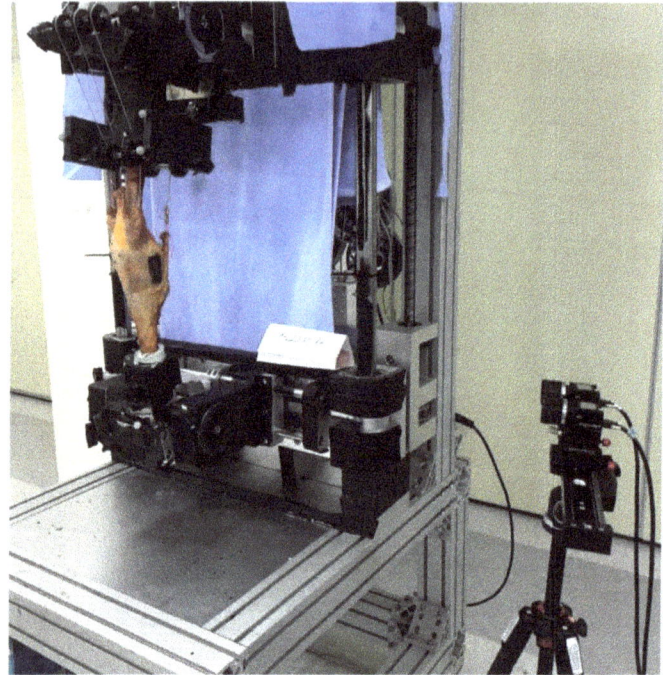

Figure 3. Experimental setup for biomechanical testing. A high-resolution digital camera was installed 1 m from the specimen, which was mounted onto a customized knee squatting simulator system.

Statistical Analysis

Data are presented as means ± standard deviations. Paired t-tests were used to determine whether the mean and peak MCL strains differed between native and post-TKA knee specimens. The Shapiro–Wilk test confirmed that this data set was normally distributed. The variables subjected to multiple between-group comparisons included the mean, peak, and distribution of MCL strain, which were analyzed using repeated-measures ANOVA, followed by the Bonferroni corrected post hoc test in order to protect against multiple comparison bias. In addition, paired t-tests were used to determine differences in the distribution of MCL strain at 9 ROIs between native and BCS TKA knee specimens. Data analysis was performed using SPSS software for Windows (ver. 26.0; IBM Corp., Armonk, NY, USA). $p < 0.05$ was considered to indicate statistical significance. A priori power analysis based on the results of our previous study of changes in the MCL strain in native knees was performed to determine the necessary sample size to achieve sufficient statistical power. Using a two-sided hypothesis test at an alpha level of 0.05 and power of 80%, 7 knees were required to detect a 5% difference. A 5% change was considered biomechanically meaningful since ligament damage occurs at 5% strain [27].

3. Results

Guided-motion BCS TKA restored the mean and peak MCL strain to the levels present in native knees during knee flexion. Guided-motion BCS TKA provided mean strain measurements similar to the levels in native knees at all flexion angles [Mean (SD) native vs. J2 BCS mean MCL strain (%) at 15°, 2.4 (1.5) vs. 3.5 (1.1), $p = 0.96$; at 30°, 3.7 (2.7) vs. 5.2 (2.4), $p = 0.43$; at 45°, 4.5 (3.0) vs. 6.0 (3.0), $p = 0.48$; at 60°, 5.1 (3.1) vs. 6.6 (3.7), $p = 0.56$; at 75°, 5.4 (3.4) vs. 7.1 (4.4), $p = 0.64$; at 90°, 5.6 (3.5) vs. 7.6 (5.2), $p = 0.72$; at 105°, 5.9 (3.7) vs. 8.0 (5.7), $p = 0.88$; at 120°, 5.9 (3.9) vs. 8.2 (5.9), $p = 0.80$] (Figure 4). The peak strains at one-fourth of the MCL area were similar between guided-motion BCS TKA and native knees [Mean (SD) native vs. J2 BCS peak MCL strain (%) at 15°, 5.3 (4.3) vs. 7.7 (3.4), $p = 0.32$; at 30°, 11.5 (10.9) vs. 14.3 (13.9), $p = 0.87$; at 45°, 14.6 (11.1) vs. 17.2 (16.7), $p = 0.92$; at 60°, 17.3 (11.4) vs. 19.1 (17.3), $p = 0.96$; at 75°, 18.6 (12.0) vs. 20.6 (17.5), $p = 0.99$; at 90°, 19.4 (12.5) vs. 21.3 (17.4), $p = 0.93$; at 105°, 20.3 (12.3) vs. 21.4 (16.4), $p = 0.70$; at 120°, 20.6 (12.0) vs. 20.8 (14.2), $p = 0.94$] (Figure 5).

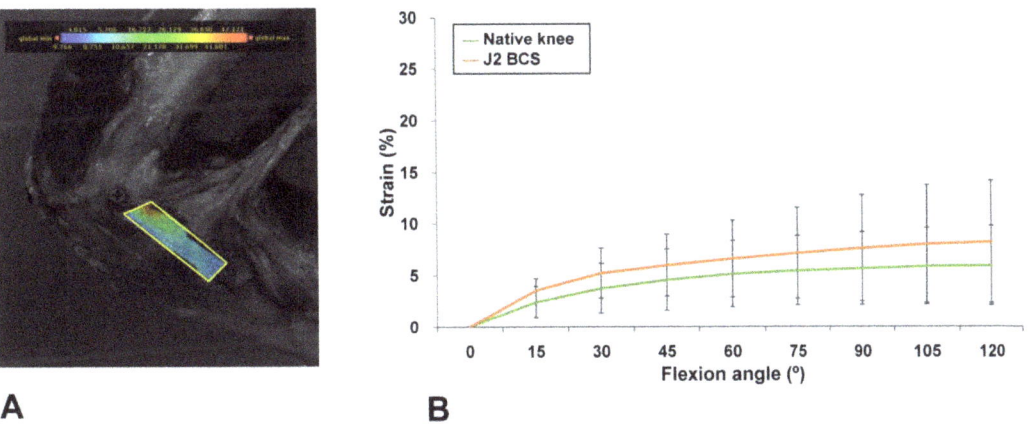

Figure 4. Area for mean MCL strain measurements (**A**) and comparisons of mean MCL strain between native and BCS TKA knees (**B**). The mean strain after BCS TKA was similar to the mean strain in native knees at all flexion angles. Error bars indicate standard deviations. The correspondence between color and strain is shown in the color bar.

Guided-motion BCS TKA restored the native knee MCL strain distribution. Significant strain differences between guided-motion BCS TKA and native knees were observed in 1 of the 9 ROIs (i.e., at M2). In this ROI, strain was higher after guided-motion BCS TKA than in native knees only at ≤30° of flexion [Mean (SD) native vs. J2 BCS MCL strain at M2 (%) at 15°, 0.69 (0.21) vs. 2.4 (0.4), $p = 0.048$; at 30°, 0.74 (0.30) vs. 2.9 (0.6), $p = 0.024$; at 45°, 1.3 (0.4) vs. 3.2 (0.7), $p = 0.12$; at 60°, 1.7 (0.5) vs. 3.4 (0.9), $p = 0.32$; at 75°, 1.9 (0.6) vs. 3.7 (1.2), $p = 0.72$; at 90°, 2.0 (0.7) vs. 3.9 (1.5), $p = 0.93$; at 105°, 2.0 (0.7) vs. 4.3 (1.9), $p = 0.99$; at 120°, 1.9 (0.7) vs. 4.6 (2.0), $p = 0.94$] (Figure 6).

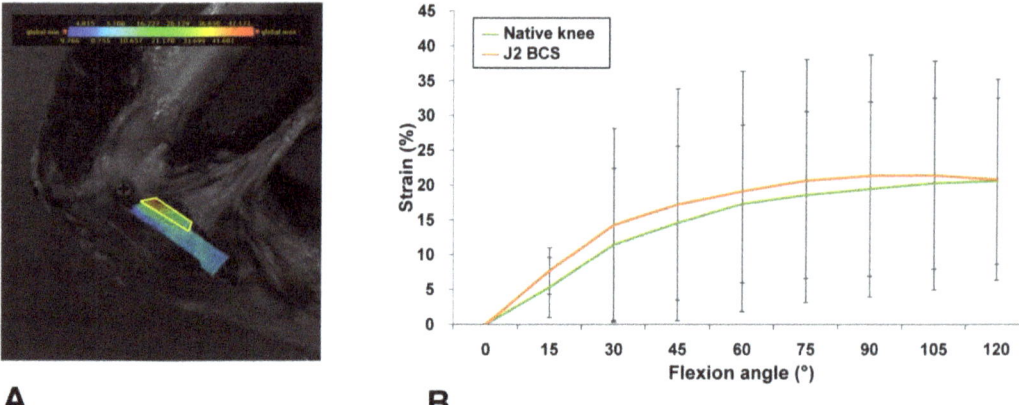

Figure 5. Area for peak MCL strain measurements (**A**) and comparisons of peak MCL strain between native and BCS TKA knees (**B**). The peak strain was measured at one-fourth of the entire MCL area, including the highest MCL strain portion. The peak MCL strain after BCS TKA was similar to the peak MCL strain of native knees at all flexion angles. Error bars indicate standard deviations. The correspondence between color and strain is shown in the color bar.

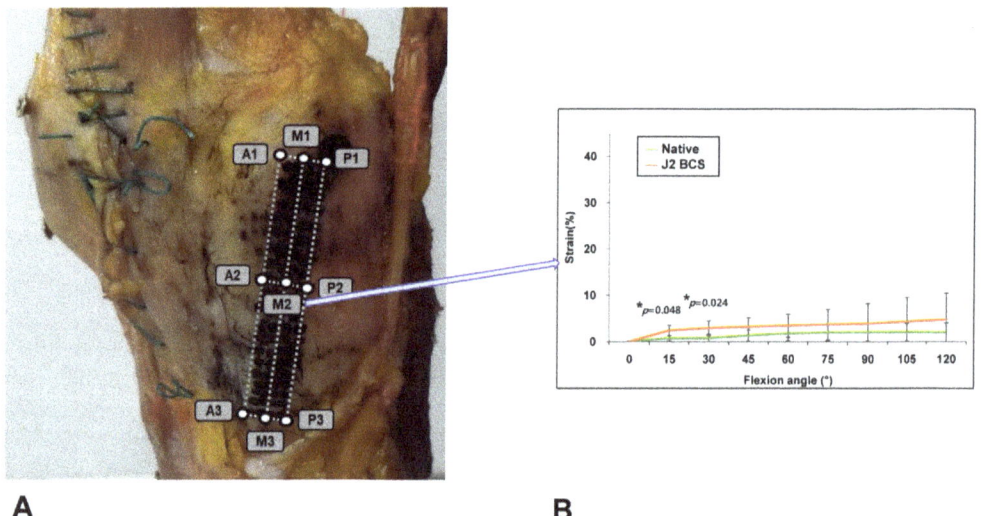

Figure 6. MCL strain distribution. Division of the MCL into 9 regions of interest (ROIs). The MCL was divided vertically into three segments labeled from front to back as anterior (A), middle (M), and posterior (P), and horizontally into three regions numbered 1–3 from top to bottom (**A**). Similar MCL strain was observed at 8 of 9 ROIs at all flexion angles; higher MCL strain after BCS TKA was observed at region M2 during early flexion, compared to native knees. (**B**) Error bars indicate standard deviations. Significant differences ($p < 0.05$) are marked with asterisks.

4. Discussion

Despite improvements in TKA design, most TKA systems sacrifice the ACL, which may lead to suboptimal satisfaction and function. Guided-motion BCS TKA replicates the normal knee motion by promoting kinematics and anterior-posterior stability. Enhanced stability after guided-motion BCS TKA may normalize the soft tissue tension that contributes the perception of a normal knee. In this cadaveric study, we compared MCL strain between native and post-BCS TKA knees using a video extensometer to determine whether guided-motion BCS TKA restores MCL strain to the level found in native knees.

Our findings suggest that guided-motion BCS TKA normalizes MCL strain. In this study, no significant differences were observed in the mean and peak strain measurements between native and guided-motion BCS-TKA knees at any flexion angle. The MCL provides restraint against anterior tibial translation in ACL-deficient knees [28]. Multiple previous studies have reported that MCL strain was significantly higher in post-TKA knees than in native knees [14,15,18] and postoperative MCL laxity was also higher in post-TKA knees than in native knees [16,17]. Our findings, when taken into account with previous studies, suggest that guided-motion BCS TKA successfully restored MCL strain to the level found in native knees. Additionally, free nerve endings that serve as a nociceptive system were reported to be the most commonly observed mechanoreceptors in the MCL [29]. Our findings, when taken into account with this anatomical detail, suggest that guided-motion BCS TKA may provide more normal feelings of the knee, which is strongly associated with patient satisfaction [11,12,30]. However, future studies that evaluate the MCL strain thresholds necessary to perceive the differences between normal and prosthetic knees are needed. Our findings also indicated that the standard deviations of the peak MCL strain were much higher than those of the mean MCL strain. One plausible explanation is that the difference in measuring area may affect MCL strain. In this study, the mean MCL strain was determined by measuring the strain over the whole MCL area and the peak MCL strain was found at one-fourth of the entire MCL area, and the distribution of MCL strain was evaluated at each of ROIs. Therefore, the surface strains measured at a smaller area, such as the peak MCL strain and strain at ROIs, are more susceptible to specimen-specific anatomical conditions, such as the bone contour underneath the measured MCL area and the soft tissues connected soft tissues to the MCL, than those measured at the entire MCL.

The results of the present study suggest that guided-motion BCS TKA can normalize the MCL strain distribution pattern. We found that guided-motion BCS TKA restored the strain to the level generated in native knee at 8 of 9 ROIs. Higher MCL strain was found at 1 ROI in the mid-portion of the MCL during flexion at $\leq 30°$. A previous cadaveric study discovered significantly higher strain after conventional ACL-deficient mechanically aligned TKA, compared to native knees, at all flexion angles in the proximal mid to posterior portion of the MCL [18]. Similar to the findings of previous studies, the current results suggest that guided-motion BCS TKA was able to better restore the native MCL strain pattern than conventional TKA. Considering the role of the MCL in neurosensory feedback, patients undergoing BCS TKA may experience greater perception of a normal knee, compared to patients who undergo conventional TKA. Yet, further studies evaluating the relationship between MCL strain and neurosensory feedback changes are required.

There were several noteworthy limitations in this cadaveric study. First, the specimen preparation and testing environment may not have replicated natural conditions and normal squatting loads and patterns. Properties of the MCL may have been changed following rigorous soft tissue balancing, which could have affected the measured surface strain. Additionally, we used muscle loads from previous cadaveric studies investigating knee squatting motions, to simulated physiological loads [23,24], but these loading parameters were too small to simulate in a normal-weight person. This should be considered before extrapolating our cadaveric test findings to real clinical scenarios. Second, we only tested guided-motion BCS TKA implants without comparing them to conventional ACL-deficient TKA implants. Thus, we compared our data with previous studies that investigated conventional mechanically aligned TKA. Third, it is difficult to determine the clinical relevance of our findings because both the threshold of MCL strain that triggers nociception and the cut-off strain value for mechanical failure in the human knee are unknown. Finally, video extensometer analyses have some inherent limitations in terms of image processing, such as poor resolution and quality, as well as distortion of the digital image. Nevertheless, this novel, non-contact analysis technique eliminates the need for strain gauge implantation, thereby reducing the risk of changes to ligament properties. Despite its limitations, this cadaveric study is the first to report MCL strain measurements using a video extensometer after guided-motion BCS TKA. Therefore, our results provide valuable information regarding MCL strain patterns following guided-motion BCS TKA.

5. Conclusions

Our study demonstrates that guided-motion BCS TKA restores the amount and distribution of MCL strain to the levels found in native knees during knee flexion. These findings may explain the perception of a normal knee after guided-motion BCS TKA, rather than conventional ACL-deficient TKA.

Author Contributions: Conceptualization, I.J.K. and D.L.; Data curation, I.J.K., D.-S.K., H.-J.C., M.K. and D.L.; Formal analysis, I.J.K., Y.D.K., J.K. and N.C.; Funding acquisition, I.J.K. and D.L.; Resources, D.-S.K. and H.-J.C.; Software, M.K., J.H.C. and D.L.; Investigation, D.-S.K., H.-J.C., M.K., J.H.C., D.L. and I.J.K.; Supervision, D.L. and I.J.K.; Validation, I.J.K.; Visualization, I.J.K., D.-S.K. and D.L.; Writing—original draft, D.-S.K. and I.J.K.; Writing—review and editing, N.C., D.-S.K., D.L., J.K. and I.J.K. All authors have read and agreed to the published version of the manuscript.

Funding: This work was supported by the National Research Foundation of Korea (NRF) grant funded by the Korea government (MSIT) (No. 2019 R1F1A 1057842 and No. 2017M3A9E9073545).

Institutional Review Board Statement: This cadaveric study was exempt from the institutional review board of our institution because it did not involve human subjects.

Informed Consent Statement: Written informed consent for use of the cadavers and consent for use of future research on the related materials were provided by all donors or authorized representatives.

Data Availability Statement: All data are presented in the article. Instrumental readings are available upon request from the corresponding author.

Acknowledgments: We thank Smith & Nephew, Korea for providing the surgical instruments used in this study. We also thank Su Gu Chai, B.S. and Seung Jun Lee, P.R.S., at Smith & Nephew, Korea, Ki Joon Yoo, B.A., Jae Young Sung, B.S., and Hyunggu Han, B.A., of Daon HealthCare, Korea, for their assistance in the test. We also thank the cadaver donors and their families.

Conflicts of Interest: The authors declare no conflict of interest. The funders had no role in the design of the study; in the collection, analyses, or interpretation of data; in the writing of the manuscript; or in the decision to publish the results.

References

1. Bourne, R.B.; Chesworth, B.M.; Davis, A.M.; Mahomed, N.N.; Charron, K.D. Patient satisfaction after total knee arthroplasty: Who is satisfied and who is not? *Clin. Orthop. Relat. Res.* **2010**, *468*, 57–63. [CrossRef]
2. Nam, D.; Nunley, R.M.; Barrack, R.L. Patient dissatisfaction following total knee replacement: A growing concern? *Bone Jt. J.* **2014**, *96*, 96–100. [CrossRef]
3. Choi, Y.J.; Seo, D.K.; Lee, K.W.; Ra, H.J.; Kang, H.W.; Kim, J.K. Results of total knee arthroplasty for painless, stiff knees. *Knee Surg. Relat. Res.* **2020**, *32*, 61. [CrossRef]
4. Kim, J.; Min, K.D.; Lee, B.I.; Kim, J.B.; Kwon, S.W.; Chun, D.I.; Kim, Y.B.; Seo, G.W.; Lee, J.S.; Park, S.; et al. Comparison of functional outcomes between single-radius and multi-radius femoral components in primary total knee arthroplasty: A meta-analysis of randomized controlled trials. *Knee Surg. Relat. Res.* **2020**, *32*, 52. [CrossRef]
5. Park, C.H.; Song, S.J. Sensor-Assisted Total Knee Arthroplasty: A Narrative Review. *Clin. Orthop. Surg.* **2021**, *13*, 1–9. [CrossRef]
6. Pawar, P.; Naik, L.; Sahu, D.; Bagaria, V. Comparative Study of Pinless Navigation System versus Conventional Instrumentation in Total Knee Arthroplasty. *Clin. Orthop. Surg.* **2021**, *13*, 358–365. [CrossRef]
7. Christen, B.; Kopjar, B. Second-generation bi-cruciate stabilized total knee system has a lower reoperation and revision rate than its predecessor. *Arch. Orthop. Trauma Surg.* **2018**, *138*, 1591–1599. [CrossRef]
8. Grieco, T.F.; Sharma, A.; Dessinger, G.M.; Cates, H.E.; Komistek, R.D. In Vivo Kinematic Comparison of a Bicruciate Stabilized Total Knee Arthroplasty and the Normal Knee Using Fluoroscopy. *J. Arthroplast.* **2018**, *33*, 565–571. [CrossRef]
9. Christen, B.; Neukamp, M.; Aghayev, E. Consecutive series of 226 journey bicruciate substituting total knee replacements: Early complication and revision rates. *BMC Musculoskelet. Disord.* **2014**, *15*, 395. [CrossRef]
10. Hommel, H.; Wilke, K. Good Early Results Obtained with a Guided-Motion Implant for Total Knee Arthroplasty: A Consecutive Case Series. *Open Orthop. J.* **2017**, *11*, 51–56. [CrossRef]
11. Iriuchishima, T.; Ryu, K. Bicruciate Substituting Total Knee Arthroplasty Improves Stair Climbing Ability When Compared with Cruciate-Retain or Posterior Stabilizing Total Knee Arthroplasty. *Indian J. Orthop.* **2019**, *53*, 641–645. [CrossRef]

12. Kono, K.; Inui, H.; Tomita, T.; Yamazaki, T.; Taketomi, S.; Sugamoto, K.; Tanaka, S. Bicruciate-stabilised total knee arthroplasty provides good functional stability during high-flexion weight-bearing activities. *Knee Surg. Sport. Traumatol. Arthrosc.* **2019**, *27*, 2096–2103. [CrossRef]
13. Takubo, A.; Ryu, K.; Iriuchishima, T.; Tokuhashi, Y. Comparison of Muscle Recovery Following Bi-cruciate Substituting versus Posterior Stabilized Total Knee Arthroplasty in the Asian Population. *J. Knee Surg.* **2017**, *30*, 725–729. [CrossRef]
14. Delport, H.; Labey, L.; De Corte, R.; Innocenti, B.; Vander Sloten, J.; Bellemans, J. Collateral ligament strains during knee joint laxity evaluation before and after TKA. *Clin. Biomech.* **2013**, *28*, 777–782. [CrossRef]
15. Delport, H.; Labey, L.; Innocenti, B.; De Corte, R.; Vander Sloten, J.; Bellemans, J. Restoration of constitutional alignment in TKA leads to more physiological strains in the collateral ligaments. *Knee Surg. Sport. Traumatol. Arthrosc.* **2015**, *23*, 2159–2169. [CrossRef]
16. Koh, I.J.; Chalmers, C.E.; Lin, C.C.; Park, S.B.; McGarry, M.H.; Lee, T.Q. Posterior stabilized total knee arthroplasty reproduces natural joint laxity compared to normal in kinematically aligned total knee arthroplasty: A matched pair cadaveric study. *Arch. Orthop. Trauma Surg.* **2021**, *141*, 119–127. [CrossRef]
17. Koh, I.J.; Lin, C.C.; Patel, N.A.; Chalmers, C.E.; Maniglio, M.; Han, S.B.; McGarry, M.H.; Lee, T.Q. Kinematically aligned total knee arthroplasty reproduces more native rollback and laxity than mechanically aligned total knee arthroplasty: A matched pair cadaveric study. *Orthop. Traumatol. Surg. Res.* **2019**, *105*, 605–611. [CrossRef]
18. Lim, D.; Kwak, D.S.; Kim, M.; Kim, S.; Cho, H.J.; Choi, J.H.; Koh, I.J. Kinematically aligned total knee arthroplasty restores more native medial collateral ligament strain than mechanically aligned total knee arthroplasty. *Knee Surg. Sports Traumatol. Arthrosc.* **2022**, *30*, 2815–2823. [CrossRef]
19. Pan, B.; Tian, L. Advanced video extensometer for non-contact, real-time, high-accuracy strain measurement. *Opt. Express* **2016**, *24*, 19082–19093. [CrossRef]
20. Villegas, D.F.; Maes, J.A.; Magee, S.D.; Donahue, T.L. Failure properties and strain distribution analysis of meniscal attachments. *J. Biomech.* **2007**, *40*, 2655–2662. [CrossRef]
21. Zavatsky, A.B. A kinematic-freedom analysis of a flexed-knee-stance testing rig. *J. Biomech.* **1997**, *30*, 277–280. [CrossRef] [PubMed]
22. Wickiewicz, T.L.; Roy, R.R.; Powell, P.L.; Edgerton, V.R. Muscle architecture of the human lower limb. *Clin Orthop Relat Res* **1983**, *179*, 275–283. [CrossRef]
23. Hofer, J.K.; Gejo, R.; McGarry, M.H.; Lee, T.Q. Effects of kneeling on tibiofemoral contact pressure and area in posterior cruciate-retaining and posterior cruciate-sacrificing total knee arthroplasty. *J. Arthroplast.* **2012**, *27*, 620–624. [CrossRef]
24. Powers, C.M.; Lilley, J.C.; Lee, T.Q. The effects of axial and multi-plane loading of the extensor mechanism on the patellofemoral joint. *Clin. Biomech.* **1998**, *13*, 616–624. [CrossRef] [PubMed]
25. Koh, I.J.; Kwak, D.S.; Kim, T.K.; Park, I.J.; In, Y. How effective is multiple needle puncturing for medial soft tissue balancing during total knee arthroplasty? A cadaveric study. *J. Arthroplast.* **2014**, *29*, 2478–2483. [CrossRef] [PubMed]
26. LaPrade, R.F.; Engebretsen, A.H.; Ly, T.V.; Johansen, S.; Wentorf, F.A.; Engebretsen, L. The anatomy of the medial part of the knee. *J. Bone Jt. Surg. Am. Vol.* **2007**, *89*, 2000–2010. [CrossRef]
27. Provenzano, P.P.; Heisey, D.; Hayashi, K.; Lakes, R.; Vanderby, R., Jr. Subfailure damage in ligament: A structural and cellular evaluation. *J. Appl. Physiol.* **2002**, *92*, 362–371. [CrossRef]
28. Sullivan, D.; Levy, I.M.; Sheskier, S.; Torzilli, P.A.; Warren, R.F. Medial restraints to anterior-posterior motion of the knee. *J. Bone Jt. Surg. Am. Vol.* **1984**, *66*, 930–936. [CrossRef]
29. Cabuk, H.; Kusku Cabuk, F. Mechanoreceptors of the ligaments and tendons around the knee. *Clin. Anat.* **2016**, *29*, 789–795. [CrossRef]
30. West, J.A.; Scudday, T.; Anderson, S.; Amin, N.H. Clinical outcomes and patient satisfaction after total knee arthroplasty: A follow-up of the first 50 cases by a single surgeon. *J. Int. Med. Res.* **2019**, *47*, 1667–1676. [CrossRef]

Article

Accuracy of the Tibial Component Alignment by Extramedullary System Using Simple Radiographic References in Total Knee Arthroplasty

Jin-Ho Cho, Jun Young Choi and Sung-Sahn Lee *

Department of Orthopedic Surgery, Ilsan Paik Hospital, Inje University School of Medicine, Goyang-si 10380, Korea
* Correspondence: sungsahnlee@gmail.com; Tel.: +82-31-910-7301

Abstract: *Background and Objectives*: The tibial component alignment is an important issue for the longevity of total knee arthroplasty (TKA). The purpose of our study was to investigate the usefulness of proximal tibial references determined by pre-operative radiography and intraoperative C-arm-guided hip and ankle center marking for the extramedullary guided tibial cut in mild (<10°) and severe (≥10°) varus knee TKA. *Materials and Methods*: A total of 150 consecutive patients (220 cases) who underwent total knee arthroplasty who were recruited from July 2011 to April 2017 were reviewed retrospectively. Before surgery, the proximal tibial reference point and medio-lateral cut thickness difference were identified. Then, hip and ankle centers were checked using a C-arm intensifier intraoperatively. The hip–knee–ankle (HKA) alignment and medial proximal tibial angle (MPTA) were assessed pre-operatively and post-operatively. More than 3° varus or valgus of HKA alignment or tibial component angle was defined as an outlier. *Results*: Mean follow-up duration was 26.9 months. Among 220 cases, 111 cases are classified as mild varus group and 109 cases are classified as severe varus group. The HKA alignment is significantly improved ($p < 0.001$). The average tibial component angle after surgery was 90.1°. A total of 21 cases (9.5%) and 3 cases (1.4%) are classified as outliers of HKA alignment and MPTA, respectively. Among MPTA outliers, one case is in the mild varus group and two cases are in the in severe varus group ($p = 0.62$). *Conclusion*: Measurement of proximal tibial radiographic references and checking the C-arm-guided intraoperative hip and ankle center could be helpful to obtain the favorable coronal position of the tibial component in the extramedullary guided tibial cut.

Keywords: total knee arthroplasty; tibial component alignment; radiographic references; extramedullary system

1. Introduction

Kinematic alignment was recently investigated as an alternative to mechanically aligned total knee arthroplasty (TKA) [1]. Several studies demonstrate that kinematically aligned TKA shows similar or better clinical outcomes due to less disruption of the native soft tissue envelope [2,3]. As a similar theoretical background, some studies show that slight under-corrected TKA results in better clinical outcomes than neutrally aligned TKA [4]. However, many studies suggest that post-operative coronal alignment is associated with implant survival; in particular, tibial component varus position is strongly correlated to implant loosening [5–7].

To enhance post-operative alignment, the computer navigation instruments or patient-specific implants (PSI) can be used [8–10]. However, these devices are not always available and have additional costs, therefore, many surgeons perform conventional jig-based TKA—intramedullary guided distal femoral cut and extramedullary guided proximal tibia cut. Various anatomical landmarks (extensor hallucis longus, dorsal pedis artery, intermalleolar point, anterior tibial border, intercondylar eminence) are used as a reference for extramedullary alignment to enhance tibial component coronal alignment [11–13]. Thippana et al. [14] reported that using the line that connects the proximal tibial reference point defined by pre-operative radiography and ankle center was helpful to set the extramedullary guide. In addition to this landmark, we thought pre-determined proximal tibial medio-lateral (ML) cut thickness difference by radiograph (Figure 1) and the intraoperative C-arm-intensifier-guided hip and ankle center marking method are helpful to enhance tibial component position.

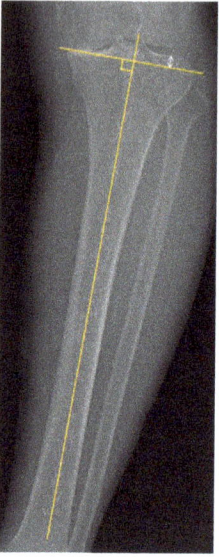

Figure 1. Proximal tibial medio-lateral (ML) cut thickness difference. The lines were drawn (1) along the anatomical axis of the tibia and (2) perpendicular to first line (starting from medial condylar edge). The *white arrow line* indicates proximal tibial 'ML cut thickness difference'.

The purpose of this study was (1) to investigate the usefulness of proximal tibial references determined by pre-operative radiography and intraoperative C-arm-guided hip and ankle center marking, and (2) to compare radiographic measurements between the patients with pre-operative mild varus (<10°) and severe varus (≥10°) deformity. It was hypothesized that favorable coronal alignment of the tibial component might be shown by this method, regardless of the severity of pre-operative varus deformity.

2. Materials and Methods

2.1. Patients

This study is a retrospectively designed study. From July 2011 to April 2017, the patients who underwent primary TKA surgery with the same method for degenerative osteoarthritis with varus deformity were reviewed. The exclusion criteria were as follows: patients who (1) followed up for less than 1 year, (2) had undergone other previous bony procedure, such as osteotomy, and (3) diagnosed systemic arthritis such as rheumatoid arthritis. The enrolled patients were divided into mild varus group (<10°) and severe varus group (≥10°). based on pre-operative hip–knee–ankle (HKA) alignment as the definition of previous studies [15,16]. Written informed consents were obtained from all patients before enrolling them in the study. This study was approved by the IRB of the authors' affiliated institutions (ISPAIK 2019-02-014 at 20 February 2019).

2.2. Radiographic and Clinical Assessment

We analyzed the HKA alignment taken from the pre-operative and 1 year follow-up low extremity whole radiography [17,18]. As in previous studies, more than 3° varus or valgus of HKA alignment was defined as an outlier [4,19]. The medial proximal tibial angle (MPTA) is the medial angle of intersection between the anatomical axis of the tibia and the horizontal axis of the proximal tibia (pre-operative measurement) or tibial component (post-operative measurement). Refs. [20,21] are same as HKA alignment, more than 3° varus or valgus of tibial component angle was defined as an outlier [4,19]. The tibial slope was also measured as previously described [22,23] (Figure 2).

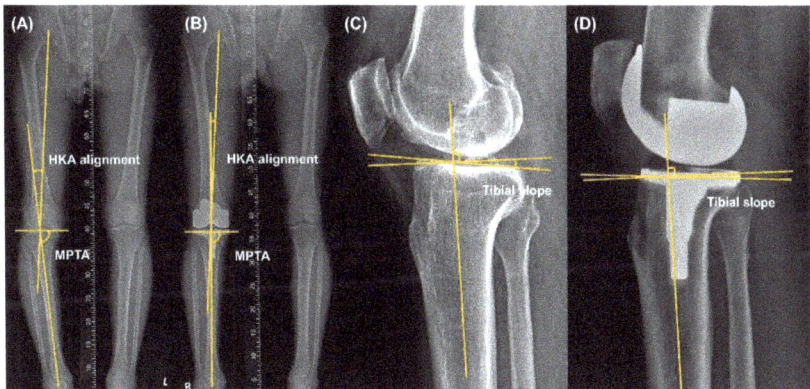

Figure 2. Measurement of the pre- and post-operative hip–knee–ankle (HKA) alignment, medial proximal tibial angle (MPTA, (**A**,**B**)) and tibial slope (**C**,**D**).

All radiographs were measured using Marosis software (INFINITT Healthcare, Seoul, Korea). The radiographs were evaluated by two independent orthopedic surgeons specializing in knee arthroplasty, who did not participate in the current study, to verify inter-observer reliability. The intra-observer reliability was checked by having the observers repeat the same measurements 6 weeks later. Intraclass correlation coefficients (ICCs) were used for intra-observer and inter-observer reliabilities.

The clinical parameters of pre-operation and last follow-up were evaluated by the following clinical scores: Hospital for Special Surgery (HSS) score [24] and Western Ontario Mac-Master University (WOMAC) Index [25,26]. In addition, the operative time and incision size were analyzed.

2.3. Pre-Operative Planning

Pre-operative tibial anteroposterior (AP) view was used to verify the proximal tibial reference point. The proximal tibial reference point is determined as the meeting point between the tibial anatomical axis and the proximal tibial joint line. Of the enrolled cases, all proximal tibial reference points existed between the center of intercondylar eminence and the lateral tibial spine. These points were classified as 3 zones—the center of intercondylar eminence, lateral tibial spine, and in-between (Figure 3).

The perpendicular line to the tibial anatomical axis was drawn from the edge of medial tibial condyle. The ML cut thickness difference of proximal tibia was measured (Figure 1).

2.4. Intraoperative Planning

After induction of anesthesia to the patients, the ankle center and hip center should be assessed under a C-arm intensifier to apply the pre-operative planning before draping. A long rod (High tibia osteotomy alignment rod, DePuy Synthes, Raynham, MA, USA) was used to confirm the hip center and ankle center. The patient was placed in a metal pelvic stabilizer with the mobile peg, so that the measured position did not change during surgery [27]. The hip center was marked with a mobile peg, and the end of the long rod was marked in the patient's ankle using a marking pen (Figure 4).

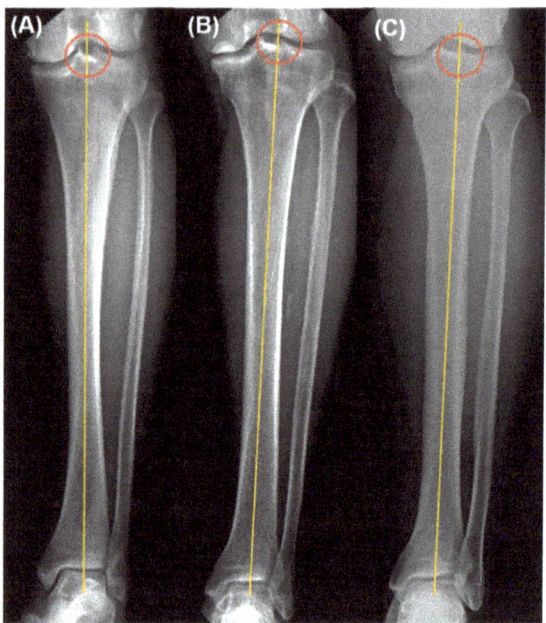

Figure 3. Proximal tibial reference point. These points were classified as 3 zones—(**A**) the center of intercondylar eminence, (**B**) in-between, and (**C**) lateral tibial spine.

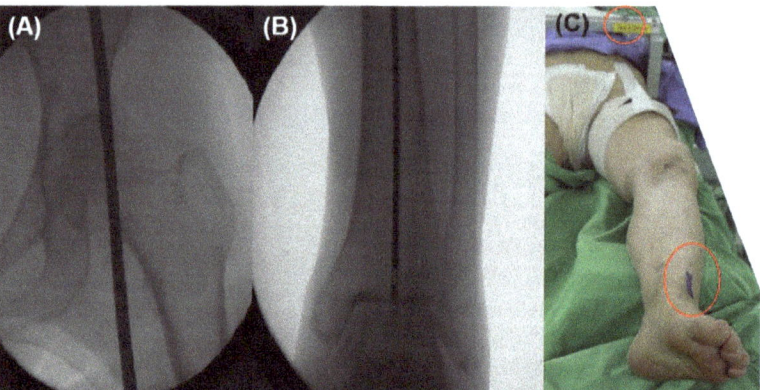

Figure 4. Marking hip and ankle centers. (**A**,**B**) Check hip and ankle centers using a metal rod under C-arm intensifier. (**C**) A hip center was marked using mobile peg in a pelvic stabilizer and an ankle center was marked with a marking pen.

2.5. Operative Procedure

All surgeries were performed by the senior author. In all cases, posterior, stabilized TKA implant was used (LEGION, Smith & Nephew, London, UK). Skin incision and medial parapatellar arthrotomy were performed. Both cruciate ligaments were removed from their femoral and tibial attachment sites and osteophytes were removed. Then, the intramedullary guided femoral cut was performed.

Extramedullary guided tibia cut was performed using pre- and intra-operatively checked references. The cartilages of lateral tibial condyle were removed. Extramedullary tibial cutting apparatus was installed using the proximal tibial reference point and marked ankle center. After that, we checked the ML thickness difference was similar between radiographic and intraoperative measurements using a cut thickness gauge.

After tibial cut and trial component insertion, marked ankle center and hip center should be connected by flexible cable (we used the cable-connecting electrocautery device) to check the tibial component coronal position and lower limb alignment. A proximal tibial cut was re-performed if the tibial component position was not perpendicular to cable (Figure 5).

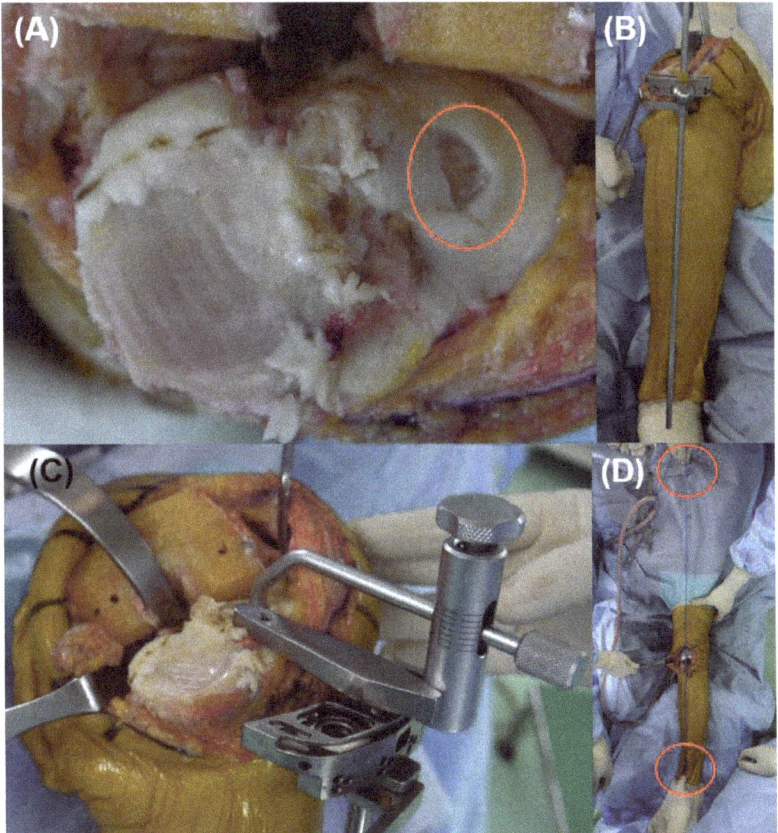

Figure 5. Operative procedure. (**A**) Gentle peeling of cartilage of the lateral condyle for precise intraoperative measurement. (**B,C**) Application of tibial cutting apparatus according to the 'proximal tibial reference point', 'ankle center', and pre-operatively measured medio-lateral cut thickness difference. (**D**) Check the limb and component coronal alignment using cable method.

After the surgery, full weight-bearing was allowed. Then, after the removal of drains, a range of motion exercises and quadriceps strengthening exercises were started.

2.6. Statistical Analyses

The intraclass correlation coefficient was used to quantify both inter-observer and intra-observer reliabilities for radiographic assessment. A descriptive analysis was performed for all the variables, including calculation of the mean and standard deviation. Data normality was tested using a *Kolmogorov–Smirnov test*. The *paired T-test* was used to compare between the pre-operative and post-operative parameters. The *Student's T-test* for continuous variables and chi-square tests for categorical variables were used to compare the parameters between mild varus group and severe varus group.

Statistical analyses were performed using SPSS software, version 18 (IBM Corp., Armonk, NY, USA). Statistical significance was determined as a *p*-value less than 0.05 for all analyses.

3. Results

A total 266 consecutive patients who underwent primary TKA surgery with the same method for degenerative osteoarthritis with varus deformity were reviewed. Among them, 80 patients were excluded who were followed up for less than 1 year. A total of 26 patients were excluded who previously underwent high tibial osteotomy or surgery for fracture. Ten patients who were diagnosed with rheumatoid arthritis were excluded. Finally, 150 patients (220 cases) were enrolled in the present study (Table 1). Among 220 cases, 111 cases are classified as mild varus group (<10°) and 109 cases are classified as severe varus group (≥10°).

Table 1. Demographic and preoperative radiographic parameters in 220 cases.

Age, year [a]	70.55 ± 7.21
Sex, male:female	46:174
Direction, right:left	107:113
Proximal tibial reference point	
Center	157 (71.4%)
In-between	24 (10.9%)
Lateral tibial spine	39 (17.7%)

[a] Values are presented as mean ± standard deviation (range).

Mean follow-up duration was 26.9 months. Inter-observer and intra-observer ICCs show good agreement regarding radiographic measurement reliability (>0.80). The HKA alignment is significantly decreased ($p < 0.001$). The average tibial component angle after surgery is 90.1°. A total of 21 cases (9.5%) and 3 cases (1.4%) are classified as an outlier of HKA alignment and tibial component angle, respectively. The average tibial slope before surgery is 9.3° and after surgery is 3.2° ($p < 0.001$). The average incision size is 12.3 cm and the average operative time is 75.1 min. The post-operative clinical outcomes including HSS score and WOMAC index are significantly improved compared to pre-operative values ($p < 0.05$) (Table 2).

Table 2. Comparison of clinical and radiographic data between pre- and post-operation.

	Pre-Operation	Post-Operation	*p* Value
HKA alignment, °	10.4 ± 6.4	1.9 ± 1.7	<0.001
MPTA, °	83.9 ± 3.3	90.1 ± 0.9	<0.001
Tibial slope, °	9.3 ± 4.4	3.2 ± 2.1	<0.001
HSS score	38.7 ± 11.9	77.7 ± 9.9	<0.001
WOMAC index	68.0 ± 7.1	28.2 ± 5.4	<0.001

HKA: hip–knee–ankle, MPTA: medial proximal tibial angle, HSS: Hospital for Special Surgery, WOMAC: Western Ontario Mac-Master University.

The severe varus group shows significantly more post-operative HKA alignment outliers than the mild varus group (mild varus group—6 cases (5.4%), severe varus group—15 cases (13.8%), $p = 0.04$, Table 3). The pre-operative MPTA is significantly greater in the mild varus group ($p < 0.001$). However, the post-operative MPTA outliers did not show statistical significance (mild varus group—one case (0.9%), severe varus group—two cases (1.5%), $p = 0.62$).

Table 3. Comparison of measurements between mild varus group and severe varus group.

	Mild Varus Group (<10°)	Severe Varus Group (≥10°)	p Value
Number of cases	111	109	
Age	70.2 ± 7.0	70.8 ± 7.4	0.517
Direction (R:L)	57:54	50:59	0.422
Pre-operative HKA alignment (°)	5.7 ± 2.5	15.0 ± 5.8	**<0.001**
Post-operative HKA alignment (°)	1.4 ± 1.7	2.4 ± 2.1	**<0.001**
HKA alignment outliers, n (%)	6 (5.4%)	15 (13.8%)	**0.04**
Pre-operative MPTA (°)	85.1 ± 2.9	82.7 ± 3.1	**<0.001**
Post-operative MPTA (°)	90.2 ± 0.8	90.1 ± 1.0	0.654
MPTA outliers, n (%)	1 (0.9%)	2 (1.5%)	0.62
Pre-operative tibial slope (°)	8.8 ± 4.5	9.9 ± 4.3	0.065
Post-operative tibial slope (°)	3.1 ± 2.0	3.4 ± 2.3	0.394

HKA: hip–knee–ankle, MPTA: medial proximal tibial angle.

4. Discussion

The principal finding of our study is that a favorable coronal position of the tibial component could be obtained by using preplanned proximal tibial radiographic references and intraoperative synchronizing. The severe varus group shows similar outliers of tibial component coronal position, but significantly more outliers of HKA alignment compared to the mild varus group.

Computer navigation instruments or patient-specific instruments (PSI) are helpful in post-operative limb and implant alignment [8,9]. Cheng et al. investigated the efficacy of computer-navigation-assisted surgery by meta-analysis of 41 randomized controlled trials [8]. They report that malalignment of >3° from neutral alignment in the HKA alignment occurs in fewer patients in the computer-navigation-assisted group than in the conventional group (12.2% vs. 28.3%, respectively). Schotanus et al. conduced a meta-analysis of comparison between PSI-assisted and conventional TKA [9]. They demonstrate that MRI-based PSIs show a 19% decline in outliers compared to conventional TKAs. However, these devices are not always available and have additional cost, therefore, many surgeons perform conventional jig-based TKA. Both extramedullary and intramedullary guided cut can be used, and show similar results [28,29]. However, the intramedullary system shows less accuracy in patients with tibial bowing or post-traumatic deformities [30]. The installation of extramedullary tibia cutting instruments depends on anatomical landmarks, which include intercondylar eminence, center of tibial plateau, posterior cruciate ligament, and tibial tuberosity for the proximal side, and anterior tibialis tendon, extensor hallucis longus, dorsal pedis, and intermalleolar center for the distal side [11–13,31]. These landmarks may not be palpable, and the surgeon's experience is important to obtain an accurate tibial component position. We suggest that additional radiographic references (proximal tibial reference point, ML cut thickness difference) and intraoperative hip and ankle center marking by C-arm intensifier could enhance the tibial component coronal position. These additional references and center markings provide an accurate location of the extramedullary instrument and allow a second chance to check limb and component alignment after trial insertion. It is well-known that high-grade pre-operative varus deformity is associated with residual post-operative varus alignment [32]. In the current study, the severe varus group shows more HKA alignment outliers than the mild varus group, which is concurrent with previous studies. However, MPTA outliers are not significantly different between both groups. Previous studies suggest that the increasing severity of pre-operative varus deformity is associated with complex bone cuts to restore a neutral mechanical alignment [1,33]. According to our findings, we think our methods aid in obtaining tibial component neutral alignment, regardless of the severity of pre-operative varus deformity.

Proximal tibial reference points of all cases exist between the center of intercondylar eminence and the lateral tibial spine in the current study. Kim et al. [34] suggest that lateral intercondylar spine rather than the center of intercondylar eminence should be used as a reference for the proximal tibial side in extramedullary guided tibial cut, in order to obtain a neutral component position. We agreed that routine use of the center of intercondylar eminence as a proximal reference point has a chance to highlight the varus position of the tibial component. However, we think an individualized proximal tibial reference point is better than routine use of lateral intercondylar spine. A further comparative study is needed to find the most reliable reference point of the proximal tibia.

This study has several limitations. First, it was not a comparative study with other methods. Second, the follow-up period was relatively short, and further studies are needed to evaluate implant survival. Third, there is not enough discussion on femur cutting with emphasis on increasing the accuracy of tibia cutting. Forth, we only focused on correcting coronal malalignment, and we need to discuss the correction technique for the sagittal plane as well. Fifth, in addition to the bone cutting, the collateral ligament and soft tissue were involved in the gap-balancing, but there was not sufficient information regarding this.

5. Conclusions

The measurement of proximal tibial radiographic references and checking C-arm-guided intraoperative hip and ankle centers could be helpful in obtaining a favorable coronal position of the tibial component for the extramedullary guided tibial cut in TKA.

Author Contributions: Conceptualization, J.-H.C. and S.-S.L.; methodology, J.-H.C. and S.-S.L.; validation, J.-H.C. and J.Y.C.; formal analysis, J.Y.C. and S.-S.L.; investigation, J.Y.C. and S.-S.L.; data curation, J.Y.C. and S.-S.L.; writing—original draft preparation, J.-H.C. and S.-S.L.; writing—review and editing, J.-H.C. and S.-S.L.; visualization, J.-H.C. and J.Y.C.; supervision, J.-H.C. and S.-S.L.; project administration, J.-H.C. and S.-S.L. All authors have read and agreed to the published version of the manuscript.

Funding: This research received no external funding.

Institutional Review Board Statement: The protocol used to evaluate radiographic findings and intraoperative navigation data was approved by our institution's investigational review board. (ISPAIK 2019-02-014 at 20 February 2019).

Informed Consent Statement: Informed consent was obtained from all individual participants included in the study.

Data Availability Statement: Not applicable.

Conflicts of Interest: The authors declare no conflict of interest.

References

1. Lee, Y.S.; Howell, S.M.; Won, Y.Y.; Lee, O.S.; Lee, S.H.; Vahedi, H.; Teo, S.H. Kinematic alignment is a possible alternative to mechanical alignment in total knee arthroplasty. *Knee Surg. Sports Traumatol. Arthrosc.* **2017**, *25*, 3467–3479. [CrossRef] [PubMed]
2. Yoon, J.R.; Han, S.B.; Jee, M.K.; Shin, Y.S. Comparison of kinematic and mechanical alignment techniques in primary total knee arthroplasty: A meta-analysis. *Medicine* **2017**, *96*, e8157. [CrossRef] [PubMed]
3. Young, S.W.; Walker, M.L.; Bayan, A.; Briant-Evans, T.; Pavlou, P.; Farrington, B. The Chitranjan, S. Ranawat Award: No Difference in 2-year Functional Outcomes Using Kinematic versus Mechanical Alignment in TKA: A Randomized Controlled Clinical Trial. *Clin. Orthop. Relat. Res.* **2017**, *475*, 9–20. [CrossRef] [PubMed]
4. Vanlommel, L.; Vanlommel, J.; Claes, S.; Bellemans, J. Slight undercorrection following total knee arthroplasty results in superior clinical outcomes in varus knees. *Knee Surg. Sports Traumatol. Arthrosc.* **2013**, *21*, 2325–2330. [CrossRef] [PubMed]
5. Ritter, M.A.; Davis, K.E.; Meding, J.B.; Pierson, J.L.; Berend, M.E.; Malinzak, R.A. The effect of alignment and BMI on failure of total knee replacement. *J. Bone Joint Surg. Am.* **2011**, *93*, 1588–1596. [CrossRef]
6. Liu, H.X.; Shang, P.; Ying, X.Z.; Zhang, Y. Shorter survival rate in varus-aligned knees after total knee arthroplasty. *Knee Surg. Sports Traumatol. Arthrosc.* **2016**, *24*, 2663–2671. [CrossRef]
7. Li, Z.; Esposito, C.I.; Koch, C.N.; Lee, Y.Y.; Padgett, D.E.; Wright, T.M. Polyethylene Damage Increases with Varus Implant Alignment in Posterior-stabilized and Constrained Condylar Knee Arthroplasty. *Clin. Orthop. Relat. Res.* **2017**, *475*, 2981–2991. [CrossRef]
8. Cheng, T.; Zhao, S.; Peng, X.; Zhang, X. Does computer-assisted surgery improve postoperative leg alignment and implant positioning following total knee arthroplasty? A meta-analysis of randomized controlled trials? *Knee Surg. Sports Traumatol. Arthrosc.* **2012**, *20*, 1307–1322. [CrossRef]
9. Schotanus, M.G.M.; Thijs, E.; Heijmans, M.; Vos, R.; Kort, N.P. Favourable alignment outcomes with MRI-based patient-specific instruments in total knee arthroplasty. *Knee Surg. Sports Traumatol. Arthrosc.* **2018**, *26*, 2659–2668. [CrossRef]

10. Kim, K.; Kim, J.; Lee, D.; Lim, S.; Eom, J. The Accuracy of Alignment Determined by Patient-Specific Instrumentation System in Total Knee Arthroplasty. *Knee Surg. Relat. Res.* **2019**, *31*, 19–24. [CrossRef]
11. Akagi, M.; Oh, M.; Nonaka, T.; Tsujimoto, H.; Asano, T.; Hamanishi, C. An anteroposterior axis of the tibia for total knee arthroplasty. *Clin. Orthop. Relat. Res.* **2004**, *420*, 213–219. [CrossRef] [PubMed]
12. Reed, M.R.; Bliss, W.; Sher, J.L.; Emmerson, K.P.; Jones, S.M.; Partington, P.F. Extramedullary or intramedullary tibial alignment guides: A randomised, prospective trial of radiological alignment. *J. Bone Joint Surg. Br.* **2002**, *84*, 858–860. [CrossRef] [PubMed]
13. Cinotti, G.; Sessa, P.; D'Arino, A.; Ripani, F.R.; Giannicola, G. Improving tibial component alignment in total knee arthroplasty. *Knee Surg. Sports Traumatol. Arthrosc.* **2015**, *23*, 3563–3570. [CrossRef]
14. Thippana, R.K.; Kumar, M.N. Lateralization of Tibial Plateau Reference Point Improves Accuracy of Tibial Resection in Total Knee Arthroplasty in Patients with Proximal Tibia Vara. *Clin. Orthop. Surg.* **2017**, *9*, 458–464. [CrossRef] [PubMed]
15. Puliero, B.; Favreau, H.; Eichler, D.; Adam, P.; Bonnomet, F.; Ehlinger, M. Total knee arthroplasty in patients with varus deformities greater than ten degrees: Survival analysis at a mean ten year follow-up. *Int. Orthop.* **2019**, *43*, 333–341. [CrossRef]
16. Rahm, S.; Camenzind, R.S.; Hingsammer, A.; Lenz, C.; Bauer, D.E.; Farshad, M.; Fucentese, S.F. Postoperative alignment of TKA in patients with severe preoperative varus or valgus deformity: Is there a difference between surgical techniques? *BMC Musculoskelet. Disord.* **2017**, *18*, 272. [CrossRef]
17. Thienpont, E.; Parvizi, J. A New Classification for the Varus Knee. *J. Arthroplast.* **2016**, *31*, 2156–2160. [CrossRef]
18. Kang, B.Y.; Lee, D.K.; Kim, H.S.; Wang, J.H. How to achieve an optimal alignment in medial opening wedge high tibial osteotomy? *Knee Surg. Relat. Res.* **2022**, *34*, 3. [CrossRef]
19. Lee, S.S.; Kwon, K.B.; Lee, Y.I.; Moon, Y.W. Navigation-Assisted Total Knee Arthroplasty for a Valgus Knee Improves Limb and Femoral Component Alignment. *Orthopedics* **2019**, *42*, e253–e259. [CrossRef]
20. Piovan, G.; Farinelli, L.; Screpis, D.; Iacono, V.; Povegliano, L.; Bonomo, M.; Auregli, L.; Zorzi, C. Distal femoral osteotomy versus lateral unicompartmental arthroplasty for isolated lateral tibiofemoral osteoarthritis with intra-articular and extra-articular deformity: A propensity score-matched analysis. *Knee Surg. Relat. Res.* **2022**, *34*, 34. [CrossRef]
21. Makiev, K.G.; Vasios, I.S.; Georgoulas, P.; Tilkeridis, K.; Drosos, G.; Ververidis, A. Clinical significance and management of meniscal extrusion in different knee pathologies: A comprehensive review of the literature and treatment algorithm. *Knee Surg. Relat. Res.* **2022**, *34*, 35. [CrossRef] [PubMed]
22. Lee, H.W.; Park, C.H.; Bae, D.K.; Song, S.J. How much preoperative flexion contracture is a predictor for residual flexion contracture after total knee arthroplasty in hemophilic arthropathy and rheumatoid arthritis? *Knee Surg. Relat. Res.* **2022**, *34*, 20. [CrossRef]
23. Lee, J.M.; Ha, C.; Jung, K.; Choi, W. Clinical Results after Design Modification of Lospa Total Knee Arthroplasty System: Comparison between Posterior-Stabilized (PS) and PS Plus Types. *Clin. Orthop. Surg.* **2022**, *14*, 236–243. [CrossRef]
24. Insall, J.N.; Ranawat, C.S.; Aglietti, P.; Shine, J. A comparison of four models of total knee-replacement prostheses. *J. Bone Joint Surg. Am.* **1976**, *58*, 754–765. [CrossRef] [PubMed]
25. Stucki, G.; Meier, D.; Stucki, S.; Michel, B.A.; Tyndall, A.G.; Dick, W.; Theiler, R. Evaluation of a German version of WOMAC (Western Ontario and McMaster Universities) Arthrosis Index. *Z Rheumatol.* **1996**, *55*, 40–49.
26. Maniar, R.N.; Bhatnagar, N.; Bidwai, R.; Dhiman, A.; Chanda, D.; Sanghavi, N. Comparison of Patellofemoral Outcomes between Attune and PFC Sigma Designs: A Prospective Matched-Pair Analysis. *Clin. Orthop. Surg.* **2022**, *14*, 96–104. [CrossRef]
27. Seo, J.G.; Moon, Y.W.; Park, S.H.; Kang, H.M.; Kim, S.M. How precise is the identification of the center of the femoral head during total knee arthroplasty? *Acta Orthop.* **2012**, *83*, 53–58. [CrossRef] [PubMed]
28. Dennis, D.A.; Channer, M.; Susman, M.H.; Stringer, E.A. Intramedullary versus extramedullary tibial alignment systems in total knee arthroplasty. *J. Arthroplast.* **1993**, *8*, 43–47. [CrossRef]
29. Teter, K.E.; Bregman, D.; Colwell, C.W., Jr. Accuracy of intramedullary versus extramedullary tibial alignment cutting systems in total knee arthroplasty. *Clin. Orthop. Relat. Res.* **1995**, *321*, 106–110. [CrossRef]
30. Ko, P.S.; Tio, M.K.; Ban, C.M.; Mak, Y.K.; Ip, F.K.; Lam, J.J. Radiologic analysis of the tibial intramedullary canal in Chinese varus knees: Implications in total knee arthroplasty. *J. Arthroplast.* **2001**, *16*, 212–215. [CrossRef]
31. Nishikawa, K.; Mizu-uchi, H.; Okazaki, K.; Matsuda, S.; Tashiro, Y.; Iwamoto, Y. Accuracy of Proximal Tibial Bone Cut Using Anterior Border of Tibia as Bony Landmark in Total Knee Arthroplasty. *J. Arthroplast.* **2015**, *30*, 2121–2124. [CrossRef] [PubMed]
32. Oh, S.M.; Bin, S.I.; Kim, J.Y.; Lee, B.S.; Kim, J.M. Impact of preoperative varus deformity on postoperative mechanical alignment and long-term results of "mechanical" aligned total knee arthroplasty. *Orthop. Traumatol. Surg. Res.* **2019**, *105*, 1061–1066. [CrossRef] [PubMed]
33. Ahn, J.H.; Back, Y.W. Comparative Study of Two Techniques for Ligament Balancing in Total Knee Arthroplasty for Severe Varus Knee: Medial Soft Tissue Release vs. Bony Resection of Proximal Medial Tibia. *Knee Surg. Relat. Res.* **2013**, *25*, 13–18. [CrossRef] [PubMed]
34. Kim, S.M.; Kim, K.W.; Cha, S.M.; Han, K.Y. Proximal tibial resection in varus-deformed tibiae during total knee arthroplasty: An in vitro study using sawbone model. *Int. Orthop.* **2015**, *39*, 429–434. [CrossRef]

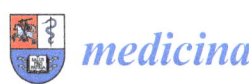

Article

Topical Tranexamic Acid Can Be Used Safely Even in High Risk Patients: Deep Vein Thrombosis Examination Using Routine Ultrasonography of 510 Patients

Yong Bum Joo [1], Young Mo Kim [1], Byung Kuk An [1], Cheol Won Lee [1], Soon Tae Kwon [2] and Ju-Ho Song [3,*]

[1] Department of Orthopedic Surgery, Chungnam National University Hospital, Chungnam National University College of Medicine, Daejeon 35015, Republic of Korea
[2] Department of Radiology, Chungnam National University Hospital, Chungnam National University College of Medicine, Daejeon 35015, Republic of Korea
[3] Department of Orthopedic Surgery, Chungnam National University Sejong Hospital, Chungnam National University College of Medicine, Sejong 30099, Republic of Korea
* Correspondence: skypillar0221@gmail.com; Tel.:+82-44-995-4798

Abstract: *Background and Objectives*: Previous studies regarding tranexamic acid (TXA) in total knee arthroplasty (TKA) investigated only symptomatic deep vein thrombosis (DVT), or did not include high risk patients. The incidence of DVT including both symptomatic and asymptomatic complications after applying topical TXA has not been evaluated using ultrasonography. *Materials and Methods*: The medical records of 510 patients who underwent primary unilateral TKA between July 2014 and December 2017 were retrospectively reviewed. Because TXA was routinely applied through the topical route, those who had a history of venous thromboembolism, myocardial infarction, or cerebral vascular occlusive disease, were not excluded. Regardless of symptom manifestation, DVT was examined at 1 week postoperatively for all patients using ultrasonography, and the postoperative transfusion rate was investigated. The study population was divided according to the use of topical TXA. After the two groups were matched based on the propensity scores, the incidence of DVT and the transfusion rate were compared between the groups. *Results*: Of the 510 patients, comprising 298 patients in the TXA group and 212 patients in the control group, DVT was noted in 22 (4.3%) patients. Two patients had DVT proximal to the popliteal vein. After propensity score matching (PSM), 168 patients were allocated to each group. In all, 11 patients in the TXA group and seven patients in the control group were diagnosed with DVT, which did not show a significant difference ($p = 0.721$). However, the two groups differ significantly in the transfusion rate ($p < 0.001$, 50.0% in the TXA group, 91.7% in the control group). *Conclusions*: The incidence of DVT, whether symptomatic or asymptomatic, was not affected by the use of topical TXA. The postoperative transfusion rate was reduced in the TXA group. Topical TXA could be applied safely even in patients who had been known to be at high risk.

Keywords: tranexamic acid; venous thromboembolism; total knee arthroplasty; transfusion

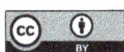

1. Introduction

Total knee arthroplasty (TKA) leads to substantial blood loss and poses a risk of transfusion [1,2]. Because allogenic blood transfusion is associated with several complications, such as allergic reactions and metabolic imbalances [3,4], surgeons have made an effort to reduce postoperative blood loss. The use of tranexamic acid (TXA), a synthetic amino acid derivative of lysine which prevents fibrin degradation [5–8], has been proven efficacious in reducing blood loss after TKA, and thus the rate of allogenic transfusion [9–11].

A substantial body of research has endorsed the efficacy and safety of TXA [2,8,12,13]. However, previous studies often excluded patients with medical comorbidities that were associated with postoperative thromboembolism. There remains a concern that TXA may increase the risk of thromboembolic complications [14–17]. In particular, patients undergoing TKA are prone to deep vein thrombosis (DVT) because surgical trauma and tourniquet application accelerate local fibrinolytic activity [18]. The incidence of DVT after arthroplasty has been investigated based on manifested symptoms in most studies [19–21]; thus, the incidence would only indicate the tip of the iceberg [22,23].

The topical use of TXA has an equivalent effect in reducing the transfusion rate after TKA, compared to intravenous (IV) use. Recent guidelines published by the American Association of Hip and Knee Surgeon (AAHKS) stated that the strong supporting evidence for use of TXA in high risk patients was lacking [24]. At our institution, topical TXA was applied without restrictions in high risk patients, such as those who had history of venous thromboembolism, myocardial infarction, or cerebral vascular occlusive disease. This study aimed to determine whether the use of topical TXA affected the true incidence of DVT using ultrasonography, regardless of symptom manifestation.

2. Materials and Methods

Medical records of 510 patients who underwent primary unilateral TKA between July 2014 and December 2017 were retrospectively reviewed after approval was obtained from our institutional review board. Because TXA was routinely applied through the topical route after September 2015, those who had history of venous thromboembolism, myocardial infarction, cerebral vascular occlusive disease, or cancer [25], were not excluded. The study population was divided according to the use of topical TXA.

2.1. Study Intervention

All TKAs were performed by two senior surgeons with the same surgical principle and prosthesis (Scorpio NRG, Stryker, Mahwah, NJ, USA). In the TXA group, 3.0 g of TXA in 100 mL of saline solution was applied directly into the knee joint cavity while suturing. An intra-articular drain was left for 48 h postoperatively. After the removal of drains, a range of motion exercise and walker-aided ambulation were encouraged. For DVT prophylaxis, intermittent pneumatic compression device was routinely used and a low molecular weight heparin was injected for 1 week after surgery [26,27]. There was no long-term anticoagulant therapy, regardless of the groups.

2.2. Study Design and Propensity Score Matching

DVT was examined using ultrasonography (Philips HD15, Bothwell, WA, USA) by two experienced radiologists. Lower extremity ultrasonography was performed at 1 week postoperatively for all patients, regardless of symptom manifestation. Proximal DVT was defined as the thrombosis that occurred proximal to the popliteal vein, and distal DVT was defined as the thrombosis of the anterior and tibial, peroneal, gastrocnemial, and soleal veins.

Postoperative transfusion records were reviewed, and the transfusion rate was compared according to the use of TXA. The necessity for transfusion was determined based on the guidelines by the National Institutes of Health Consensus Conference: hemoglobin level < 8.0 g/dL, or hemoglobin level < 10.0 g/dL with intolerable anemic symptoms or any anemia-related organ dysfunctions.

The two groups were matched at a 1:1 ratio based on propensity score [28]. The relevant variables were applied in a logistic regression analysis to calculate propensity scores. The incidence of DVT and the transfusion rate were compared between the groups after propensity score matching (PSM).

2.3. Statistical Analysis

The sample size of each group (168 patients) was confirmed by post hoc analysis to achieve a power of 96% to reject the null hypothesis with regard to the incidence of DVT, with a significance level of 0.05. Post hoc power analysis was performed using G*Power (Version 3.1.7, Franz Faul, Christian-Albrechts-Universitätzu Kiel, Kiel, Germany).

The propensity score variables included age, sex, body mass index (BMI), American Society of Anesthesiologists (ASA) score, smoking, hypertension, diabetes mellitus, chronic kidney disease, arrhythmia, blood profiles (platelet count, prothrombin time (PT), and activated partial thromboplastin time (aPTT)), and medical comorbidities (cerebrovascular accident, myocardial infarction, other thromboembolism, and cancer). Propensity scores were matched using one-to-one nearest neighbor matching with no replacement and no caliper width. The matched patients were selected randomly to avoid a potential bias that came from an imbalance in the number of patients between the groups. After PSM, intergroup comparison of each variable was performed to confirm the validity of the matching. Categorical variables including the incidence of DVT and the transfusion rate were analyzed by Chi-square test when the expected value of the cell was 5 or more in at least 80% of the cells; otherwise, Fisher exact test was used. Continuous variables were analyzed by t test. All statical analyses were performed using the R software version 4.1.1 (R foundation for Statistical Computing, Vienna, Austria), with a p value < 0.05 considered statistically significant.

3. Results

A total of 510 patients with a mean age of 69.8 ± 7.6 years (range, 53–86 years) were followed up for 39.6 ± 23.5 months (range, 12–86 months). There were 298 patients in the TXA group and 212 patients in the control group (Table 1). Overall, DVT was noted in 22 (4.3%) patients, with two patients having DVT proximal to the popliteal vein. Computed tomography pulmonary angiography was performed in those patients, and none of them showed pulmonary embolism. No patients exhibited symptoms for DVT. The odds ratio of topical TXA was 1.03 (95% confidence interval 0.43–2.45).

Table 1. Patient characteristics between the TXA and the control groups before PSM.

	Overall	Topical TXA		p Value
		TXA Group (n = 298)	Control Group (n = 212)	
Age, y	69.8 ± 7.6	70.1 ± 8.0	69.6 ± 7.3	0.527
Male/Female, n	74/436	44/254	30/182	0.899
BMI, kg/m^2	26.3 ± 3.8	26.4 ± 4.0	26.1 ± 3.5	0.355
ASA score	2.2 ± 0.4	2.2 ± 0.4	2.2 ± 0.4	0.623
Smoking, n	35	15	20	0.074
Hypertension, n	344	199	145	0.703
Diabetes mellitus, n	119	55	64	0.002
Chronic kidney disease, n	33	19	14	0.926
Arrhythmia, n	23	13	10	0.856
Blood profiles				
Platelet count, 10^3/μL	247.3 ± 73.7	248.4 ± 75.5	245.7 ± 71.1	0.683
PT, INR	1.0 ± 0.4	1.0 ± 0.6	1.0 ± 0.2	0.790
aPTT, sec	32.8 ± 4.8	32.6 ± 5.4	33.0 ± 2.4	0.416
Medical comorbidities				
Cerebrovascular accident, n	35	18	17	0.478
Myocardial infarction, n	48	27	21	0.760
Other thromboembolism, n	22	11	11	0.508
Cancer, n	14	9	5	0.787

TXA, tranexamic acid; PSM, propensity score matching; BMI, body mass index; ASA, American Society of Anesthesiologists; PT, prothrombin time; INR, international normalized ratio; aPTT, activated partial thromboplastin time.

After PSM, 168 patients were allocated to each group (Table 2). In all, 11 patients in the TXA group and seven patients in the control group were diagnosed with DVT. One patient in each group had DVT proximal to the popliteal vein. There was no significant difference in the incidence of DVT between the groups (p = 0.721). A total of 84 (50.0%) patients in the TXA group and 154 (91.7%) patients received allogenic transfusion, which did not show a significant difference between the groups (p < 0.001; Table 3).

Table 2. Patient characteristics between the TXA and the control groups after PSM.

	Overall	Topical TXA		p Value
		TXA Group (n = 168)	Control Group (n = 168)	
Age, y	69.7 ± 7.6	69.3 ± 7.2	70.0 ± 8.0	0.447
Male/Female, n	43/293	20/148	23/145	0.744
BMI, kg/m^2	26.3 ± 3.7	26.2 ± 3.8	26.4 ± 3.5	0.529
ASA score	2.2 ± 0.4	2.2 ± 0.4	2.2 ± 0.4	0.547
Smoking, n	22	9	13	0.388
Hypertension, n	222	112	110	0.908
Diabetes mellitus, n	70	33	37	0.687
Chronic kidney disease, n	26	14	12	0.689
Arrhythmia, n	17	7	10	0.620
Blood profiles				
Platelet count, 10^3/μL	248.0 ± 67.4	246.5 ± 65.0	249.4 ± 69.9	0.697
PT, INR	1.0 ± 0.5	1.0 ± 0.7	1.0 ± 0.3	0.954
aPTT, sec	32.8 ± 5.2	32.7 ± 6.2	32.9 ± 4.1	0.662
Medical comorbidities				
Cerebrovascular accident, n	26	11	15	0.541
Myocardial infarction, n	32	14	18	0.578
Other thromboembolism, n	18	10	8	0.809
Cancer, n	7	3	4	0.702

TXA, tranexamic acid; PSM, propensity score matching; BMI, body mass index; ASA, American Society of Anesthesiologists; PT, prothrombin time; INR, international normalized ratio; aPTT, activated partial thromboplastin time.

Table 3. Comparison of outcomes between the TXA group and the control group.

	TXA Group (n = 168)	Control Group (n = 168)	p Value
DVT			0.721
Distal to the popliteal vein	10	6	
Proximal to the popliteal vein	1	1	
Transfusion	84	154	<0.001

TXA, tranexamic acid; DVT, deep vein thrombosis.

4. Discussion

The primary finding of the present study was that topical TXA did not increase the incidence of DVT that was evaluated using ultrasonography. In this study, postoperative ultrasonography was performed in all patients to find both symptomatic and asymptomatic thrombosis, which could be the source of other serious complications such as pulmonary thromboembolism and cerebral infraction. The incidence of DVT represented the potential risk of TXA that could trigger systemic coagulation. This study proved that topical TXA reduced postoperative transfusion rate in TKA, which is consistent with previous studies [12,18,29].

It is surprising that concerns over the safety of TXA has not been fully addressed, given that TXA is a widely used modality to reduce the risk of transfusion after TKA. Based on recent guidelines by AAHKS, the recommendation for use of TXA in high risk patients is limited due to a lack of strong evidence [24]. There have been several randomized controlled trials (RCT) or level 1 studies investigating the efficacy and safety of TXA; however, those studies excluded high risk patients [13–15,29–31]. In their notable study, Whiting et al. performed a retrospective review of 1002 total joint arthroplasty patients with ASA score ≥ 3 to evaluate the outcomes of high risk patients who received TXA [19]. They found no differences in 30-day postoperative symptomatic thromboembolic events and postoperative transfusion rate. However, a concern regarding the potential procoagulant effect of TXA still remained because only symptomatic events were assessed. Besides, the indication of TXA was different among surgeons in their study, which would cause selection bias. Sabbag et al. also reviewed 1262 primary total hip or knee arthroplasty patients with a history of DVT [21]. There was no difference in the incidence of recurrent DVT between patients who received TXA and those who did not receive TXA. However, asymptomatic DVT and medical comorbidities could not be investigated in detail because the study was based on total joint registry data.

Another remarkable study by Jules-Elysee et al. compared local and systemic levels of thrombogenic markers and TXA between IV TXA group and topical TXA group [32]. They collected peripheral and wound blood samples, measuring levels of plasmin-anti-plasmin (PAP, a measure of fibrinolysis), prothrombin fragment 1.2 (PF1.2, a marker of thrombin generation), and TXA. The authors recommended a single dose of IV TXA because no major difference was found in the mechanism of action, coagulation, and fibrinolytic profile between topical TXA and a single dose of IV TXA. However, postoperative (1 and 4 h after tourniquet release) systemic PF1.2 levels were higher than intraoperative levels in both IV TXA group and topical TXA group. The procoagulant effect of TXA cannot be ruled out although TXA was not the only reason of increased PF1.2 levels. In the present study, the incidence of DVT was investigated as an indicator of thromboembolic complications by topical TXA.

This study proved the efficacy of topical TXA in reducing the transfusion rate after TKA. The AAHKS guidelines stated that a superior method of administration could not be identified [24]. The aforementioned study by Jules-Elysee et al. concluded that a single dose of IV TXA was preferable to topical TXA because of its convenience without making a significant difference in coagulation profile, compared to the latter. However, the safety of IV TXA in high risk patients has not been strictly tested. Based on the present study, topical TXA could be considered in high risk patients undergoing TKA.

Several limitations should be noted. First, the retrospective nature of this study brought potential bias. The ideal design in examining the effects of TXA would be RCT. However, as in the previous RCT studies [18,29,32], including high risk patients in the study population would face an ethical issue. Although this study was based on retrospective data, PSM was applied to minimize the possible confounding effects. Second, this study showed relatively high transfusion rates, compared to other studies [19,29]. Because our hospital is the only tertiary referral center in the region, TKA patients often have multiple comorbidities that necessitate low threshold of transfusion. This can be the reason of the high transfusion rates. Third, DVT might have occurred after ultrasonographic examination that was performed at 1 week postoperatively. However, the delayed thrombosis can hardly be attributed to TXA, considering the short half-life of it.

5. Conclusions

The incidence of DVT, whether symptomatic or asymptomatic, was not affected by the use of topical TXA. Postoperative transfusion rate was reduced in the TXA group. Topical TXA could be applied safely even in patients who had been known to be at high risk.

Author Contributions: Conceptualization, J.-H.S.; data curation, B.K.A., C.W.L. and S.T.K.; writing—original draft, Y.B.J.; Writing—review and editing, Y.M.K.; supervision, Y.M.K.; statistical analysis, J.-H.S. All authors have read and agreed to the published version of the manuscript.

Funding: This work was supported by research fund of Chungnam National University.

Institutional Review Board Statement: The study was conducted in accordance with the Declaration of Helsinki, and approved by the Institutional Review Board of Chungnam National University Hospital (No. 2021-09-084, 5 February 2021).

Informed Consent Statement: Patient consent was waived due to the retrospective nature of the study.

Data Availability Statement: The manuscript has associated data, which will be deposited in repositories if necessary.

Conflicts of Interest: The authors declare no conflict of interest.

References

1. Moráis, S.; Ortega-Andreu, M.; Rodríguez-Merchán, E.C.; Padilla-Eguiluz, N.G.; Pérez-Chrzanowska, H.; Figueredo-Zalve, R.; Gómez-Barrena, E. Blood transfusion after primary total knee arthroplasty can be significantly minimised through a multimodal blood-loss prevention approach. *Int. Orthop.* **2014**, *38*, 347–354. [CrossRef] [PubMed]
2. Fillingham, Y.A.; Ramkumar, D.B.; Jevsevar, D.S.; Yates, A.J.; Shores, P.; Mullen, K.; Bini, S.A.; Clarke, H.D.; Schemitsch, E.; Johnson, R.L.; et al. The Efficacy of Tranexamic Acid in Total Knee Arthroplasty: A Network Meta-Analysis. *J. Arthroplast.* **2018**, *33*, 3090–3098.e1. [CrossRef]
3. Spahn, D.R. Anemia and patient blood management in hip and knee surgery: A systematic review of the literature. *Anesthesiology* **2010**, *113*, 482–495. [CrossRef]
4. Sehat, K.; Evans, R.; Newman, J. How much blood is really lost in total knee arthroplasty? Correct blood loss management should take hidden loss into account. *Knee* **2000**, *7*, 151–155. [CrossRef]
5. Wong, J.; Abrishami, A.; El Beheiry, H.; Mahomed, N.N.; Roderick Davey, J.; Gandhi, R.; Syed, K.A.; Hasan, S.M.O.; De Silva, Y.; Chung, F. Topical application of tranexamic acid reduces postoperative blood loss in total knee arthroplasty: A randomized, controlled trial. *J. Bone Jt. Surg. Am.* **2010**, *92*, 2503–2513. [CrossRef]
6. Patel, J.N.; Spanyer, J.M.; Smith, L.S.; Huang, J.; Yakkanti, M.R.; Malkani, A.L. Comparison of intravenous versus topical tranexamic acid in total knee arthroplasty: A prospective randomized study. *J. Arthroplast.* **2014**, *29*, 1528–1531. [CrossRef]
7. Alshryda, S.; Sarda, P.; Sukeik, M.; Nargol, A.; Blenkinsopp, J.; Mason, J.M. Tranexamic acid in total knee replacement: A systematic review and meta-analysis. *J. Bone Jt. Surg. Br.* **2011**, *93*, 1577–1585. [CrossRef] [PubMed]
8. Fillingham, Y.A.; Ramkumar, D.B.; Jevsevar, D.S.; Yates, A.J.; Shores, P.; Mullen, K.; Bini, S.A.; Clarke, H.D.; Schemitsch, E.; Johnson, R.L.; et al. The Safety of Tranexamic Acid in Total Joint Arthroplasty: A Direct Meta-Analysis. *J. Arthroplast.* **2018**, *33*, 3070–3082.e1. [CrossRef] [PubMed]
9. Wind, T.C.; Barfield, W.R.; Moskal, J.T. The effect of tranexamic acid on blood loss and transfusion rate in primary total knee arthroplasty. *J. Arthroplast.* **2013**, *28*, 1080–1083. [CrossRef]
10. Huang, F.; Wu, D.; Ma, G.; Yin, Z.; Wang, Q. The use of tranexamic acid to reduce blood loss and transfusion in major orthopedic surgery: A meta-analysis. *J. Surg. Res.* **2014**, *186*, 318–327. [CrossRef]
11. Bagsby, D.T.; Samujh, C.A.; Vissing, J.L.; Empson, J.A.; Pomeroy, D.L.; Malkani, A.L. Tranexamic Acid Decreases Incidence of Blood Transfusion in Simultaneous Bilateral Total Knee Arthroplasty. *J. Arthroplast.* **2015**, *30*, 2106–2109. [CrossRef] [PubMed]
12. Xiong, H.; Liu, Y.; Zeng, Y.; Wu, Y.; Shen, B. The efficacy and safety of combined administration of intravenous and topical tranexamic acid in primary total knee arthroplasty: A meta-analysis of randomized controlled trials. *BMC Musculoskelet. Disord.* **2018**, *19*, 321. [CrossRef]
13. Yang, Z.-G.; Chen, W.-P.; Wu, L.-D. Effectiveness and safety of tranexamic acid in reducing blood loss in total knee arthroplasty: A meta-analysis. *J. Bone Jt. Surg. Am.* **2012**, *94*, 1153–1159. [CrossRef]
14. Alvarez, J.C.; Santiveri, F.X.; Ramos, I.; Vela, E.; Puig, L.; Escolano, F. Tranexamic acid reduces blood transfusion in total knee arthroplasty even when a blood conservation program is applied. *Transfusion* **2008**, *48*, 519–525. [CrossRef]
15. Kagoma, Y.K.; Crowther, M.A.; Douketis, J.; Bhandari, M.; Eikelboom, J.; Lim, W. Use of antifibrinolytic therapy to reduce transfusion in patients undergoing orthopedic surgery: A systematic review of randomized trials. *Thromb. Res.* **2009**, *123*, 687–696. [CrossRef]
16. Onodera, T.; Majima, T.; Sawaguchi, N.; Kasahara, Y.; Ishigaki, T.; Minami, A. Risk of deep venous thrombosis in drain clamping with tranexamic acid and carbazochrome sodium sulfonate hydrate in total knee arthroplasty. *J. Arthroplast.* **2012**, *27*, 105–108. [CrossRef]
17. Sukeik, M.; Alshryda, S.; Haddad, F.S.; Mason, J.M. Systematic review and meta-analysis of the use of tranexamic acid in total hip replacement. *J. Bone Jt. Surg. Br.* **2011**, *93*, 39–46. [CrossRef] [PubMed]
18. Roy, S.P.; Tanki, U.F.; Dutta, A.; Jain, S.K.; Nagi, O.N. Efficacy of intra-articular tranexamic acid in blood loss reduction following primary unilateral total knee arthroplasty. *Knee Surg. Sports Traumatol. Arthrosc.* **2012**, *20*, 2494–2501. [CrossRef]
19. Whiting, D.R.; Gillette, B.P.; Duncan, C.; Smith, H.; Pagnano, M.W.; Sierra, R.J. Preliminary results suggest tranexamic acid is safe and effective in arthroplasty patients with severe comorbidities. *Clin. Orthop. Relat. Res.* **2014**, *472*, 66–72. [CrossRef]
20. Duncan, C.M.; Gillette, B.P.; Jacob, A.K.; Sierra, R.J.; Sanchez-Sotelo, J.; Smith, H.M. Venous thromboembolism and mortality associated with tranexamic acid use during total hip and knee arthroplasty. *J. Arthroplast.* **2015**, *30*, 272–276. [CrossRef]
21. Sabbag, O.D.; Abdel, M.P.; Amundson, A.W.; Larson, D.R.; Pagnano, M.W. Tranexamic Acid Was Safe in Arthroplasty Patients With a History of Venous Thromboembolism: A Matched Outcome Study. *J. Arthroplast.* **2017**, *32*, S246–S250. [CrossRef] [PubMed]
22. Sasanuma, H.; Sekiya, H.; Takatoku, K.; Takada, H.; Sugimoto, N.; Hoshino, Y. Efficient strategy for controlling postoperative hemorrhage in total knee arthroplasty. *Knee Surg. Sports Traumatol. Arthrosc.* **2011**, *19*, 921–925. [CrossRef] [PubMed]
23. Zhang, H.; Chen, J.; Chen, F.; Que, W. The effect of tranexamic acid on blood loss and use of blood products in total knee arthroplasty: A meta-analysis. *Knee Surg. Sports Traumatol. Arthrosc.* **2012**, *20*, 1742–1752. [CrossRef]

24. Fillingham, Y.A.; Ramkumar, D.B.; Jevsevar, D.S.; Yates, A.J.; Bini, S.A.; Clarke, H.D.; Schemitsch, E.; Johnson, R.L.; Memtsoudis, S.G.; Sayeed, S.A.; et al. Tranexamic Acid Use in Total Joint Arthroplasty: The Clinical Practice Guidelines Endorsed by the American Association of Hip and Knee Surgeons, American Society of Regional Anesthesia and Pain Medicine, American Academy of Orthopaedic Surgeons, Hip Society, and Knee Society. *J. Arthroplast.* **2018**, *33*, 3065–3069. [CrossRef]
25. Canonico, M.E.; Santoro, C.; Avvedimento, M.; Giugliano, G.; Mandoli, G.E.; Prastaro, M.; Franzone, A.; Piccolo, R.; Ilardi, F.; Cameli, M.; et al. Venous Thromboembolism and Cancer: A Comprehensive Review from Pathophysiology to Novel Treatment. *Biomolecules* **2022**, *12*, 259. [CrossRef] [PubMed]
26. Russell, R.D.; Huo, M.H. Apixaban and rivaroxaban decrease deep venous thrombosis but not other complications after total hip and total knee arthroplasty. *J. Arthroplast.* **2013**, *28*, 1477–1481. [CrossRef] [PubMed]
27. Kim, Y.-H.; Kulkarni, S.S.; Park, J.-W.; Kim, J.-S. Prevalence of Deep Vein Thrombosis and Pulmonary Embolism Treated with Mechanical Compression Device After Total Knee Arthroplasty in Asian Patients. *J. Arthroplast.* **2015**, *30*, 1633–1637. [CrossRef] [PubMed]
28. Austin, P.C. An Introduction to Propensity Score Methods for Reducing the Effects of Confounding in Observational Studies. *Multivar. Behav. Res.* **2011**, *46*, 399–424. [CrossRef]
29. Seo, J.-G.; Moon, Y.-W.; Park, S.-H.; Kim, S.-M.; Ko, K.-R. The comparative efficacies of intra-articular and IV tranexamic acid for reducing blood loss during total knee arthroplasty. *Knee Surg. Sports Traumatol. Arthrosc.* **2013**, *21*, 1869–1874. [CrossRef] [PubMed]
30. Henry, D.A.; Carless, P.A.; Moxey, A.J.; O'Connell, D.; Stokes, B.J.; Fergusson, D.A.; Ker, K. Anti-fibrinolytic use for minimising perioperative allogeneic blood transfusion. *Cochrane Database Syst. Rev.* **2011**, CD001886. [CrossRef]
31. Shiga, T.; Wajima, Z.; Inoue, T.; Sakamoto, A. Aprotinin in major orthopedic surgery: A systematic review of randomized controlled trials. *Anesth. Analg.* **2005**, *101*, 1602–1607. [CrossRef]
32. Jules-Elysee, K.M.; Tseng, A.; Sculco, T.P.; Baaklini, L.R.; McLawhorn, A.S.; Pickard, A.J.; Qin, W.; Cross, J.R.; Su, E.P.; Fields, K.G.; et al. Comparison of Topical and Intravenous Tranexamic Acid for Total Knee Replacement: A Randomized Double-Blinded Controlled Study of Effects on Tranexamic Acid Levels and Thrombogenic and Inflammatory Marker Levels. *J. Bone Jt. Surg. Am.* **2019**, *101*, 2120–2128. [CrossRef]

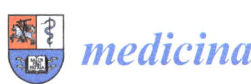

Article

Continuous Cold Flow Device Following Total Knee Arthroplasty: Myths and Reality

Michele Coviello [1,*,†], Antonella Abate [2,†], Francesco Ippolito [2], Vittorio Nappi [2], Roberto Maddalena [2], Giuseppe Maccagnano [3,*], Giovanni Noia [3] and Vincenzo Caiaffa [2]

[1] Orthopaedic and Trauma Unit, Department of Basic Medical Sciences, Neurscience and Sense Organs, School of Medicine, AOU Consorziale Policlinico, University of Bari "Aldo Moro", Piazza Giulio Cesare 11, 70124 Bari, Italy
[2] Orthopaedic and Traumatology Unit, "Di Venere" Hospital, Via Ospedale di Venere, 1, 70131 Bari, Italy
[3] Orthopaedics Unit, Department of Clinical and Experimental Medicine, Faculty of Medicine and Surgery, University of Foggia, Policlinico Riuniti di Foggia, 71122 Foggia, Italy
* Correspondence: michelecoviello91@gmail.com (M.C.); g.maccagnano@gmail.com (G.M.); Tel.: +39-338-9652261 (G.M.)
† These authors contributed equally to this work.

Abstract: *Background and Objectives*: To assess the effect of continuous cold flow (CCF) therapy on pain reduction, opioid consumption, fast recovery, less perioperative bleeding and patient satisfaction in patients undergoing a total knee arthroplasty. *Materials and Methods*: Patients affected by knee osteoarthritis between September 2020 and February 2022 were enrolled in this case-control study. Patients were randomly divided into two groups (n = 50, each): the study group received postoperative CCF therapy while the control group was treated by cold pack (gel ice). The CCF device is a computer-assisted therapy with continuous cold fluid, allowing a selective distribution, constant and uniform, of cold or hot on the areas to be treated. In both groups, pre- and postoperative evaluations at 6, 24, 72 h and at the fifth day were conducted using Visual Analogic Scale (VAS), opioid consumption, passive range of motion, preoperative hematocrit, total blood loss by Gross formula, transfusion requirement and patient satisfaction questionnaire. *Results*: One hundred patients, 52 women (52%), were included in the study. Reduction of pain, opioid consumption and increase in passive range of movement were statistically significantly demonstrated in the study group on the first and third days. Patients were satisfied with adequate postoperative pain management due to CCF therapy (p = 0.01) and they would recommend this treatment to others (p = 0.01). *Conclusions*: A continuous cold flow device in the acute postoperative setting after total knee arthroplasty is associated with pain reduction and improving early movement. Patients were almost satisfied with the procedure. The management of perioperative pain control could improve participation in the early rehabilitation program as demonstrated by the increase in ROM, psychological satisfaction and reduction in opioid use.

Keywords: continuous cold flow therapy; cryotherapy; total knee arthroplasty; pain; opioids consumption; patient satisfaction

Citation: Coviello, M.; Abate, A.; Ippolito, F.; Nappi, V.; Maddalena, R.; Maccagnano, G.; Noia, G.; Caiaffa, V. Continuous Cold Flow Device Following Total Knee Arthroplasty: Myths and Reality. *Medicina* **2022**, *58*, 1537. https://doi.org/10.3390/medicina58111537

Academic Editors: Yong In and In Jun Koh

Received: 6 September 2022
Accepted: 24 October 2022
Published: 27 October 2022

Publisher's Note: MDPI stays neutral with regard to jurisdictional claims in published maps and institutional affiliations.

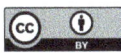

Copyright: © 2022 by the authors. Licensee MDPI, Basel, Switzerland. This article is an open access article distributed under the terms and conditions of the Creative Commons Attribution (CC BY) license (https://creativecommons.org/licenses/by/4.0/).

1. Introduction

Total knee arthroplasty (TKA) is a widely accepted and successful procedure for end-stage arthritis. However, being a major orthopedic intervention, it is accompanied by tissue damage and an inflammatory response, manifesting as local swelling and edema [1,2], reduced range of motion (ROM), stiffness and reduced quadriceps strength [3,4]. Acute postoperative period after TKA may be quite challenging; patients may experience pain, swelling, restricted knee joint excursion, nausea or vomiting, and potential blood loss. A painful acute postoperative period may affect the so called fast track recovery [3], with patient discomfort and long-term effects on knee function [5,6].

Pain is often severe in the early postoperative period, impeding rehabilitation [7]. Multimodal approaches to obtain pain control, throughout advances in anesthetic technique and narcotics administration, is not always sufficient to promote early rehabilitation and is often associated with side effects, such as nausea, vomiting, sedation, pruritus, hypotension, and respiratory depression, which can limit activity, result in longer hospital stays, increase morbidity, and reduce patients' satisfaction [8,9].

Cold therapy for pain reduction is an accepted and frequently used treatment in daily practice after trauma or surgery. It involves the application of cold to the skin surrounding the injured soft tissues and in joint surgery is supposed to reduce the intraarticular temperature [10] (Figure 1). It is supposed to reduce the local blood flow by vasoconstriction, swelling, and pain experience by slowing the conduction of nerve signals [11,12].

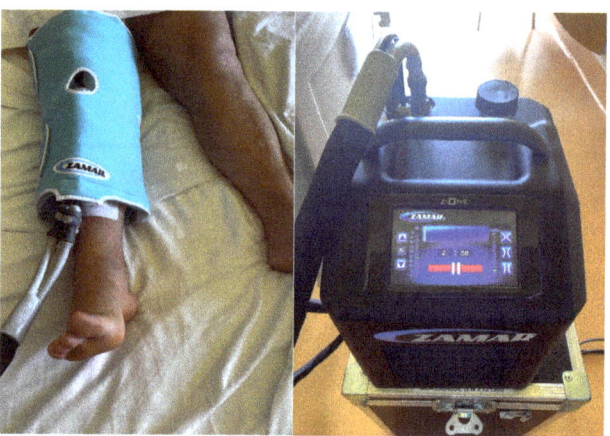

Figure 1. Application of cryotherapy pad on a patient.

Several cold therapeutic options are available, including first generation cold therapy, such as crushed ice in a plastic bag; second generation cold therapy with circulating ice water with or without compression; and third generation advanced computer-assisted devices with continuous controlled cold therapy. The advantage of these latter devices is the possibility of temperature modulation with cooling at a specific and continuous temperature (generally 5–11°) for a prolonged time. These devices also allow a progressive increase in the temperature before stopping the treatment to avoid secondary cold-induced vasodilatation, and they are not needed to be periodically filled with cold water or ice [13].

Even though some studies show excellent results regarding computer-assisted continuous cold flow therapy, the quality of the available literature is not convincing and level I evidence is still missing [14].

The main aim of this study is to assess the effect of continuous cold flow therapy on pain reduction, opioid consumption, ROM recovery, less perioperative bleeding and patient satisfaction in patients undergoing a TKA.

2. Materials and Methods

This is a prospective, case-control, monocenter study, validated by the Ethics Committee (protocol number: 10/CE/2020—1 June 2020) and performed in accordance with the ethical standards laid down in the 1964 Declaration of Helsinki. All the patients involved in the study gave their informed consent prior to their inclusion in the study.

The patients who were scheduled to undergo primary TKA replacement for grade IV gonarthrosis due to a proven painful knee osteoarthritis, who need to obtain pain relief and improve function, who were able and willing to follow instructions, were enrolled and treated at the Di Venere Hospital of Bari between September 2020 and February 2022.

The patients were divided into two groups using a predefined program (http://www.randomization.com, accessed on 1 September 2020). After surgery, the circulating nurse reviewed the random numbers list. The study group was represented by patients who were treated with postoperative continuous cold flow (CCF) therapy; the control group included patients treated with a cold pack (gel ice) postoperatively.

The inclusion criteria were primary knee osteoarthritis, age between 40 and 81, body mass index (BMI) between 20 and 29.9 and chronic history (for at least 4 months) of knee joint pain.

The exclusion criteria were inflammatory diseases, infection, coagulopathy, previous knee surgery, history of deep vein thrombosis or pulmonary embolism, rheumatoid arthritis, pregnancy and patients who were not able to understand and complete the procedure due to cognitive dysfunction or language barrier.

The sample size as a prospective study was calculated using a pain score tested by visual analogic scale (VAS), referring to previous paper values on the same treatment protocol [15] as primary endpoint. Using a standard deviation of 0.6-point [16,17], we estimated that we would need 23 participants in each group to detect a statistically significant differences at an α level of 0.05 and power level of 80%.

Between September 2020 and February 2022, one hundred and twelve patients with grade IV gonarthrosis were evaluated for eligibility for the present study. Four patients had previous surgery of the knee, four patients participated in another study, two were living in another country, one declined to participate, and one other patient had reprieved the operation. Therefore, they were excluded from the study. Subsequently, 100 patients were included. An overview of the number of patients recruited, enrolled and analyzed in this work is presented in Figure 2 in the manner recommended by consolidated standards of the Strengthening the Reporting of Observational Studies in Epidemiology (STROBE) guidelines [18].

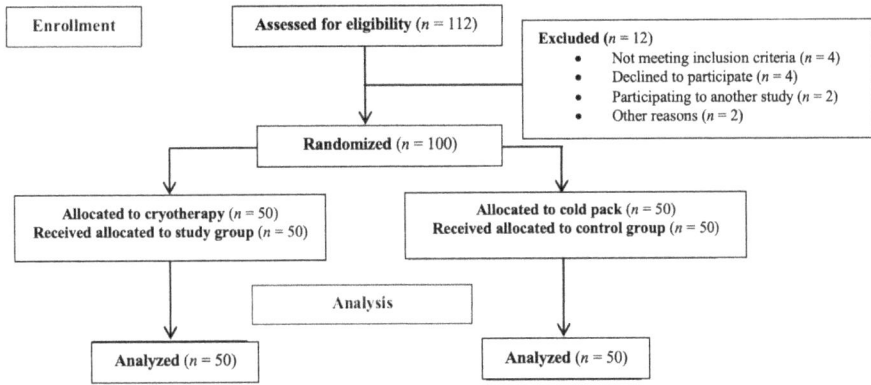

Figure 2. Diagram of the number of patients enrolled and analyzed in this study using STROBE guidelines.

For each patient, the following data were recorded: age; sex; BMI; side of surgery; American Society of Anesthesiologists score (ASA) [19], surgical time; VAS (visual analogic scale) (X), opioid consumption; passive range of motion (ROM); preoperative hematocrit; total blood loss (using the formula described by Gross [7], transfusion requirement and patient satisfaction questionnaire.

Data were recorded at the following times: T0 (before the surgical procedure); T1 (six-hours post-surgery); T2 (24 h post-surgery); T3 (72 h post-surgery) and T4 (fifth day post-surgery).

Opioid consumption was measured as number of tablets, tramadol (50 mg), used in the postoperative days. All patients received standard pain therapy with acetaminophen

1 g every 12 h, ketorolac tromethamine 30 mg and daily low molecular heparin injections (Fondaparinux, Arixtra, Glaxo-SmithKline, Brentford, Middlesex, UK) as thrombosis prophylaxis up to 4 weeks after surgery.

Passive range of motion as functional recovery was measured by the same operator for each patient using an orthopedic protractor.

Blood loss was evaluated only at T2 using the formula described by Gross.

$$\text{Total blood volume} = \frac{\text{Preoperative hematocrit} - \text{postoperative day 1 hematocrit}}{\text{Average hematocrit between preoperative and postoperative day 1}}$$

Transfusion requirement was evaluated as the number of blood transfusions during hospitalization (transfusion trigger was set at 8.0 g/dL of hemoglobin).

Patient satisfaction was assessed via questionnaire. Participants reported their overall satisfaction by placing an X on a 10-cm line (from 0 (extremely unsatisfied) to 10 (extremely satisfied)). The distance was measured in centimeters from the beginning of the line to the center of the patient's X, using a ruler with 1-mm increments. Participants were also asked to recommend the method of cooling, answering "yes" or "not".

According to a standardized protocol, patients received antibiotic prophylaxis with cefazolin 2 g and premedication 2 h before operation with acetaminophen 1 g. Patients were operated under spinal anesthetic treatment by one experienced knee surgeon (VC), performing a minimum of 150 TKA procedures annually. Patients were operated on using a midline anterior incision with a medial parapatellar arthrotomy and with the use of dedicated instruments for the implantation of a cemented Postero-Stabilized (PS) TKA [20] (Zimmer Biomet, Warsaw, IN, USA). No tourniquet was used during surgery. Before skin closure, hemostasis was controlled using diathermia. The wound margins were infiltrated with 140 cc ropivacaine (0.2%) as local infiltration anesthesia (LIA). No adrenaline was used during LIA, since it was shown that adrenaline could be omitted from the LIA-mixture [21]. A wound drain was used. All wounds were closed with a barbed suture wire. The surgical wound was covered with a hydrocolloid dressing (Aquacel® Surgical, ConvaTec Inc., Reading, UK) for 7 days and a compressive dressing was applied in the operating room. A strict urinary nurse-led bladder scan management protocol was used for the prevention of postoperative urinary retention [22]. All patients were planned to be discharged on the fifth day after surgery.

The study group received advanced cooling devices. The machine used (Zamar Z-one MG465A, Croatia, Balkans) was dedicated to each patient during the entire period of hospital stay. It is a computer-assisted continuous cold flow therapy allowing a selective distribution, constant and uniform of cold or hot, on the areas to be treated. Patients cooled the affected knee according to a fixed protocol.

The application started the day before surgery for 3 h and repeated within 6 h post-operation for 3 h. Then it was applied for 3 h respectively in the morning and in the afternoon, during the five postoperative days.

Temperature was set at 5° as efficient CCF therapy requires cooling the skin and achieving reduction in pain according to Chesterton et al. [1]. Compression was granted at the minimum level to avoid discomfort.

In the control group patients received 15 min cold pack (conserved at −17°) treatment with two cold packs anterior and one posterior to the knee within 6 h post-operation and then repeated at 2 and 4 h after surgery. The following days patients received the same cold pack 15 min after each physiotherapy session (10 am and 3 pm). Cold packs were also permitted as requested during the night. No compression was applied.

Thereafter the same rehabilitation program was employed for all patients, consisting of full weight bearing and active range of motion exercises at day of surgery. A continuous passive motion device was used twice a day.

As a primary endpoint, pain was quantified using the VAS scale with scores ranging from 0 (no pain) to 10 (worst imaginable pain).

The functional recovery, pain management, blood loss and patient satisfaction were assessed as a secondary endpoint.

A prospective clinical study was conducted. The data were collected and analyzed using SPSS (v 23; IBM® Inc., Armonk, NY, USA). Descriptive statistics were calculated for the overall sample and for follow-up. Categorical variables were presented as numbers or percentages. Continuous variables were presented as mean and standard deviation. Due to the non-homogeneous distribution of the values using the Kolmogorov–Smirnov test ($p > 0.05$), non-parametric tests were considered. To compare the average values between the groups at the same times, the U Mann–Whitney test or Fischer's test were used, when appropriate. To compare the value within the same group at different times, the Wilcoxon test or Related-Samples Friedman's test Two-Way Analysis of Variance were used. To demonstrate the correlation between the CCF device and variables, a multiple regression model was then fitted. For all the tests, a p-value of less than 0.05 was considered to be statistically significant.

The data presented in this study are available on request from the corresponding author.

3. Results

One hundred consecutive patients treated with TKA were enrolled in this study and allocated into two groups, with 50 cases in each group. We compared the study and control group at recruitment (Table 1). No statistical differences emerged between groups.

Table 1. Main data of the study.

Preoperative Features	Study Group	Control Group	p-Value
Age (year)	66.56 ± 6.78	65.76 ± 6.23	0.63
Gender (female)	27 (54%)	25 (50%)	0.84
BMI (Kg/m^2)	28.50 ± 4.32	27.82 ± 3.47	0.56
Side (left)	23 (46%)	21 (42%)	0.84
ASA Classification			0.86
I	20 (40%)	18 (36%)	
II	16 (32%)	14 (28%)	
III	11 (22%)	13 (26%)	
IV	3 (6%)	5 (10%)	
Preoperative hematocrit (%)	38.82 ± 3.67	39.73 ± 3.87	0.16
Surgical time (min)	57.09 ± 15.04	58.16 ± 15.46	0.70

(One hundred patients; U Mann–Whitney and Fischer's test; data are presented as mean ± standard deviation or number and percentage; BMI: Body Mass Index; ASA: American Society of Anesthesiologists score).

None of the patients experienced any skin complications due to the CCF therapy or gel ice. None of patients needed revision surgery due to infection and mechanical relaxation in the early period. Neither intraoperative nor postoperative complication was recorded.

The VAS scores before and after surgery were noted for each time. No difference was shown preoperatively. The study group recorded lower values if compared with control, but only at one day postoperatively was the difference statistically significant ($p = 0.01$, Table 2 and Figure 3).

Table 2. Differences in pain and opioid treatment between groups.

VAS		Study Group	Control Group	*p*-Value
	T0	9.00 ± 0.47	9.06 ± 0.49	0.52
	T1	6.39 ± 1.23	6.20 ± 1.12	0.46
	T2	5.09 ± 0.94	5.69 ± 1.08	**0.01**
	T3	4.06 ± 0.89	4.21 ± 0.72	0.51
	T4	3.48 ± 0.68	3.57 ± 0.64	0.52
Opioid consumption				
	T1 (mg)	8 (400)	9 (450)	1.00
	T2 (mg)	17 (850)	32 (1600)	**0.01**
	T3 (mg)	9 (450)	19 (950)	**0.05**
	T4 (mg)	11 (550)	14 (700)	0.64
	Total (mg)	45 (2250)	74 (3700)	**0.02**

(One hundred patients; U Mann–Whitney test for VAS and Fischer's test for opioid consumption; data are presented as mean ± standard deviation or number of tablets tramadol and equivalent mg; VAS: visual analogic scale).

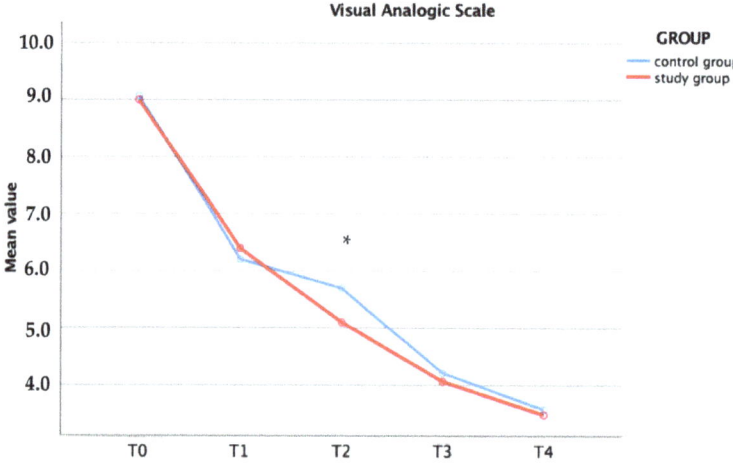

Figure 3. Visual analogic scale within each group (* $p = 0.01$).

In the study group a reduction in opioid consumption was demonstrably statistically significant in the first- and third-days postoperative. Overall, there was a lower consumption in the study group than in the control ($p = 0.02$, Table 2).

Descriptive values and comparison results of passive knee range of motion values are given in Table 3. It was found that the difference between preoperative and postoperative knee flexion measurements was significantly improved in both groups ($p = 0.01$ in both groups using Two-Way Analysis of Variance) and the differences between the groups were changed one- and three-day postoperative.

Table 3. Differences in passive range of motion, total blood loss using Gross formula and patient satisfaction between groups.

Passive ROM (°)		Study Group	Control Group	p-Value
	T0	84.40 ± 7.14	83.48 ± 7.02	0.55
	T2	111.57 ± 7.04	105.49 ± 11.24	**0.01**
	T3	110.94 ± 7.52	107.39 ± 7.89	**0.01**
	T4	108.84 ± 6.07	108.22 ± 6.61	0.64
Total blood loss (Gross formula)				
	T2	1.03 ± 0.42	1.06 ± 0.55	0.86
Number of transfusions		4 (8%)	5 (10%)	0.50
Patient satisfaction (cm)		8.55 ± 0.36	6.05 ± 0.58	**0.01**
Patient who recommended "yes"		43 (86%)	31 (62%)	**0.01**

(One hundred patients; U Mann–Whitney test and Fischer's test; data are presented as mean ± standard deviation or number and percentage; ROM: range of motion).

No statistically significant difference was found between the groups regarding blood loss and transfusion number (Table 3).

Patients treated with CCF therapy were more satisfied than the control group (Table 3).

The multiple linear regression models showed postoperative VAS score and opioid consumption were influenced by CCF therapy rather than other preoperative variables (Table 4).

Table 4. Multiple linear regression models for postoperative VAS and opioid consumption.

	VAS			Opioid Consumption		
	B	95% CI	p-Value	B	95% CI	p-Value
Intercept	7.50		<0.01	0.915		0.05
Group (cryotherapy)	−0.62	−1.04 −0.20	<0.01	−0.31	−0.50 −0.11	<0.01
Age	−0.01	−0.04 0.02	0.57	0.01	−0.01 0.03	0.15
Sex (female)	−0.25	−0.93 0.41	0.45	0.12	−0.19 0.44	0.44
Left knee	0.53	−0.14 1.20	0.12	−0.21	−0.52 0.10	0.18
BMI	−0.01	−0.06 0.05	0.93	−0.02	−0.05 0.01	0.12
ASA Classification	−0.01	−0.24 0.22	0.96	−0.07	−0.17 0.04	0.22
Preoperative hematocrit	−0.01	−0.07 0.04	0.69	−0.01	−0.03 0.02	0.72
Surgical time	−0.01	−0.02 0.01	0.32	−0.01	−0.01 0.01	0.69
Total blood loss	−0.20	−0.63 0.25	0.39	−0.01	−0.21 0.20	0.99

(BMI: Body Mass Index).

4. Discussion

After a major orthopedic surgical procedure, such as TKA, pain control is imperative to promote rapid recovery and collaboration to the rehabilitation program. Nowadays, specific pathways of care, including enhanced recovery after surgery (ERAS), have been introduced. It has been proposed these pathways, along with multimodal analgesia, have reduced the length of hospital stay (LOS) for patients undergoing TKA [23]. Analgesic options for TKA include pre-emptive analgesia, local infiltration, systemic analgesics (opioids, non-opioids, and patient-controlled analgesia), epidural analgesia and, more recently, femoral nerve block [24]. It has been postulated that peripheral nerve blocks provide intense, site-specific analgesia and are associated with a lower incidence of side effects when compared with many other modalities of postoperative analgesia [25]. Another approach to reduce pain and promote recovery consisted of cooling obtained by a different kind of CCF therapy approach [26,27]. However, consensus has not successfully been reached on the better modality, its efficiency and scheme of application.

The most important finding in our study is that postoperative computer assisted CCF therapy is effective in pain control after TKA and associated with reduction in analgesic use during the early postoperative period. It is also associated with a major passive ROM during the first two days and with a great grade of patient satisfaction. We enrolled a larger study population if compared to power analysis due to the possibility of patient refusal and to strengthen the results.

Significant reduction in VAS was observed only at T2 (24 h), however there was a reduction in VAS after every cooling session in the study group. Similar to these findings, pain reductions in the acute postoperative phase were reported [7,28,29]. Inflammatory conditions secondary to surgery cause most of the perceived pain in the immediate postoperative period after knee replacement. Additionally, patients undergoing knee surgery have already suffered pain for a long period secondary to established central nervous system sensitization. It seems to be intuitive that any approach aimed to reduce pain should be pursued to avoid risk of development of chronic pain [30]. Bech et al. found no superiority in reducing pain compared with traditional icing. Cooling reduces the tissue metabolic rate and relieves inflammation by suppressing enzymatic activity and preventing secondary tissue damage, reducing muscle tissue spasm [31].

Consumption of analgesic was also investigated in this study. In our paper the consumption of additional opioids as rescue medication was up to two times greater in the control group than in the study group. However, this trend was significant only in the first two postoperative days, with these days being the worst period for pain management.

The incremented use of opioids can slow a patient's rehabilitation program due to side effects (nausea, vomiting, headache, constipation). A slower rehabilitation can be associated with retarded discharge and increased costs [32].

Su et al. [33] showed a lower consumption of opioids in a multicenter RCT. In another recent systematic review and meta-analysis of 11 RCT, Addie et al. [28] showed no benefits for analgesic use. Thienpont et al. [14], on the contrary, found no difference in VAS and morphine use in their RCT. They shared Algafly's conviction that a decreased nerve conduction velocity resulting in better pain tolerance can explain the local anesthetic effect of intense cooling [11]. However, this is merely a temporary measure that disappears after ice removal.

The CCF therapy is crucial and ensures that the knee ROM movements start in the early postoperative period. There were studies reporting that the CCF therapy affects the knee movement gap in a positive way in the early postoperative period [34–36]. In our study passive ROM at first and second postoperative day was better in the cold compression group. Su et al. found no differences for ROM or functional testing between a cryopneumatic device and ice packs [33]. Kullemberg et al. [12] and Holmstrom et al. [37] reported that cold compression was more efficient than epidural analgesia with better ROM, reducing hospital stay.

Patients reported high satisfaction rate with postoperative cooling and were likely to recommend icing device. Less pain could substantiate this validation. The high level of satisfaction may also be associated to greater patient contact with the staff conduction device function and periodic skin and dressing check. The psychological aspect plays a key role in rehabilitation [38]. Only two patients reported that the device was uncomfortable and that some nurses appeared not to be sure how to apply it.

Blood loss evaluation is a key point to justify routine use of a cold flow device, considering its additional costs. Reduction in blood loss and blood transfusion may reduce costs associated with TKA. Additionally, blood transfusion is associated with an increased rate of periprosthetic infection. In our study we found that the total blood loss measured by Gross formula in the postoperative period in the study group was lower than in the control group; however, non-statistically significant values were observed in total blood loss. Kuyucu et al. [26] also did not find significant difference in blood loss between their study groups. Ruffilli et al. [7] carefully evaluated blood loss throughout drain output, blood loss with Gross formula, transfusion requirements, and did not find any difference between their study groups. Contradictory results have been found by several authors regarding visible and real blood loss [37,39]. This could be explained by the fact that CCF therapy may cause an immediate reduction of bleeding by vasoconstriction and compression but later lead to a cold-induced vasodilatation and interfere with secondary hemostasis [40]. Hemostasis and coagulation are biochemical reactions that are most efficient at basal body temperature. Computed control of temperature progressive increase before cryotherapy removal should be considered to reduce secondary vasodilatation and blood loss [41]. Karaduman et al. found the Hb levels measured in the ice pack group were lower than those in experimental groups treated with CCF therapy in the postoperative period. They also sustained that postoperative CCF therapy was effective in reducing blood loss. However, preoperative CCF therapy application had no significant effect [15].

The evaluation method of blood loss could explain the difference in results in the literature. We decided to use the formula described by Gross et al. [42] for blood loss calculation after arthroplasty surgery, which is one of the most popular among surgeons. However, the Gross equation does not involve Hb-related factors. Actual blood loss and anemia are revealed by the calculated perioperative volume and the changing in hematocrit [42]. This could consist of a limitation of this method and additional evaluation of Hb values and drainage blood loss should be considered.

The novelty of this study is the careful analysis of the patient's outcomes combined with their satisfaction. Psychological well-being improves clinical outcomes and makes the patient prone to better physiotherapy [38].

Our study has several strengths. This was performed in one single center, one single experienced surgeon performed all surgeries using the same surgical approach, one type of anesthesia, implant, pain and rehabilitation program. The self-reported patient satisfaction questionnaire is an additional element considering the importance of a fast-track recovery plan in replacement surgery.

However, some limitations must be considered. The sample size could be increased. Better evaluation of blood loss throughout alternative formula, including Hb values, should be adopted. Another limitation is that patients were evaluated only during the hospital stay so it cannot draw definitive long-term conclusions about CCF therapy efficacy.

5. Conclusions

Continuous cold flow devices in the acute postoperative setting after TKA are associated with pain reduction and improving early ROM. Although reduction in blood loss throughout the Gross formula was observed, no significant differences were found. Patients were almost satisfied with the procedure and should recommend it to improve perioperative pain control and participation to the early rehabilitation program due to lower opioid consumption and higher passive ROM.

Author Contributions: Conceptualization, M.C.; data curation, M.C.; writing—original draft preparation, A.A., V.N. and F.I.; writing—review and editing, G.M. and G.N.; supervision, R.M. and V.C. All authors have read and agreed to the published version of the manuscript.

Funding: This research received no external funding.

Institutional Review Board Statement: The study was conducted according to the guidelines of the Declaration of Helsinki and approved by the Ethics Committee (protocol number: 10/CE/2020—1 June 2020).

Informed Consent Statement: Informed consent was obtained from all subjects involved in the study. Written informed consent has been obtained from the patient(s) to publish this paper if applicable.

Data Availability Statement: The data presented in this study are available on request from the corresponding author.

Conflicts of Interest: The authors declare no conflict of interest.

References

1. Chesterton, L.S.; Foster, N.E.; Ross, L. Skin temperature response to cryotherapy. *Arch. Phys. Med. Rehabil.* **2002**, *83*, 543–549. [CrossRef]
2. Sehat, K.R.; Evans, R.L.; Newman, J.H. Hidden blood loss following hip and knee arthroplasty. Correct management of blood loss should take hidden loss into account. *J. Bone Joint Surg. Br.* **2004**, *86*, 561–565. [CrossRef] [PubMed]
3. Adie, S.; Naylor, J.M.; Harris, I.A. Cryotherapy after Total Knee Arthroplasty. *J. Arthroplast.* **2010**, *25*, 709–715. [CrossRef] [PubMed]
4. Holm, B.; Husted, H.; Kehlet, H.; Bandholm, T. Effect of knee joint icing on knee extension strength and knee pain early after total knee arthroplasty: A randomized cross-over study. *Clin. Rehabil.* **2012**, *26*, 716–723. [CrossRef] [PubMed]
5. Bourne, R.B.; McCalden, R.W.; MacDonald, S.J.; Mokete, L.; Guerin, J. Influence of Patient Factors on TKA Outcomes at 5 to 11 Years Followup. *Clin. Orthop. Relat. Res.* **2007**, *464*, 27–31. [CrossRef]
6. Barry, S.; Wallace, L.; Lamb, S. Cryotherapy after total knee replacement: A survey of current practice. *Physiother. Res. Int.* **2003**, *8*, 111–120. [CrossRef] [PubMed]
7. Ruffilli, A.; Castagnini, F.; Traina, F.; Corneti, I.; Fenga, D.; Giannini, S.; Faldini, C. Temperature-Controlled Continuous Cold Flow Device after Total Knee Arthroplasty: A Randomized Controlled Trial Study. *J. Knee Surg.* **2017**, *30*, 675–681. [CrossRef] [PubMed]
8. Trueblood, A.; Manning, D.W. Analgesia following total knee arthroplasty. *Curr. Opin. Orthop.* **2007**, *18*, 76–80. [CrossRef]
9. White, P.F. The Changing Role of Non-Opioid Analgesic Techniques in the Management of Postoperative Pain. *Anesth. Analg.* **2005**, *101*, S5–S22. [CrossRef] [PubMed]
10. Martin, S.S.; Spindler, K.P.; Tarter, J.W.; Detwiler, K.B. Does Cryotherapy Affect Intraarticular Temperature after Knee Arthroscopy? *Clin. Orthop. Relat. Res.* **2002**, *400*, 184–189. [CrossRef]
11. Algafly, A.A.; George, K.P.; Herrington, L. The effect of cryotherapy on nerve conduction velocity, pain threshold and pain tolerance * Commentary. *Br. J. Sports Med.* **2007**, *41*, 365–369. [CrossRef] [PubMed]
12. Kullenberg, B.; Ylipää, S.; Söderlund, K.; Resch, S. Postoperative Cryotherapy After Total Knee Arthroplasty. *J. Arthroplast.* **2006**, *21*, 1175–1179. [CrossRef] [PubMed]
13. Saito, N.; Horiuchi, H.; Kobayashi, S.; Nawata, M.; Takaoka, K. Continuous local cooling for pain relief following total hip arthroplasty. *J. Arthroplast.* **2004**, *19*, 334–337. [CrossRef] [PubMed]
14. Thijs, E.; Schotanus, M.G.M.; Bemelmans, Y.F.L.; Kort, N.P. Reduced opiate use after total knee arthroplasty using computer-assisted cryotherapy. *Knee Surg. Sport. Traumatol. Arthrosc.* **2019**, *27*, 1204–1212. [CrossRef] [PubMed]
15. Karaduman, Z.O.; Turhal, O.; Turhan, Y.; Orhan, Z.; Arican, M.; Uslu, M.; Cangur, S. Evaluation of the Clinical Efficacy of Using Thermal Camera for Cryotherapy in Patients with Total Knee Arthroplasty: A Prospective Study. *Medicina* **2019**, *55*, 661. [CrossRef]
16. Moretti, L.; Maccagnano, G.; Coviello, M.; Cassano, G.D.; Franchini, A.; Laneve, A.; Moretti, B. Platelet Rich Plasma Injections for Knee Osteoarthritis Treatment: A Prospective Clinical Study. *J. Clin. Med.* **2022**, *11*, 2640. [CrossRef] [PubMed]
17. Wang, X.; Ji, X. Sample Size Estimation in Clinical Research. *Chest* **2020**, *158*, S12 S20. [CrossRef] [PubMed]
18. von Elm, E.; Altman, D.G.; Egger, M.; Pocock, S.J.; Gøtzsche, P.C.; Vandenbroucke, J.P. The Strengthening the Reporting of Observational Studies in Epidemiology (STROBE) statement: Guidelines for reporting observational studies. *J. Clin. Epidemiol.* **2008**, *61*, 344–349. [CrossRef] [PubMed]
19. Ryan, S.P.; Politzer, C.; Green, C.; Wellman, S.; Bolognesi, M.; Seyler, T. Albumin Versus American Society of Anesthesiologists Score: Which Is More Predictive of Complications Following Total Joint Arthroplasty? *Orthopedics* **2018**, *41*, 354–362. [CrossRef]
20. Moretti, L.; Coviello, M.; Rosso, F.; Calafiore, G.; Monaco, E.; Berruto, M.; Solarino, G. Current Trends in Knee Arthroplasty: Are Italian Surgeons Doing What Is Expected? *Medicina* **2022**, *58*, 1164. [CrossRef]
21. Schotanus, M.G.M.; Bemelmans, Y.F.L.; van der Kuy, P.H.M.; Jansen, J.; Kort, N.P. No advantage of adrenaline in the local infiltration analgesia mixture during total knee arthroplasty. *Knee Surg. Sport. Traumatol. Arthrosc.* **2017**, *25*, 2778–2783. [CrossRef] [PubMed]
22. Kort, N.P.; Bemelmans, Y.; Vos, R.; Schotanus, M.G.M. Low incidence of postoperative urinary retention with the use of a nurse-led bladder scan protocol after hip and knee arthroplasty: A retrospective cohort study. *Eur. J. Orthop. Surg. Traumatol.* **2018**, *28*, 283–289. [CrossRef] [PubMed]
23. Hasan, M.N.; Saleem, S.A.; Rehman Rao, S.; Wasim, M.H.; Durrani, N.A.; Naqvi, S.A. Comparison of the Efficacy of Continuous Femoral Nerve Block with Epidural Analgesia for Postoperative Pain Relief after Unilateral Total Knee Replacement. *Cureus* **2022**, *14*. [CrossRef]
24. Vishwanatha, S.; Kalappa, S. Continuous femoral nerve blockade versus epidural analgesia for postoperative pain relief in knee surgeries: A randomized controlled study. *Anesth. Essays Res.* **2017**, *11*, 599. [CrossRef]

25. Danninger, T. Perioperative pain control after total knee arthroplasty: An evidence based review of the role of peripheral nerve blocks. *World J. Orthop.* **2014**, *5*, 225. [CrossRef]
26. Kuyucu, E.; Bülbül, M.; Kara, A.; Koçyiğit, F.; Erdil, M. Is cold therapy really efficient after knee arthroplasty? *Ann. Med. Surg.* **2015**, *4*, 475–478. [CrossRef]
27. Jamison, R.N.; Ross, M.J.; Hoopman, P.; Griffin, F.; Levy, J.; Daly, M.; Schaffer, J.L. Assessment of Postoperative Pain Management: Patient Satisfaction and Perceived Helpfulness. *Clin. J. Pain* **1997**, *13*, 229–236. [CrossRef]
28. Adie, S.; Kwan, A.; Naylor, J.M.; Harris, I.A.; Mittal, R. Cryotherapy following total knee replacement. *Cochrane Database Syst. Rev.* **2012**, *9*. [CrossRef]
29. Farrar, J.T.; Young, J.P.; LaMoreaux, L.; Werth, J.L.; Poole, M.R. Clinical importance of changes in chronic pain intensity measured on an 11-point numerical pain rating scale. *Pain* **2001**, *94*, 149–158. [CrossRef]
30. Latremoliere, A.; Woolf, C.J. Central Sensitization: A Generator of Pain Hypersensitivity by Central Neural Plasticity. *J. Pain* **2009**, *10*, 895–926. [CrossRef] [PubMed]
31. Bech, M.; Moorhen, J.; Cho, M.; Lavergne, M.R.; Stothers, K.; Hoens, A.M. Device or Ice: The Effect of Consistent Cooling Using a Device Compared with Intermittent Cooling Using an Ice Bag after Total Knee Arthroplasty. *Physiother. Can.* **2015**, *67*, 48–55. [CrossRef] [PubMed]
32. Duellman, T.J.; Gaffigan, C.; Milbrandt, J.C.; Allan, D.G. Multi-modal, pre emptive analgesia decreases the length of hospital stay following total joint arthroplasty. *Orthopedics* **2009**, *32*, 167. [PubMed]
33. Su, E.P.; Perna, M.; Boettner, F.; Mayman, D.J.; Gerlinger, T.; Barsoum, W.; Randolph, J.; Lee, G. A prospective, multi-center, randomised trial to evaluate the efficacy of a cryopneumatic device on total knee arthroplasty recovery. *J. Bone Joint Surg. Br.* **2012**, *94-B*, 153–156. [CrossRef] [PubMed]
34. Morsi, E. Continuous-flow cold therapy after total knee arthroplasty. *J. Arthroplast.* **2002**, *17*, 718–722. [CrossRef] [PubMed]
35. Pritchard, K.A.; Saliba, S.A. Should Athletes Return to Activity After Cryotherapy? *J. Athl. Train.* **2014**, *49*, 95–96. [CrossRef]
36. Scharf, H.-P. CORR Insights®: Does Advanced Cryotherapy Reduce Pain and Narcotic Consumption After Knee Arthroplasty? *Clin. Orthop. Relat. Res.* **2014**, *472*, 3424–3425. [CrossRef]
37. Holmström, A.; Härdin, B.C. Cryo/Cuff Compared to Epidural Anesthesia After Knee Unicompartmental Arthroplasty. *J. Arthroplast.* **2005**, *20*, 316–321.
38. Maccagnano, G.; Solarino, G.; Pesce, V.; Vicenti, G.; Coviello, M.; Nappi, V.S.; Giannico, O.V.; Notarnicola, A.; Moretti, B. Plate vs reverse shoulder arthroplasty for proximal humeral fractures: The psychological health influence the choice of device? *World J. Orthop.* **2022**, *13*, 297–306. [CrossRef]
39. Healy, W.L.; Seidman, J.; Pfeifer, B.A.; Brown, D.G. Cold compressive dressing after total knee arthroplasty. *Clin. Orthop. Relat. Res.* **1994**, 143–146. Available online: https://europepmc.org/article/med/7907012 (accessed on 1 September 2022).
40. Forsyth, A.L.; Zourikian, N.; Valentino, L.A.; Rivard, G.E. The effect of cooling on coagulation and haemostasis: Should "Ice" be part of treatment of acute haemarthrosis in haemophilia? *Haemophilia* **2012**, *18*, 843–850. [CrossRef] [PubMed]
41. Hughes, S.F.; Hendricks, B.D.; Edwards, D.R.; Maclean, K.M.; Bastawrous, S.S.; Middleton, J.F. Total hip and knee replacement surgery results in changes in leukocyte and endothelial markers. *J. Inflamm.* **2010**, *7*, 2. [CrossRef]
42. Gao, F.-Q.; Li, Z.-J.; Zhang, K.; Sun, W.; Zhang, H. Four Methods for Calculating Blood-loss after Total Knee Arthroplasty. *Chin. Med. J.* **2015**, *128*, 2856–2860. [CrossRef] [PubMed]

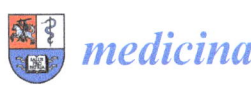

Article

Optimal Release Timing of Drain Clamping to Reduce Postoperative Bleeding after Total Knee Arthroplasty with Intraarticular Injection of Tranexamic Acid

Myung-Ku Kim, Sang-Hyun Ko, Yoon-Cheol Nam, Yoon-Sang Jeon, Dae-Gyu Kwon and Dong-Jin Ryu *

Department of Orthopaedic Surgery, Inha University Hospital, Incheon 22332, Korea
* Correspondence: mdryu24@naver.com; Tel.: +82-10-7161-3684; Fax: +82-32-890-2387

Abstract: *Background and Objectives*: Intraarticular injection of tranexamic acid (IA-TXA) plus drain-clamping is a preferred method of reducing bleeding after total knee arthroplasty (TKA). However, no consensus has been reached regarding the timing of the clamping. The purpose of this study was to determine the optimum duration of drain-clamping after TKA with IA-TXA. *Materials and Methods*: We retrospectively reviewed 151 patients that underwent unilateral TKA with IA-TXA plus drain-clamping for 30 min, 2 h, or 3 h. The total drained volume was reviewed as the primary outcome, and hematocrit (Hct) reductions, estimated blood loss (EBL), transfusion rates, and wound complications were reviewed as secondary outcomes. *Results*: The mean total drained volume, Hct reduction, and EBL were significantly less in the 3 h group than in the 30 min group. Between the 2 h and 3 h groups, there was no statistical difference in the mean total drained volume, Hct reduction, or EBL. The proportion of patients who drained lesser than 300 mL was high in the 3 h group. No significant intergroup difference was observed for transfusion volume, transfusion rate, and wound related complications. *Conclusions*: In comparison of the IA-TXA plus drain-clamping after TKA, there was no difference in EBL between the 2 h group and the 3 h group, but the amount of drainage volume was small in the 3 h group.

Keywords: total knee arthroplasty; tranexamic acid; clamping time; transfusion; estimated blood loss

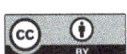

1. Introduction

Total knee arthroplasty (TKA) is a major orthopedic surgical procedure used to treat end-stage osteoarthritic knees, and it has good clinical and functional outcomes [1]. However, TKA is associated with significant blood loss, and 18% to 67% of patients require a blood transfusion, which is associated with poor outcomes such as allergic reaction, extended hospitalization, thromboembolic events, and mortality [2–4]. For these reasons, various methods such as a tourniquet application, drain clamping, epinephrine or tranexamic acid (TXA), and fibrin sealant have been proposed to reduce blood loss [5–11].

TXA is a hemostatic substance that inhibits fibrinolysis, providing a pharmacological option to reduce blood loss. Previous studies have reported that intraarticular TXA (IA-TXA) combined with drain clamping is a more effective mean of preventing blood loss than drain clamping alone [12–16]. Liao et al. conducted a meta-analysis of the results of seven different studies and confirmed the efficacy of IA-TXA plus drain-clamping [16]. However, in this meta-analysis, little data were available for clamping times between 1 and 4 h, and it remains controversial (1 h: Onodera et al. [17], Mutsuzaki et al. [18]; 2 h: Sa-Ngasoongsong et al. [11,19]; 3 h: Chareancholvanich et al. [20]; 4 h: Wang et al. [21], Wu et al. [22]).

To the best of our knowledge, no study has compared blood loss with respect to drain-clamping time after TKA with IA-TXA. Accordingly, the present study was performed to determine an optimum drain-clamping time after TKA with IA-TXA by comparing blood loss and complication rates for different drain-clamping times. In this study, total drained volume was reviewed as the primary outcome and hematocrit (Hct) reductions, estimated blood loss (EBL), transfusion rates, and wound complications were reviewed as secondary outcomes.

2. Materials and Methods

This study was approved by our Institutional Review Board (IRB No. INHAUH 2020-03-035 at 20 April 2020). The requirement for informed consent was waived due to the retrospective nature of the study. The medical and surgical records of 151 patients that underwent TKA surgery at our hospital from January 2017 to December 2019 were retrospectively reviewed. According to our database, 328 patients underwent TKA surgery after being diagnosed with knee osteoarthritis. However, 177 patients were excluded after applying the following exclusion criteria: simultaneous bilateral TKA; concomitant operation; TKA with lateral retinacular release; TKA with patella resurfacing; use of an extended stem; a diagnosis of secondary osteoarthritis; a neurologic disorder; and the receipt of medications, such as antiplatelet or anticoagulant medications, likely to interfere with findings.

The 151 study subjects were allocated to 3 groups according to clamping time; that is, Group A ($n = 60$) had a clamping time of 30 min, Group B ($n = 42$) had a clamping time of 2 h, and Group C ($n = 49$) had a clamping time of 3 h. A schematic of the patient selection is presented in Figure 1.

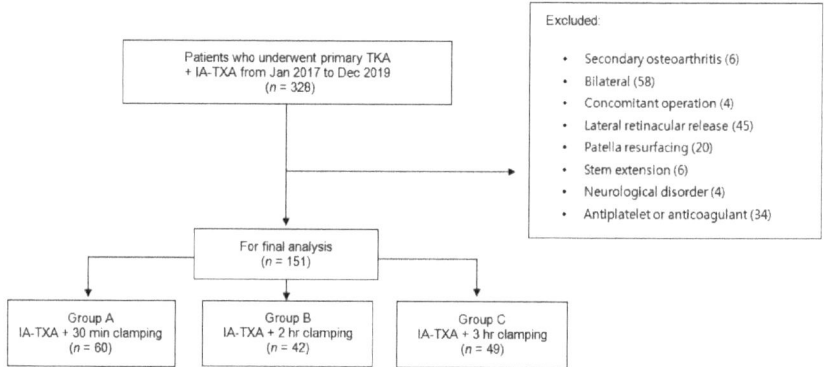

Figure 1. Flowchart of patient selection for this study.

2.1. Operation Procedures

All patients underwent TKA by a single senior surgeon (MKK) and were provided with the same procedures and post-operative managements, except clamping time. Spinal anesthesia was used in most cases (93.4%), except for patients in whom spinal anesthesia was impossible due to severe degenerative deformation of the spine. In the supine position, a standard mid-line skin incision was made using a medial parapatellar approach after applying a pneumatic tourniquet at 350 mmHg. The same implant system (Persona-Zimmer Biomet, Warsaw, IN, USA) with cement fixation (Optipac 80, Biomet Orthopaedics GmbH, Dietikon, Switzerland) was applied to all patients, and a 3.2 mm drainage tube and a BAROVAC (400 mL, Sewoon Medical, Seoul, Republic of Korea, negative pressure 90 mmHg) comprised the drainage system. IA-TXA (3 g/30 cc + normal saline 70 cc) was administered immediately after joint capsule closure [23,24]; 1-0 Vicryl simple interrupted sutures were used for joint capsules and tendons, and 3-0 Vicryl simple running sutures were used for synovium. After subcutaneous and skin closures with 2-0 Vicryl and skin staples, respectively, we confirmed no leakage. An aseptic compression dressing was applied using an elastic bandage. Drains were clamped off in a timely manner.

2.2. Postoperative Management

All case-patients received the same perioperative management, including preemptive medications. Anti-embolism stockings and intermittent pneumatic compression were applied in all cases to prevent deep vein thrombosis (DVT) or pulmonary thromboembolism (PTE). In addition, anticoagulant (rivaroxaban, Xarelto®, 10 mg) was given from postoperative days (POD) 3 to 14. Patients with a hemoglobin level of <7 g/dL received a unit of packed red blood cells (RBCs), and patients that maintained a hemoglobin level between 7 and 9 g/dL received a unit of packed RBCs postoperatively [25]. All patients performed weight-bearing exercise (using a walker), active thigh lifting exercise, passive range of motion (ROM) exercise, and cryotherapy from POD 1 to 14 in consultant with the Department of Rehabilitation.

2.3. Perioperative Laboratory Factors and Hemodynamic Factors

Because of massive irrigation during TKA, blood loss under anesthesia cannot be measured appropriately. We used Nadler's formula adjusted for height and body weight using Mercuriali's formula to calculate blood volume from preoperative and POD 5 hematocrit values [26,27]. Mercuriali's and Nadler's formulae are as follows.

$$EBL = \text{Blood volume} \times (Hct_{preop} - Hct_{5 \text{ days postoperative}}) + \text{volume of transfused RBCs}$$
$$\text{Blood volume in men (L)} = \text{Height (m)}^3 \times 0.367 + \text{Body weight (kg)} \times 0.032 + 0.604$$
$$\text{Blood volume in women (L)} = \text{Height (m)}^3 \times 0.356 + \text{Body weight (kg)} \times 0.033 + 0.183$$

2.4. Outcomes Measurement

Total drained volume was reviewed as the primary outcome. Drainage amounts were recorded at 24 and 48 h postoperatively, and all drains were removed at 48 h postoperatively. For secondary outcomes, we measured Hct reduction and EBL with Hct value at preoperation and POD 5. The transfusion rate was calculated by counting the number of patients who received a transfusion after surgery.

2.5. Complications

Complications such as DVT and PTE were evaluated closely because they can occur during clamping. From POD 2, surgical wounds were monitored to evaluate superficial infections and wound complications such as major bruises, oozing, hemarthrosis, subcutaneous hematoma, and blisters. Wounds were assessed up to POD 12 to evaluate possible superficial or deep wound infections. Major bruises were defined as bruises that extended >5 cm around wounds. Oozing was defined when three or more gauzes were soaked with blood.

2.6. Statistical Analysis

Results are presented as means ± standard deviations for continuous variables and as numbers and relative frequencies for categorical variables. Groups were compared using one-way analysis of variance (ANOVA) for quantitative data or Pearson's chi-squared test for qualitative data. The test of significance was conducted on IBM SPSS Statistics for Windows version 25.0 (IBM Corp., Armonk, NY, USA), and statistical significance was accepted for p-values < 0.05. A post hoc power analysis was performed among the three groups using the G power 3.1 software (JMP., Lane Cove, NSW, Australia). The statistical power was 0.9505, which means that the number of subjects and the results were significant.

3. Results

3.1. Patient Demographics

Age, gender, surgery side, height, weight, blood volume, anesthesia method, and preoperative Hct level before surgery are presented in Table 1. No significant difference was found between these variables in the three groups (all $p > 0.05$).

Table 1. The patients' preoperative characteristics data.

	Time of Clamp Release			
Characteristics	30 min (n = 60)	1 h (n = 42)	2 h (n = 49)	p-Value
Age at surgery (year) [a]	70.9 ± 6.8	71.8 ± 7.9	69.9 ± 7.5	0.517
Gender [b]				0.805
Female	47 (78.3%)	31 (73.8%)	36 (73.5%)	
Male	13 (21.7%)	11 (26.2%)	13 (26.5%)	
Side [b]				0.453
Right	33 (55.0%)	18 (42.9%)	26 (53.1%)	
Left	27 (45.0%)	24 (57.1%)	23 (46.9%)	
Height (cm) [a]	160.7 ± 4.7	161.6 ± 5.5	159.4 ± 8.2	0.429
Weight (kg) [a]	62.2 ± 5.6	60.9 ± 7.8	60.5 ± 8.1	0.614
Blood volume (L) [a]	3.78 ± 0.38	3.81 ± 0.54	3.74 ± 0.62	0.947
Anesthesia [b]				0.666
General anesthesia	5 (8.3%)	3 (7.1%)	2 (4.1%)	
Spinal anesthesia	55 (91.7%)	39 (92.9%)	47 (95.9%)	
Preoperative Hct level (%) [a]	37.3 ± 3.7	37.6 ± 3.0	38.5 ± 3.5	0.425

Hct: Hematocrit. [a] Data presented as mean ± standard deviation. [b] Data presented as number of patients having that condition (percentage of this group).

3.2. Drainage Amount

Mean total drainage amounts at 48 h postoperatively in groups A, B, and C were 332.3 ± 100.2, 286.4 ± 127.9, and 255.8 ± 84.5 mL, respectively ($p = 0.001$). Group C had a significantly lower amount than group A ($p = 0.001$), but no significant difference was observed between groups A and B ($p = 0.09$) or groups B and C ($p = 0.495$) (Table 2). The proportions of patients in the three groups with a drainage amount < 300 mL were 36.6%, 59.6%, and 79.6%, respectively. Notably, as clamping time increased, the percentage of patients with a drainage amount of <300 mL also increased (Figure 2).

Table 2. Blood loss and blood transfusion outcome in three groups.

Variable	Time of Clamp Release			p-Value			
	30 min (n = 60)	2 h (n = 42)	3 h (n = 49)	Over-All Significance	30 min vs. 2 h	30 min vs. 3 h	2 h vs. 3 h
Drain amount (mL) [a]							
24 h	240.2 ± 92.6	183.8 ± 96.9	143.2 ± 82.5	0.001	0.236	<0.001	0.185
48 h	130.1 ± 65.5	103.2 ± 65.5	81.3 ± 53.8	0.010	0.046	0.021	>0.999
Total	332.3 ± 100.2	286.4 ± 127.9	255.8 ± 84.5	0.001	0.09	0.001	0.495
Decreasing Hct (%) [a]	10.8 ± 2.3	8.7 ± 2.0	6.6 ± 2.2	<0.001	<0.001	<0.001	<0.001
EBL (mL) [a]	513.6 ± 276.3	396.7 ± 212.5	280.6 ± 182.0	<0.001	0.085	<0.001	0.112
Transfusion							
Transfusion volume (mL)	106.7 ± 253.7	66.7 ± 174.8	32.7 ± 137.5	0.146			
Transfusion rate [b]	9 (16.7%)	4 (9.5%)	2 (4.1%)	0.165			

[a] Data presented as mean ± standard deviation. [b] Data presented as number of patients having that condition (percentage of this group). Statistical significance was determined by one-way ANOVA followed by Scheffe's post hoc analysis.

3.3. Total Blood Loss

Mean EBL calculated using Mercuriali's and Nadler's formulae was higher in Group A than in the other groups ($p \leq 0.001$) (Table 2). Mean EBL showed a decreasing tendency as clamping time increased.

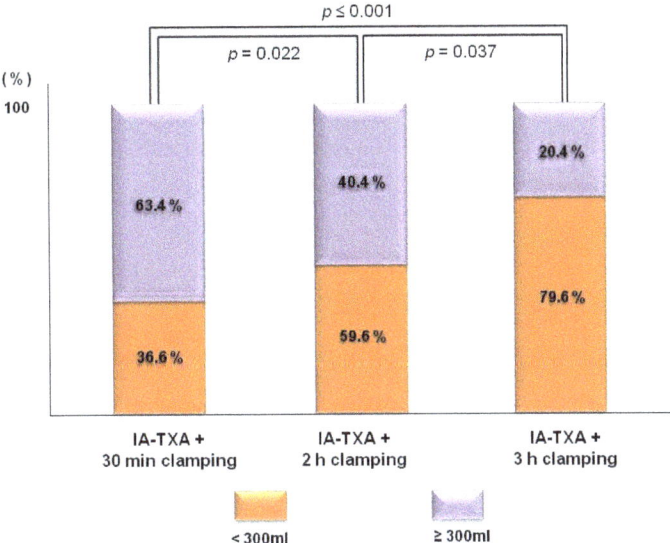

Figure 2. Percentages of patients with drainage volumes of <300 mL. Percentages of patients with a drainage volume of <300 mL increased with drainage time.

3.4. Need for Transfusion

Regarding the need for transfusion, results showed a tendency similar to EBL and drainage amounts. Mean transfusion volume was highest in group A and tended to decrease with clamping time. Transfusion rates showed a similar tendency and were 16.7, 9.5, and 4.0% in groups A, B, and C, respectively.

3.5. Complications

No deep vein thrombosis or superficial infection occurred. Wound complications were categorized as major bruises, hemarthrosis, subcutaneous hematomas, and blisters, but no significant intergroup difference was observed (Table 3).

Table 3. Complications.

Variable	Time of Clamp Release			p-Value
	30 min (n = 60)	2 h (n = 42)	3 h (n = 49)	
Deep vein thrombosis	0 (0%)	0 (0%)	0 (0%)	0.999
Superficial infection	0 (0%)	0 (0%)	0 (0%)	0.999
Wound complications [a]	6 (10.0%)	4 (9.5%)	5 (10.2%)	0.994
Major bruise	1 (1.7%)	2 (4.8%)	1 (2.0%)	0.600
Hemarthrosis	3 (5.0%)	2 (4.8%)	3 (6.1%)	0.951
Subcutaneous hematoma	1 (1.7%)	0 (0%)	1 (2.0%)	0.667
Blisters	1 (1.7%)	0 (0%)	1 (2.0%)	0.667

[a] Data presented as number of patients having that condition (percentage of this group). Data presented as number (%). Statistical significance was determined by Pearson's chi-squared test.

4. Discussion

Previous studies have reported that IA-TXA combined with drain clamping effectively prevents blood loss after TKA [12–16]. However, to our knowledge, no study has determined the optimum timing of drain clamp release. In the present study, TKA with IA-TXA plus drain clamping for 3 h resulted in a significant blood loss reduction compared to clamping for 30 min. Between the 2 h and 3 h groups, although there were no statistical differences, the proportion of patients who drained a lower volume than 300 mL was high in the 3 h group. No significant intergroup difference was observed for complication rates. Blood loss is an important postoperative consideration that must be considered after TKA. Bleeding into soft tissues surrounding the knee increases pain, stiffness, and length of recovery following surgery [28]. TXA application has recently become one of the most popular methods for reducing blood loss and transfusion requirements. TXA is an antifibrinolytic agent and was discovered in 1962. It prevents the formation of plasmin, inhibiting the breakdown of fibrin clots and decreasing bleeding. Although TXA has been administered intramuscularly, intravenously, and intraarticularly, it is being increasingly administered locally due to theoretically lower rates of systemic effects, including those related to thromboembolic disease [13,23,24,29]. However, due to safety concerns regarding PTE, interest is growing in the use of TXA as an IA agent in TKA. In the present study, we decided to use IA-TXA to reduce blood loss after TKA.

IA-TXA with drain-clamping reduces blood loss in TKA compared to IA-TXA without clamping [16]. This method is considered effective for reducing bleeding by forming a tamponade before opening. Prior studies have examined many methods, such as the intermittent method and specific timed drain clamping after surgery to reduce blood loss postoperatively [18,20–22]. However, no study has determined the optimum timing of drain clamp release after TKA with TXA. Liao et al. [16] conducted a systematic review and meta-analysis on the efficacy of TXA plus drain-clamping in TKA and concluded that this technique reduced blood loss and the need for transfusion. However, the seven clinical studies [11,17–22] included in their meta-analysis [16] were conducted using different clamping times (1 h: Onodera et al. [17], Mutsuzaki et al. [18]; 2 h: Sa-Ngasoongsong et al. [11,19]; 3 h: Chareancholvanich et al. [20]; 4 h: Wang et al. [21], Wu et al. [22]) and TXA dosages (range 250 to 1000 mg). To avoid confusion, we tried to define an effective clamping time by injecting TXA at 3 g/30 cc + 70 cc of normal saline and found EBL decreased and the percentage of patients with a drainage amount of <300 mL increased as the clamping time increased from 30 min to 3 h.

When clamping is released early, effective bleeding control cannot be achieved, i.e., longer clamping times are required to form effective tamponades. Since the half-life of TXA is 3 h, we examined the effects of clamping times up to 3 h [29]. Furthermore, it should be noted that complications such as hematoma can occur when clamping times are excessive (ca. > 4 h), as accumulations of blood in knee joints can lead to swelling, delayed wound healing, and increased risk of infection [14]. We found no significant difference between the three groups in terms of complications such as DVT, superficial infections, and wound complications.

The cytotoxic effect of IA-TXA on cartilage should be considered when the surgical intention is to preserve native cartilage tissues; its cytotoxicity may not affect total joint arthroplasties involving the removal of entire articular cartilage. Effective dosing for topical TXA ranges from 15 to 100 mg/mL. Increased exposure time to TXA at high concentrations is cytotoxic to cartilage. Because patients included in this study did not undergo patella resurfacing, we needed to minimize TXA exposure time and concentration on the articular surface and, thus, decided to use TXA at a concentration of 30 mg/mL and to limit the maximum exposure time to 3 h.

This study has several limitations. First, this is a retrospective study. Although we excluded the confounding factors that could affect bleeding tendency, a randomized control trial is needed for exact evaluation. Second, a relatively small number of cases were included in each group because all operations were performed by one surgeon in a single center. Third, postoperative blood loss was low in some patients when the surgeon was able to well identify and cauterize bleeding vessels, though vessel bleeding was carefully cauterized in all cases. Fourth, individual bleeding tendencies differ, and numerous factors can affect blood loss. However, considering the size of our cohort, we excluded factors that may have confounded results, such as a history of anticoagulant/antiplatelet medication, abnormal coagulation factors, and patients at a high risk of blood loss. Fifth, as blood loss could not be accurately measured, EBL was calculated using Mercuriali's and Nadler's formulae. However, Nadler's formula calculates blood volume based on weight and height; thus, fluid-induced body changes pre-operation to POD 5 may have introduced errors. Sixth, postoperative pain is an important evaluation factor, and blood management can affect postoperative pain. However, in this study, we focused on blood loss rather than postoperative pain. Seventh, because of the limited sample size and low prevalence of perioperative complications, this study design was insufficient to draw a clear conclusion towards complications. Thus, we performed a power analysis among the three groups using the G power 3.1 software, and the power calculated was 97.9%. Despite these limitations, we believe our findings are meaningful as they provide evidence of the optimal duration of the drain-clamp application with IA-TXA after TKA. Further, our study provides orthopedic surgeons with a rationale for how to minimize bleeding after TKA.

5. Conclusions

Temporary drain clamping after TKA with an intraarticular injection of tranexamic acid can effectively reduce EBL. Although there were no statistical differences between the groups of 2 h and 3 h in terms of blood loss, the proportion of patients who drained lesser than 300 mL was notably higher in the 3 h group. In comparison to IA-TXA plus drain-clamping after TKA, there was no difference in EBL between the 2 h group and the 3 h group, but the amount of drainage was small in the 3 h group.

Author Contributions: Conceptualization, D.-J.R., Y.-S.J. and M.-K.K.; methodology, D.-J.R., Y.-S.J. and M.-K.K.; validation, D.-J.R. and D.-G.K.; formal analysis, Y.-C.N. and S.-H.K.; investigation, Y.-C.N. and S.-H.K.; data curation, Y.-C.N. and S.-H.K.; writing—original draft preparation, D.-J.R., D.-G.K., Y.-S.J. and M.-K.K.; writing—review and editing, D.-J.R., Y.-S.J. and M.-K.K.; visualization, D.-J.R., Y.-S.J. and M.-K.K.; supervision, M.-K.K.; project administration, M.-K.K. All authors have read and agreed to the published version of the manuscript.

Funding: This study was supported by Inha University Hospital research grant.

Institutional Review Board Statement: The design and protocol of this study were reviewed and approved by the institutional review board of Inha university hospital (IRB No. INHAUH 2020-03-035). All the experiments were performed in accordance with the relevant guidelines and regulations.

Informed Consent Statement: An exemption from informed consent was obtained from the institutional review board of Inha university hospital due to its retrospective nature.

Data Availability Statement: Not applicable.

Conflicts of Interest: The authors declare that they have no conflict of interest.

References

1. Cram, P.; Lu, X.; Kates, S.L.; Singh, J.A.; Li, Y.; Wolf, B.R. Total Knee Arthroplasty Volume, Utilization, and Outcomes among Medicare Beneficiaries, 1991–2010. *JAMA* **2012**, *308*, 1227–1236. [CrossRef] [PubMed]
2. Friedman, R.; Homering, M.; Holberg, G.; Berkowitz, S.D. Allogeneic Blood Transfusions and Postoperative Infections after Total Hip or Knee Arthroplasty. *J. Bone Jt. Surg.* **2014**, *96*, 272–278. [CrossRef] [PubMed]
3. Hart, A.; Khalil, J.A.; Carli, A.; Huk, O.; Zukor, D.; Antoniou, J. Blood Transfusion in Primary Total Hip and Knee Arthroplasty. Incidence, Risk Factors, and Thirty-Day Complication Rates. *J. Bone Jt. Surg. Am. Vol.* **2014**, *96*, 1945–1951. [CrossRef] [PubMed]
4. Boutsiadis, A.; Reynolds, R.J.; Saffarini, M.; Panisset, J.-C. Factors That Influence Blood Loss and Need for Transfusion Following Total Knee Arthroplasty. *Ann. Transl. Med.* **2017**, *5*, 418. [CrossRef]
5. Li, M.M.-L.; Kwok, J.Y.-Y.; Chung, K.-Y.; Cheung, K.-W.; Chiu, K.-H.; Chau, W.-W.; Ho, K.K.-W. Prospective Randomized Trial Comparing Efficacy and Safety of Intravenous and Intra-Articular Tranexamic Acid in Total Knee Arthroplasty. *Knee Surg. Relat. Res.* **2020**, *32*, 62. [CrossRef]
6. Jang, S.; Shin, W.C.; Song, M.K.; Han, H.-S.; Lee, M.C.; Ro, D.H. Which Orally Administered Antithrombotic Agent Is Most Effective for Preventing Venous Thromboembolism after Total Knee Arthroplasty? A Propensity Score-Matching Analysis. *Knee Surg. Relat. Res.* **2021**, *33*, 10. [CrossRef]
7. Palmer, A.; Chen, A.; Matsumoto, T.; Murphy, M.; Price, A. Blood Management in Total Knee Arthroplasty: State-of-the-Art Review. *J. ISAKOS* **2018**, *3*, 358–366. [CrossRef]

8. Karam, J.A.; Bloomfield, M.R.; DiIorio, T.M.; Irizarry, A.M.; Sharkey, P.F. Evaluation of the Efficacy and Safety of Tranexamic Acid for Reducing Blood Loss in Bilateral Total Knee Arthroplasty. *J. Arthroplast.* **2014**, *29*, 501–503. [CrossRef]
9. Chen, S.; Li, J.; Peng, H.; Zhou, J.; Fang, H.; Zheng, H. The Influence of a Half-Course Tourniquet Strategy on Peri-Operative Blood Loss and Early Functional Recovery in Primary Total Knee Arthroplasty. *Int. Orthop.* **2014**, *38*, 355–359. [CrossRef]
10. Yildiz, C.; Koca, K.; Kocak, N.; Tunay, S.; Basbozkurt, M. Late Tourniquet Release and Drain Clamping Reduces Postoperative Blood Loss in Total Knee Arthroplasty. *HSS J.* **2014**, *10*, 2–5. [CrossRef]
11. Sa-ngasoongsong, P.; Channoom, T.; Kawinwonggowit, V.; Woratanarat, P.; Chanplakorn, P.; Wibulpolprasert, B.; Wongsak, S.; Udomsubpayakul, U.; Wechmongkolgorn, S.; Lekpittaya, N. Postoperative Blood Loss Reduction in Computer-Assisted Surgery Total Knee Replacement by Low Dose Intra-Articular Tranexamic Acid Injection Together with 2-Hour Clamp Drain: A Prospective Triple-Blinded Randomized Controlled Trial. *Orthop. Rev.* **2011**, *3*, e12. [CrossRef] [PubMed]
12. Marra, F.; Rosso, F.; Bruzzone, M.; Bonasia, D.; Dettoni, F.; Rossi, R. Use of Tranexamic Acid in Total Knee Arthroplasty. *Joints* **2016**, *4*, 202–213. [CrossRef] [PubMed]
13. Seo, J.-G.; Moon, Y.-W.; Park, S.-H.; Kim, S.-M.; Ko, K.-R. The Comparative Efficacies of Intra-Articular and IV Tranexamic Acid for Reducing Blood Loss during Total Knee Arthroplasty. *Knee Surg. Sports Traumatol. Arthrosc.* **2012**, *21*, 1869–1874. [CrossRef]
14. Adravanti, P.; Di Salvo, E.; Calafiore, G.; Vasta, S.; Ampollini, A.; Rosa, M.A. A Prospective, Randomized, Comparative Study of Intravenous Alone and Combined Intravenous and Intraarticular Administration of Tranexamic Acid in Primary Total Knee Replacement. *Arthroplast. Today* **2018**, *4*, 85–88. [CrossRef]
15. Zhang, Y.; Zhang, J.-W.; Wang, B.-H. Efficacy of Tranexamic Acid plus Drain-Clamping to Reduce Blood Loss in Total Knee Arthroplasty: A Meta-Analysis. *Medicine* **2017**, *96*, e7363. [CrossRef] [PubMed]
16. Liao, L.; Chen, Y.; Tang, Q.; Chen, Y.; Wang, W. Tranexamic Acid plus Drain-Clamping Can Reduce Blood Loss in Total Knee Arthroplasty: A Systematic Review and Meta-Analysis. *Int. J. Surg.* **2018**, *52*, 334–341. [CrossRef] [PubMed]
17. Onodera, T.; Majima, T.; Sawaguchi, N.; Kasahara, Y.; Ishigaki, T.; Minami, A. Risk of Deep Venous Thrombosis in Drain Clamping with Tranexamic Acid and Carbazochrome Sodium Sulfonate Hydrate in Total Knee Arthroplasty. *J. Arthroplast.* **2012**, *27*, 105–108. [CrossRef]
18. Mutsuzaki, H.; Ikeda, K. Intra-Articular Injection of Tranexamic Acid via a Drain plus Drain-Clamping to Reduce Blood Loss in Cementless Total Knee Arthroplasty. *J. Orthop. Surg. Res.* **2012**, *7*, 32. [CrossRef]
19. Sa-ngasoongsong, P.; Wongsak, S.; Chanplakorn, P.; Woratanarat, P.; Wechmongkolgorn, S.; Wibulpolprasert, B.; Mulpruek, P.; Kawinwonggowit, V. Efficacy of Low-Dose Intra-Articular Tranexamic Acid in Total Knee Replacement; a Prospective Triple-Blinded Randomized Controlled Trial. *BMC Musculoskelet. Disord.* **2013**, *14*, 340. [CrossRef]
20. Pornrattanamaneewong, C.; Narkbunnam, R.; Siriwattanasakul, P.; Chareancholvanich, K. Three-Hour Interval Drain Clamping Reduces Postoperative Bleeding in Total Knee Arthroplasty: A Prospective Randomized Controlled Trial. *Arch. Orthop. Trauma. Surg.* **2012**, *132*, 1059–1063. [CrossRef]
21. Wang, G.; Wang, D.; Wang, B.; Lin, Y.; Sun, S. Efficacy and Safety Evaluation of Intra-Articular Injection of Tranexamic Acid in Total Knee Arthroplasty Operation with Temporarily Drainage Close. *Int. J. Clin. Exp. Med.* **2015**, *8*, 14328. [PubMed]
22. Wu, Y.; Yang, T.; Zeng, Y.; Li, C.; Shen, B.; Pei, F. Clamping Drainage Is Unnecessary after Minimally Invasive Total Knee Arthroplasty in Patients with Tranexamic Acid: A Randomized, Controlled Trial. *Medicine* **2017**, *96*, e5804. [CrossRef] [PubMed]
23. Gomez-Barrena, E.; Ortega-Andreu, M.; Padilla-Eguiluz, N.G.; Pérez-Chrzanowska, H.; Figueredo-Zalve, R. Topical Intra-Articular Compared with Intravenous Tranexamic Acid to Reduce Blood Loss in Primary Total Knee Replacement: A Double-Blind, Randomized, Controlled, Noninferiority Clinical Trial. *J. Bone Jt. Surg.* **2014**, *96*, 1937–1944. [CrossRef] [PubMed]
24. Patel, J.N.; Spanyer, J.M.; Smith, L.S.; Huang, J.; Yakkanti, M.R.; Malkani, A.L. Comparison of Intravenous versus Topical Tranexamic Acid in Total Knee Arthroplasty: A Prospective Randomized Study. *J. Arthroplast.* **2014**, *29*, 1528–1531. [CrossRef]
25. Sharma, S.; Sharma, P.; Tyler, L.N. Transfusion of Blood and Blood Products: Indications and Complications. *Am. Fam. Physician* **2011**, *83*, 6.
26. Nadler, S.B.; Hidalgo, J.H.; Bloch, T. Prediction of Blood Volume in Normal Human Adults. *Surgery* **1962**, *51*, 224–232.
27. Gibon, E.; Courpied, J.-P.; Hamadouche, M. Total Joint Replacement and Blood Loss: What Is the Best Equation? *Int. Orthop.* **2013**, *37*, 735–739. [CrossRef]
28. Friedman, R.J. Limit the Bleeding, Limit the Pain in Total Hip and Knee Arthroplasty. *Orthopedics* **2010**, *33*, 11–13. [CrossRef]
29. Chen, J.Y.; Chia, S.-L.; Lo, N.N.; Yeo, S.J. Intra-Articular versus Intravenous Tranexamic Acid in Primary Total Knee Replacement. *Ann. Transl. Med.* **2015**, *3*, 33.

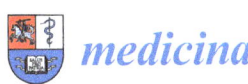

Article

Current Trends in Knee Arthroplasty: Are Italian Surgeons Doing What Is Expected?

Lorenzo Moretti [1,†], Michele Coviello [1,*,†], Federica Rosso [2], Giuseppe Calafiore [3], Edoardo Monaco [4], Massimo Berruto [5] and Giuseppe Solarino [1]

1. Orthopaedic and Trauma Unit, Department of Basic Medical Sciences, Neurscience and Sense Organs, School of Medicine, AOU Consorziale Policlinico, University of Bari "Aldo Moro", Piazza Giulio Cesare 11, 70124 Bari, Italy
2. Ordine Mauriziano, Orthopaedics and Traumatology Department, Largo Turati 62, 10128 Turin, Italy
3. Department of Orthopaedic and Trauma Surgery, Città di Parma Clinic, Piazzale Athos Maestri 5, 43123 Parma, Italy
4. Orthopedic Unit, Kirk Kilgour Sports Injury Centre, S. Andrea Hospital, University of Rome Sapienza, 00189 Rome, Italy
5. Chirurgia Articolare del Ginocchio, ASST Ospedale Gaetano Pini CTO, 20122 Milano, Italy
* Correspondence: michelecoviello91@gmail.com; Tel.: +39-3938165088
† These authors contributed equally to this work.

Abstract: Objectives: The purpose of this study is to evaluate Italian surgeons' behavior during knee arthroplasty. Materials and Methods: All orthopedic surgeons who specialized in knee replacement surgeries and were members of the Italian Society of Knee, Arthroscopy, Sport, Cartilage and Orthopedic Technologies (SIGASCOT) between January 2019 and August 2019 were asked to complete a survey on the management of knee arthroplasty. Data were collected, analyzed, and presented as frequencies and percentages. Results: One-hundred and seventy-seven surgeons completed the survey and were included in the study. Ninety-five (53.7%) surgeons were under 40 years of age. Eighty-five surgeons (48%) worked in public hospitals and 112 (63.3%) were considered "high volume surgeons", with more than 100 knee implants per year. Postero-stabilized total knee arthroplasty was the most commonly used, implanted with a fully cemented technique by 162 (91.5%) surgeons. Unicompartmental knee arthroplasty (UKA) was a rarer procedure compared to TKA, with 77% of surgeons performing less than 30% of UKAs. Most common TKA pre-operative radiological planning included complete antero-posterior (AP) weight-bearing lower limb radiographs, lateral view and patellofemoral view (used by 91%, 98.9% and 70.6% of surgeons, respectively). Pre-operative UKA radiological images included Rosenberg or Schuss views, patellofemoral view and magnetic resonance imaging (66.1%, 71.8% and 46.3% of surgeons, respectively). One hundred and thirty-two surgeons (74.6%) included an AP weight-bearing lower limb X-ray one year after surgery in the post-operative radiological follow-up. Furthermore, 119 surgeons (67.2%) did not perform a post-operative patellofemoral view because it was not considered useful for radiological follow-up. There was no uniformity in the timing and features of post-operative follow-up, with 13 different combinations. Conclusions: Italian surgeons perform TKA more commonly than UKA. Pre-operative TKA planning is quite uniform rather than UKA planning. Despite literature evidence, there is no agreement on follow-up. It may be useful to create a uniform checklist, including correct timing and exams needed. This analysis is also part of a society surgical educational project for training doctor.

Keywords: orthopedic surgeon; planning; survey; total knee arthroplasty; unicompartmental knee arthroplasty

---

1. Introduction

Total knee arthroplasty (TKA) is a very common procedure in orthopedic surgery. It has increased by 162% over the past twenty years with approximately 250,000 primary and revision arthroplasties performed each year [1]. Main indications for knee arthroplasty remain primary or secondary osteoarthritis, rheumatoid arthritis in association or not with limitation in range of movement (ROM) or deformities. Modifiable and nonmodifiable prognostic factors were associated with the rate of unsatisfied patients from 5 to 40% after TKA [2,3]. Nowadays there are several TKA designs, which can be chosen depending on the patients' age, expected activity level, pre-operative deformity and stability of the knee [4]. Particularly, different types of constraint can be used in primary TKA, from cruciate-retaining (CR) to postero-stabilized (PS) implants. There are also "high constrained" implants, such as condylar constrained, but they are normally reserved to revision TKA due to lower survivorship in primary TKA [5,6]. The first TKA designs did not include patellar implants, and they were characterized by high rate of post-operative anterior knee pain [7]. In the 1980s, patella-related complications accounted for up to 50% of complications following TKA [8]. Consequently, patellar resurfacing was introduced, but different complications were described. For these reasons, despite the number of studies, there is still some disagreement between surgeons who prefer patellar resurfacing, surgeons who never resurface the patella and surgeons who resurface it in selected cases [8–12]. In the case of degenerative arthritis involving only the medial or lateral compartment, unicompartmental knee arthroplasty (UKA) can be performed [13]. UKA needed the patient to have an intact anterior cruciate ligament and correctable knee alignment [14]. Similarly, isolated patellofemoral arthroplasty (PFA) can also be performed in selected cases with isolated patellofemoral osteoarthritis (PFOA) [15].

Both in TKA or UKA, correct pre-operative planning is mandatory to achieve a good outcome [16]. Different X-ray protocols have been described, but the most used are still the long-leg anteroposterior (AP) view for evaluation of the anatomical and mechanical axis [17–20], weight-bearing AP and lateral view of the knee and patellar view [21,22]. Magnetic resonance imaging (MRI) is usually not useful in TKA pre-operative planning, but it may be reasonable in UKA planning to evaluate cruciate ligaments status as well as cartilage status of the not-replaced compartment. Furthermore, it may also be useful in some revision surgery cases [23]. Careful pre-operative planning allowed the surgeon to predict possible difficulties or complications, need for higher constraint or specific instrumentation and it is mandatory to plan the surgeries [24]. Despite different studies on the correct pre-operative planning needed for both TKA and UKA, in practice there is still lack of uniformity. Current literature was investigated to compare our results with other large working groups, such as national registries, demonstrating similarities and differences. With regard to the Nordic Arthroplasty Register Association (NARA), that confirmed some Italian data, TKA was used as a primary implant (92%) in patients less than 65 y.o. (64%), while UKA and PFA were used less (3% and 1%, respectively) [25]. The experienced surgeons' behaviors together with new learning technologies, such as augmented reality or cadaver labs, represent the focus of young surgeons trained by orthopedic societies [26,27].

The purpose of this study is to evaluate how Italian surgeons specialized in knee replacement behave in pre-operative planning and surgery. The authors, as active members of Italian orthopedic society and as active knee surgeons, guided this analysis as a starting point for educational pathways for young surgeons.

2. Materials and Methods

All orthopedic surgeons who specialized in knee replacement surgeries and were members of the Italian Society of Knee, Arthroscopy, Sport, Cartilage and Orthopedic Technologies (SIGASCOT) were asked to complete a survey on the current management of TKA and UKA, between January 2019 and August 2019, including pre-operative planning, implants used and characteristics of follow-up. Surgeons interviewed belong to the "knee surgery" specialized group of the society with 415 members. This is represented by doctors who spend more than half of their surgery in knee procedures with both arthroplasty and arthroscopy and who have followed high specialization courses.

An online questionnaire was built using SurveyMonkey (Portland, OR, USA®), a free, open-source online survey tool. The 25 multiple choice questions were divided by subject into 5 parts: surgeons' characteristics (i.e., age, volume of surgeries), TKA data (i.e., type of insert, cementation technique), UKA data (numbers of surgeries, type of implants), data regarding the pre-operative planning and follow-up (Scheme 1). The survey required approximately 10–12 min to be completed. Results from the survey were collected electronically and anonymously using SurveyMonkey (Portland, OR, USA®). All data were analyzed using SPSS 25.0 (IBM, Armonk, NY, USA). Data were evaluated using descriptive analysis, and they were presented as frequencies and percentages. The data used to support the findings of this study are available from the corresponding author upon request.

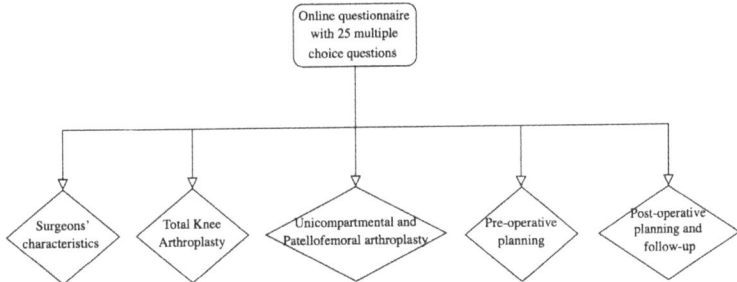

Scheme 1. Flow diagram of questionnaire.

3. Results

One hundred and seventy-seven orthopedic surgeons (42.65%) completed the survey. Table 1 reports the survey in detail. Of the respondents, 46.9% worked in semiprivate hospitals, and 53.7% were under the age of 40. The demographic data, workplace and number of total annual implants included in the study are summarized in Table 2 and Figure 1.

Table 1. Questions asked and possible responses.

	Questions	Possible Responses
1.	How old are you?	<40 y 41–55 y >55 y
2.	Where do you work, as your main activity?	Public hospital Semiprivate hospital Private hospital University hospital
3.	How many total knee arthroplasties are performed each year in the hospital you work at?	0–30 n° 31–50 n° 51–100 n° >100 n°
4.	What kind of first implant do you mainly perform?	PS CR Medial Pivot
5.	What kind of fixation do you perform?	Cemented arthroplasty Uncemented arthroplasty Hybrid arthroplasty Cemented and uncemented Cemented or uncemented

Table 1. Cont.

	Questions	Possible Responses
6.	If you answered cemented to the previous question: what type of cement?	Antibiotic cement always Antibiotic in revision surgery only Antibiotic in selected patient only Antibiotic cement never
7.	Do you perform unicompartmental knee arthroplasty? If so, compared to total arthroplasty?	None >10% 10–30% >30%
8.	If you answered NO to the previous question, explain why:	Open answer
9.	Do you perform femoropatellar arthroplasty?	Yes No
10.	Do you perform a patella arthroplasty?	Hardly ever Almost always Selected patient 90% in woman
11.	Do you perform patellar view X-ray in the preoperative study of total knee arthroplasty?	Yes No routinely
12.	Do you perform patellar view X-ray in the preoperative study of unicompartmental knee arthroplasty?	Yes No routinely
13.	Do you perform lateral view in the preoperative study?	Yes No routinely
14.	Do you perform AP weight-bearing of the whole lower limb view in the preoperative study?	Yes No routinely UKA only
15.	If you answered NO to the previous question, explain why:	Useless Organizational budget reasons Severe axis changes Major deformities Execution errors are frequent
16.	If you answered YES to the previous question, how do you request it?	Bipodalic position Monopodalic position Monopodalic for UKA
17.	Do you perform varus/valgus stress view?	Yes No
18.	Do you perform Rosenberg or Schuss views in the unicompartmental knee arthroplasty preoperative study?	Yes No
19.	Do you regularly perform preoperative planning?	Yes No
20.	Do you regularly perform MRI in the preoperative study?	Yes No UKA only
21.	One year after knee replacement surgery, do you require AP weight-bearing of the whole lower limb view?	Yes No Selected patient Pain UKA only For research only Severe axis changes

Table 1. Cont.

	Questions	Possible Responses
22.	If you answered NO to the previous question, explain why:	Useless Organizational budget reasons
		Useless if the patient has no pain Execution errors are frequent
23.	Do you regularly perform postoperative patellar view?	Yes No
24.	If so, which one?	Merchant (45° view) Ficat (30-60-90° view) Baldini (under bearing view) 30° view
25.	When do you perform postoperative radiographic follow-up (you can choose multiple answers)?	1 m 3 m 6 m 12 m
26.	Comments and advice	Open answer

(y = year, n° = number, PS = postero stabilized, CR = cruciate retaining, m = month).

Table 2. Demographic data, workplace and number of total annual implants.

How Many Total Knee Arthroplasties Are Performed Each Year in the Hospital You Work At?	<40 y	>55 y	41–55 y	Total
Semiprivate hospital	22.0%	11.3%	13.6%	**46.9%**
0–30 n°	1.1%	0.6%	0.0%	1.7%
31–50 n°	1.1%	1.7%	0.0%	2.8%
51–100 n°	2.8%	1.1%	4.0%	7.9%
>100 n°	17.0%	7.9%	9.6%	34.5%
University hospital	19.8%	1.7%	4.5%	**26.0%**
31–50 n°	4.0%	0.0%	1.1%	5.1%
51–100 n°	3.4%	0.0%	1.1%	4.5%
>100 n°	12.4%	1.7%	2.3%	16.4%
Public hospital	9.6%	4.0%	8.5%	**22.0%**
0–30 n°	0.6%	0.0%	0.6%	1.1%
31–50 n°	1.1%	0.6%	2.3%	4.0%
51–100 n°	4.0%	1.7%	2.8%	8.5%
>100 n°	4.0%	1.7%	2.8%	8.5%
Private hospital	2.3%	1.1%	1.7%	**5.1%**
0–30 n°	0.6%	0.0%	0.0%	0.6%
31–50 n°	0.0%	0.6%	0.0%	0.6%
>100 n°	1.7%	0.6%	1.7%	4.0%
Total	53.7%	18.1%	28.2%	**100.0%**

(y = year, n° = number).

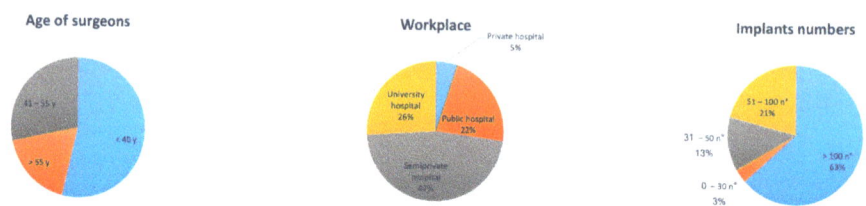

Figure 1. Demographic data, workplace and number of total annual implants. (y = year, n° = number).

With regard to total knee arthroplasty, most of the surgeons preferred a postero-stabilized (PS) (78%) cemented (91.5%) implant. Focusing on the type of cement preferred, most of the surgeons (45.2%) used antibiotic-loaded cement only in selected patients, while 35% of the surgeons always used antibiotic-loaded cement. The cruciate retaining (CR) insert was used by 20.3% of surgeons, while only 1.7% preferred the medial pivot insert. Nearly half of the surgeons preferred selected patellar resurfacing (46.3%). Data related to the TKA surgical technique are presented in Table 3.

Table 3. Total knee arthroplasty related data.

	Frequency (%)
Type of first implant	
Postero-stabilized	138 (78%)
Cruciate retaining	36 (20.3)
Medial pivot	3 (1.7)
Type of fixation	
Cemented arthroplasty	162 (91.5)
Uncemented arthroplasty	8 (4.5)
Hybrid arthroplasty	5 (2.8)
Cemented and uncemented	1 (0.6%)
Cemented or uncemented	1 (0.6%)
Type of cement	
Antibiotic in selected patient only	80 (47.6)
Antibiotic cement always	62 (36.9%)
Antibiotic cement never	23 (13.7%)
Antibiotic in revision surgery only	3 (1.8%)
Patellar resurfacing	
Selected patients	82 (46.3%)
Almost always	49 (27.7)
Hardly ever	45 (25.4%)
90% in woman	1 (0.6%)

With regard to unicompartmental knee arthroplasty (UKA) and patellofemoral arthroplasty (PFA), UKA was chosen less compared to TKA, with 40% of surgeons performing it in less than 10% of the cases, while 37.3% of surgeons performed UKA in 30% of the cases. Surgeons did not recognize a correct indication towards UKA (46.4%) and they were unfamiliar with the surgical technique (35.7%). During their activity, surgeons performed patellofemoral arthroplasty (PFA) in 36.2% of cases. UKA and PFA related data are summarized in order of frequency in Figure 2.

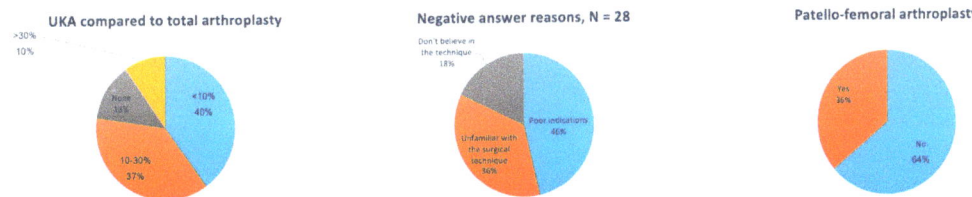

Figure 2. UKA and PFA related data. (N = number of answers).

With regard to radiological planning, characteristics of pre-operative planning were shared by most of the surgeons. For example, patellar view X-ray was required both in the total (70.6%) and in the unicompartmental knee arthroplasty (71.8%). Other routinely used radiographs were lateral view in 98.9% of cases and complete lower limb AP weight-bearing in 91% of cases. Some surgeons only used the latter for unicompartmental (1.7%) and others found it not useful (7.3%) due to its frequent execution errors (27.3%) or due to organization budget reasons (36.3%). However, in most of the cases the long-leg view was performed in bipodalic position (80.8%). Varus/valgus stress view was required only in 0.6% of cases, while Rosenberg or Schuss views in unicompartmental knee arthroplasty were requested in two thirds of cases (66.1%). The majority of surgeons recognized the importance of adequate pre-operative planning (80.2%). Regarding pre-operative MRI, 53.7% of surgeons did not require it and 37.3% required it only for UKA. Radiographic pre-operative data are summarized in order of frequency in Table 4.

Table 4. Radiographic pre-operative data.

	Frequency (%)
Patellar view X-ray in the pre-operative of TKA	
Yes	125 (70.6%)
No routinely	52 (29.4%)
Patellar view X-ray in the pre-operative of UKA	
Yes	127 (71.8%)
No routinely	50 (28.2%)
Lateral view in the pre-operative	
Yes	175 (98.9%)
No routinely	2 (1.1%)
AP weight-bearing of the whole lower limb view in the pre-operative	
Yes	161 (91%)
No routinely	13 (7.3%)
UKA only	3 (1.7%)
Negative answer reasons	N = 11
Organizational budget reasons	4 (36.3%)
Execution errors are frequent	3 (27.3%)
Useless	2 (18.2%)
Severe axis changes	1 (9.1%)
Major deformities	1 (9.1%)

Table 4. Cont.

	Frequency (%)
How do you request it?	N = 167
Bipodalic position	143 (85.6%)
Monopodalic position	16 (9.6%)
Monopodalic for UKA	8 (4.8%)
Varus/valgus stress view	
No	176 (99.4%)
Yes	1 (0.6%)
Rosenberg or Schuss views in the UKA pre-operative	
Yes	117 (66.1%)
No	60 (33.9%)
Pre-operative planning	N = 177
Yes	142 (80.2%)
No	35 (19.8%)
MRI in the pre-operative	
No	95 (53.7%)
UKA only	66 (37.3%)
Yes	16 (9%)

(TKA = total knee arthroplasty, UKA = unicompartmental knee arthroplasty, AP = antero-posterior, MRI = magnetic resonance imaging, N = number of answers).

With regard to post-operative follow-up, 74.6% of surgeons requested complete lower limb AP weight-bearing X-rays one year after knee replacement surgery. Only 23.2% did not use this view, mainly because they did not consider it useful (53,7%). Patellar view X-ray, very important in the pre-operative planning, was not required in the postoperative evaluation by 67.2% of the surgeons. When it was required, in one third of cases (32.8%), different views were performed, with the most commonly requested being the Merchant view at 45° of knee flexion (71% of the cases). The last two questions of the survey evaluated the post-operative follow-up. Unfortunately, there was no uniformity in the management of post-operative follow-up, with thirteen different combinations of timing and exams required, with none exceeding 35%. Radiographic and follow-up post-operative data are summarized in order of frequency in Table 5.

Table 5. Radiographic and follow-up post-operative data.

	Frequency (%)
AP weight-bearing of the whole lower limb view one year after surgery	
Yes	132 (74.6%)
No	41 (23.2%)
Selected patient	1 (0.6%)
Pain UKA only	1 (0.6%)
For research only	1 (0.6%)
Severe axis changes	1 (0.6%)

Table 5. Cont.

	Frequency (%)
Negative answer reasons	N = 41
Useless	22 (53.7%)
Organizational budget reasons	13 (31.7%)
Execution errors are frequent	5 (12.2%)
Useless if the patient has no pain	1 (2.4%)
Post-operative patellar view	
No	119 (67.2%)
Yes	58 (32.8%)
Kind of post-operative patellar view	N = 62
Merchant (45° view)	44 (71%)
Baldini (under bearing view)	9 (14.5)
Ficat (30–60–90° view)	8 (12.9%)
30° view	1 (1.6%)
Post-operative radiographic follow-up (months)	N = 177
1–3–6–12 m	56 (31.6%)
1–6–12 m	29 (16.4%)
3–6–12 m	27 (15.3%)
3–12 m	19 (10.7%)
1–12 m	13 (7.3%)
1 m	12 (6.8%)
3 m	8 (4.5%)
6–12 m	6 (3.4%)
1–6 m	3 (1.7%)
12 m	2 (1.1%)
1–3–6 m	1 (0.6%)
6 m	1 (0.6%)
Comments and advice	N = 2
First check-up 45 days	1 (50%)
Long plate X-ray complete AP weight-bearing radiograph	1 (50%)

(AP = antero-posterior, UKA = unicompartmental knee arthroplasty, N = number of answers).

4. Discussion

The present survey was carried out in collaboration with the Italian Society of Knee, Arthroscopy, Sport, Cartilage and Orthopedic Technologies (SIGASCOT) and members of the Italian Society of Orthopedics (SIOT). The purpose of this study was to summarize Italian surgeons' preferences in pre-operative planning, surgical technique and post-operative follow-up for TKA and UKA. The analysis of our data is the research subject of the Italian orthopedics society for educational pathway promotion for training doctors. The study was strongly supported by the society because it represents one of the starting points of training: the role of possible tutors and training centers. Every year the universities try to ensure proper education for their training doctors. The role of the societies in this educational program is to improve the choice of non-university training centers. The debate is still open regarding hospital type, the role of the tutor and the main features of the training center.

An Italian survey example carried out by the same society with an education objective was published in 2017 [27].

Survey analysis revealed a population of young surgeons who worked mainly in semi-private hospitals and with "high volume" surgeries (more than 100 arthroplasties per year) (Table 2). Italian orthopedic training was made up of various resources, such as cad-lab, face-to-face and multimedia courses, and indexed journals [27]. This training leads young surgeons to being open to innovations and continuous updating.

TKA is still one of the most common orthopedic procedures, with good reported outcomes. However, almost 20% of the patients are still unsatisfied post-operatively and there is also a considerable complication rate, including periprosthetic joint infection [28,29]. Historically, UKA and PFA were considered "at risk" procedures, with high failure rates, mainly due to poor implants and surgical techniques [15,30]. However, recently, better outcomes were reported with new implants, with lower failure rate and higher patient satisfaction compared to TKA, especially for "high volume" surgeons [31]. However, despite improvement in UKA outcomes, Italian knee surgeons still performed more TKAs compared to UKAs or PFAs. The TKA planning was uniform among the surgeons, with a prevalence of the PS-TKA over the other types of implants. Instead, the planning of the UKA has proved uneven, with a major impact of surgeon volume on planning type. Finally, the post-operative follow-up was too different in terms of timing and type of radiological examination required. Emerged data respected the current literature review with lack of standardization of UKA. Many authors have recognized the importance of standing AP, lateral, Merchant and Rosenberg, stress views and MRI for UKA focusing attention on some radiographic prognostic values, but no recommendations have yet emerged from these results [31]. Furthermore, recent literature has also shown great interest in MRI in total knee arthroplasty. Some authors demonstrated that measuring the distances of Achilles tendon from the mechanical axis of lower limb in magnetic resonance imaging of the ankle helps towards correct alignment of the components in the coronal plane. The pre-operative planning role is fundamental for the success of the arthroplasty. Correct pre-operative studies, such as X-ray or MRI, are necessary for the evaluation of the axes of the knee [32]. Additionally, a new MRI-based approach for the analysis of thigh muscles was described to improve a patient-specific rehabilitation program [33]. Computerized tomography seems to be of great importance in the use of robot surgery, as demonstrated in a 2020 ESSKA review [34]. The robotic-assisted procedure had significantly lower postoperative pain score, significantly reduced time until hospital discharge and significantly better functional scores when compared with traditional surgery [34].

Similar society analyses have been conducted in the literature. Friederich et al. [35] investigated the computer-assisted use for total knee surgery among members of the European Society of Sports Traumatology Knee Surgery and Arthroscopy (ESSKA) and the Swiss Orthopedic Society (SGO-SSO). Authors described half of surgeons using this technology and the improvement in alignment of prosthesis was the most strongly cited reason for using a navigation system. Jaap et al. [36] studied realistic expectations for recovery one year after TKA among Dutch orthopedic surgeons using a hospital for special surgery score. They concluded that greatest improvement was predicted for the items "pain relief" and "walking short distances". The British Association for Surgery of the Knee in conjunction with the James Lind Alliance investigated assessment, management and rehabilitation of patients with persistent symptoms after knee arthroplasty including patients, surgeons, anesthetists, nurses, physiotherapists and researchers. They concluded that the top ten research priorities focused on pain, infection, stiffness, health service configuration, surgical and non-surgical management strategies and outcome measures [37]. Alexander et al. [38], instead, surveyed orthopedic surgeons affiliated with the American Association of Hip and Knee Surgeons to inquire into the global impact of the COVID-19 pandemic on patient care. They described that all respondents noted their practices had been reduced and 70% of the surgeons canceled elective procedures. Our study, unlike the previous ones, examined Italian knee surgeons' behaviors. The questionnaire is completed with a pre- and post-operative analysis, including the main types of implants available. Furthermore, it is important to underline the careful selection of the interviewees, as members of a specialized group of society.

Considering the type of implants used, data from this study can be compared to different international arthroplasty registers. The Nordic Arthroplasty Register Association (NARA) confirmed some Italian data. TKA was used as a primary implant (92%) in patients younger than 65 y.o. (64%), while UKA and PFA were less used (3% and 1%, respectively). From our data, UKA was chosen in less than 10% of cases and PFA was implanted in 36.2%. NARA demonstrated that cemented fixation was used in 92% of all TKAs as in our survey (91.5%). The patella was resurfaced in 22% of cases, while our survey showed almost double the value. Hybrid fixation was used in 5% of all TKAs [25] as with our data (2.8%). Similar data emerged from the Italian register of arthroplasty (RIAP). TKA was chosen more often than UKA (83.6% and 16.4%, respectively), as emerged from our data. Cemented fixation was used in 66.9% of TKAs and 65.7% of all UKAs, slightly lower values than ours. Hybrid fixation was used in 3.4% and 6.9% of TKAs and UKAs, respectively, as with our data. Patellar resurfacing was only used in 12.1% of TKAs and 1.8% of UKAs [39]. These data seem lower than ours due to the "Selected patients" answers to question 10. This created a bias regarding the absolute value of resurfacing, masking data similar to the Italian register

In the United States in 2016, 50% of surgeons preferred postero stabilized (PS) implants, and cruciate retaining (CR) was the second design commonly used, with almost 42% of total procedures [40]. These data are in line with this study, in which PS implants are preferred by most of the surgeons. This is probably due to contraindication to CR implants, such as posterior cruciate ligament (PCL) insufficiency, significant coronal deformity, extensor mechanism deficiency, posterolateral instability and inflammatory arthritis. Moreover, PS-TKA is generally easier to perform in most surgical situations without concern for obtaining appropriate tension on the PCL [41].

Cemented TKA guarantees good clinical outcomes with a long-term survival rate of up to 99% in comparison to a survival rate of up to 97% documented in cementless TKA [6,42].

Initial total knee arthroplasty designs did not include patellar implants, in fact high rate of anterior knee pain was found following these operations [7]. Modern TKA designs have all-polyethylene patellar implants, as the older metal-backed implants had high rates of wear and loosening [43]. Despite this innovation there are still complications related to the patellar implant, so much so that patellar resurfacing has been subject to controversy for several years [44].

Different implant types were studied by researchers but not included in our survey due to their non-popularity. Sabatini et al. [45] reviewed the second generation of bicruciate-retaining TKA. They summarized that in cases of high demand, end-stage bi- or tricompartmental knee arthritis, coronal malalignment <15°, ACL integrity and minimal ROM reduction (< 5/10°), this procedure could be a valid alternative to TKA or UKA [45].

Custom TKA, as new implants, are useful in cases of anatomical and functional variability. They added asymmetry and sizes to the existing implants. Actually, our understanding of the relation between the dynamic aspects of gait and position and form of the knee implants is lacking. Custom arthroplasties could also address these conceptual and practical difficulties due to robotics and artificial intelligence [46].

New materials for use are currently being researched. Ultra-high molecular weight polyethylene (UHMWPE) is widely chosen for its biomechanical characteristics. For reducing the polyethylene wear, one of the efforts is to investigate the selection of metal materials. Jamari et al. [47] analyzed the relationship between the polyethylene and metals via finite element analysis. They described, in total hip arthroplasty, that titanium alloy is able to reduce cumulative contact pressure if compared to stainless steel and cobalt chromium molybdenum on UHMWPE [47].

As emerged from the survey, there is no uniformity in the management of postoperative follow-up, with thirteen different answers. Different studies confirmed the importance of a complete post-operative follow-up, but also in the literature there is no uniformity in timing of evaluation, with variability ranging from 3 to 6 months [15].

The novelty of this study is the careful analysis of the Italian surgical situation compared to other countries. With the high number of annual procedures, the state could play a key role in research and innovation.

This study had some limitations. The number of participants in the study was low compared to those registered with the society. The sample was not homogeneous in terms of age, location of work and number of prostheses, leading to some bias. The analysis does not consider the new technologies present in the literature such as robots, patient-specific instrument or fluoroscopy-guided surgery. On the other hand, thanks to a complete questionnaire, the study analyzes the behavior of Italian surgeons and provides society with the starting point for the educational analysis of young surgeons. Although the questionnaire was quite complete, further aspects could be investigated about the surgical technique, such as surgical time, surgical approach and others.

An analysis is currently underway with similar questions addressed to training doctors, with the aim of comparing the answers of this analysis. This second survey represents the end of the research project which will be followed by the conception of educational practical courses, together with other projects already in progress.

5. Conclusions

Despite the improvement in UKA and PFA, we conclude that TKA still remains the preferred surgical option for Italian surgeons. PS cemented implants are the most commonly used, and patellar resurfacing was selected by most of the surgeons. Pre-operative planning is consistent with those reported in the literature and there is some agreement between surgeons, especially for TKA planning. When evaluating data regarding UKA, there is less agreement in pre-operative X-ray evaluation, with some surgeons requesting MRI and some surgeons preferring stress X-rays. Similar to the literature, there is absolutely no agreement in post-operative follow-up, both in terms of timing or radiological evaluation for both TKA and UKA. Considering these data, it may also be useful to promote some educational programs for training doctors after knowing their starting point.

Author Contributions: Conceptualization, L.M.; data curation, M.C.; writing—original draft preparation, F.R., E.M. and G.C.; writing—review and editing, M.B. and M.C.; supervision, G.S. All authors have read and agreed to the published version of the manuscript.

Funding: This research received no external funding.

Institutional Review Board Statement: The study was conducted according to the guidelines of the Declaration of Helsinki and approved by the Ethics Committee of Policlinico di Bari Hospital (delib. 0207 approved on 15 September 2018).

Informed Consent Statement: Informed consent was obtained from all subjects involved in the study. Written informed consent has been obtained from the patient(s) to publish this paper if applicable.

Data Availability Statement: The data presented in this study are available on request from the corresponding author.

Conflicts of Interest: The authors declare no conflict of interest.

References

1. Miller, T.T. Imaging of knee arthroplasty. *Eur. J. Radiol.* **2005**, *54*, 164–177. [CrossRef] [PubMed]
2. Bonasia, D.E.; Palazzolo, A.; Cottino, U.; Saccia, F.; Mazzola, C.; Rosso, F.; Rossi, R. Modifiable and Nonmodifiable Predictive Factors Associated with the Outcomes of Total Knee Arthroplasty. *Joints* **2019**, *7*, 13–18. [CrossRef] [PubMed]
3. Moretti, L.; Maccagnano, G.; Coviello, M.; Cassano, G.D.; Franchini, A.; Laneve, A.; Moretti, B. Platelet Rich Plasma Injections for Knee Osteoarthritis Treatment: A Prospective Clinical Study. *J. Clin. Med.* **2022**, *11*, 2640. [CrossRef] [PubMed]

4. Brander, V.A.; Stulberg, S.D.; Adams, A.D.; Harden, R.N.; Bruehl, S.; Stanos, S.P.; Houle, T. Predicting Total Knee Replacement Pain: A Prospective, Observational Study. *Clin. Orthop. Relat. Res.* **2003**, *416*, 27–36. [CrossRef] [PubMed]
5. Vince, K.G. Prosthetic selection in total knee arthroplasty. *Am. J. Knee Surg.* **1996**, *9*, 76–82.
6. Nisar, S.; Ahmad, K.; Palan, J.; Pandit, H.; van Duren, B. Medial stabilised total knee arthroplasty achieves comparable clinical outcomes when compared to other TKA designs: A systematic review and meta-analysis of the current literature. *Knee Surg. Sports Traumatol. Arthrosc.* **2020**, *30*, 638–651. [CrossRef] [PubMed]
7. Assiotis, A.; To, K.; Morgan-Jones, R.; Pengas, I.P.; Khan, W. Patellar complications following total knee arthroplasty: A review of the current literature. *Eur. J. Orthop. Surg. Traumatol.* **2019**, *29*, 1605–1615. [CrossRef]
8. Keblish, P.A.; Varma, A.K.; Greenwald, A.S. Patellar resurfacing or retention in total knee arthroplasty. A prospective study of patents with bilateral re-placements. *J. Bone Jt. Surg. Ser. B* **1994**, *76*, 930–937. [CrossRef]
9. Barrack, R.L.M.L.; Bertot, A.J.; Wolfe, M.W.; Waldman, D.A.; Milicic, M. Patellar resurfacing in total knee arthroplasty: A prospective, randomized, double-blind study with five to seven years of follow-up. *J. Bone Jt. Surg. Am. Ser A* **2001**, *83*, 1376–1381. [CrossRef]
10. Panni, A.S.; Cerciello, S.; Del Regno, C.; Felici, A.; Vasso, M. Patellar resurfacing complications in total knee arthroplasty. *Int. Orthop.* **2013**, *38*, 313–317. [CrossRef]
11. Johnson, T.C.; Tatman, P.J.; Mehle, S.; Gioe, T.J. Revision surgery for patellofemoral problems. *Clin. Orthop. Relat. Res.* **2012**, *470*, 211–219. [CrossRef] [PubMed]
12. Roberts, D.W.; Hayes, T.D.; Tate, C.T.; Lesko, J.P. Selective patellar resurfacing in total knee arthroplasty: A prospective, randomized, double-blind study. *J. Arthroplast.* **2015**, *30*, 216–222. [CrossRef]
13. Vince, K.G.; Cyran, L.T. Unicompartmental knee arthroplasty: New indications, more complications? *J. Arthroplast.* **2004**, *19*, 9–16. [CrossRef] [PubMed]
14. Deshmukh, R.V.; Scott, R.D. Unicompartmental knee arthroplasty: Longterm results. *Clin. Orthop. Relat. Res.* **2001**, *392*, 272–278. [CrossRef]
15. Remy, F. Surgical technique in patellofemoral arthroplasty. *Orthop. Traumatol. Surg. Res.* **2019**, *105*, S165–S176. [CrossRef]
16. Kumar, N.; Yadav, C.; Raj, R.; Anand, S. How to Interpret Postoperative X-rays after Total Knee Arthroplasty. *Orthop. Surg.* **2014**, *6*, 179–186. [CrossRef]
17. Rossi, R.; Cottino, U.; Bruzzone, M.; Dettoni, F.; Bonasia, D.E.; Rosso, F. Total knee arthroplasty in the varus knee: Tips and tricks. *Int. Orthop.* **2018**, *43*, 151–158. [CrossRef]
18. Patel, D.V.; Ferris, B.D.; Aichroth, P.M. Radiological study of alignment after total knee replacement. Short radiographs or long radiographs? *Int. Orthop.* **1991**, *15*, 209–210. [CrossRef]
19. Stern, S.H.; Insall, J.N. Posterior stabilized prosthesis. Results after follow-up of nine to twelve years. *J. Bone Jt. Surg. Am.* **1992**, *74*, 980–986. [CrossRef]
20. Gujarathi, N.; Putti, A.B.; Abboud, R.J.; MacLean, J.G.B.; Espley, A.J.; Kellett, C.F. Risk of periprosthetic fracture after anterior femoral notching: A 9-year follow-up of 200 total knee arthroplasties. *Acta Orthop.* **2009**, *80*, 553–556. [CrossRef]
21. Rogers, B.A.; Thornton-Bott, P.; Cannon, S.R.; Briggs, T.W.R. Interobserver variation in the measurement of patellar height after total knee arthroplasty. *J. Bone Jt. Surgery. Br. Vol.* **2006**, *88*, 484–488. [CrossRef] [PubMed]
22. Merchant, A.C.; Mercer, R.L.; Jacobsen, R.H.; Cool, C.R. Roentgenographic analysis of patellofemoral congruence. *J. Bone Jt. Surg. Am.* **1974**, *56*, 1391–1396. [CrossRef]
23. Lachiewicz, P.F.; Henderson, R.A. Patient-specific instruments for total knee arthroplasty. *J. Am. Acad. Orthop. Surg.* **2013**, *21*, 513–518. [PubMed]
24. Tanzer, M.; Makhdom, A.M. Preoperative Planning in Primary Total Knee Arthroplasty. *J. Am. Acad. Orthop. Surg.* **2016**, *24*, 220–230. [CrossRef] [PubMed]
25. Irmola, T.; Ponkilainen, V.; Mäkelä, K.T.; Robertsson, O.; W.-Dahl, A.; Furnes, O.; Fenstad, A.M.; Pedersen, A.B.; Schrøder, H.M.; Eskelinen, A.; et al. Association between fixation type and revision risk in total knee arthroplasty patients aged 65 years and older: A cohort study of 265,877 patients from the Nordic Arthroplasty Register Association 2000–2016. *Acta Orthop.* **2020**, *92*, 91–96. [CrossRef]
26. Alpaugh, K.; Ast, M.P.; Haas, S.B. Immersive technologies for total knee arthroplasty surgical education. *Arch. Orthop. Trauma. Surg.* **2021**, *141*, 2331–2335. [CrossRef] [PubMed]
27. Losco, M.; Familiari, F.; Giron, F.; Papalia, R. Use and Effectiveness of the Cadaver-Lab in Orthopaedic and Traumatology Education: An Italian Survey. *Joints* **2017**, *05*, 197–201. [CrossRef]
28. Solarino, G.; Abate, A.; Vicenti, G.; Spinarelli, A.; Piazzolla, A.; Moretti, B. Reducing periprosthetic joint infection: What really counts? *Joints* **2015**, *3*, 208–214. [CrossRef]
29. Ratto, N.; Arrigoni, C.; Rosso, F.; Bruzzone, M.; Dettoni, F.; Bonasia, D.E.; Rossi, R. Total knee arthroplasty and infection: How surgeons can reduce the risks. *EFORT Open Rev.* **2016**, *1*, 339–344. [CrossRef]
30. Mukherjee, K.; Pandit, H.; Dodd, C.; Ostlere, S.; Murray, D. The Oxford unicompartmental knee arthroplasty: A radiological perspective. *Clin. Radiol.* **2008**, *63*, 1169–1176. [CrossRef]
31. Jennings, J.M.; Kleeman-Forsthuber, L.T.; Bolognesi, M.P. Medial Unicompartmental Arthroplasty of the Knee. *J. Am. Acad. Orthop. Surg.* **2019**, *27*, 166–176. [CrossRef] [PubMed]

32. Serbest, S.; Tiftikçi, U.; Karaaslan, F.; Tosun, H.B.; Sevinç, H.F.; Balci, M. A neglected case of giant synovial chondromatosis in knee joint. *Pan Afr. Med. J.* **2015**, *22*, 5. [CrossRef] [PubMed]
33. Tiftikçi, U.; Serbest, S.; Burulday, V. Can Achilles tendon be used as a new distal landmark for coronal tibial component alignment in total knee replacement surgery? An observational MRI study. *Ther. Clin. Risk Manag.* **2017**, *13*, 81–86. [CrossRef]
34. Batailler, C.; Fernandez, A.; Swan, J.; Servien, E.; Haddad, F.S.; Catani, F.; Lustig, S. MAKO CT-based robotic arm-assisted system is a reliable procedure for total knee arthroplasty: A systematic review. *Knee Surg. Sports Traumatol. Arthrosc.* **2020**, *29*, 3585–3598. [CrossRef] [PubMed]
35. Friederich, N.; Verdonk, R. The use of computer-assisted orthopedic surgery for total knee replacement in daily practice: A survey among ESSKA/SGO-SSO members. *Knee Surg. Sports Traumatol. Arthrosc.* **2008**, *16*, 536–543. [CrossRef]
36. van der Steen, M.C.; Janssen, R.P.A.; Reijman, M.; Tolk, J.J. Total Knee Arthroplasty: What to Expect? A Survey of the Members of the Dutch Knee Society on Long-Term Recovery after Total Knee Arthroplasty. *J. Knee Surg.* **2016**, *30*, 612–616. [CrossRef]
37. Mathews, J.A.; Kalson, N.S.; Tarrant, P.M.; Toms, A.D. Revision Knee Replacement Priority Setting Partnership steering group Top ten research priorities for problematic knee arthroplasty. *Bone Jt. J.* **2020**, *102-B*, 1176–1182. [CrossRef] [PubMed]
38. Athey, A.G.; Cao, L.; Okazaki, K.; Zagra, L.; Castelli, C.C.; Kendoff, D.O.; Kerr, J.M.; Yates, A.J.; Stambough, J.B.; Sierra, R.J. Survey of AAHKS International Members on the Impact of COVID-19 on Hip and Knee Arthroplasty Practices. *J. Arthroplast.* **2020**, *35*, S89–S94. [CrossRef]
39. Torre, M.; Carrani, E.; Ceccarelli, S.; Biondi, A.; Masciocchi, M.; Cornacchia, A. *Registro Italiano ArtroProtesi—Report Annuale 2019*; Istituto Superiore di Sanità: Rome, Italy, 2020.
40. Vaishya, R.; Agarwal, A.K.; Vijay, V. Extensor Mechanism Disruption after Total Knee Arthroplasty: A Case Series and Review of Literature. *Cureus* **2016**, *8*, e479. [CrossRef]
41. Song, S.J.; Park, C.H.; Bae, D.K. What to Know for Selecting Cruciate-Retaining or Posterior-Stabilized Total Knee Arthroplasty. *Clin. Orthop. Surg.* **2019**, *11*, 142–150. [CrossRef]
42. Papas, P.V.; Congiusta, D.; Cushner, F.D. Cementless versus Cemented Fixation in Total Knee Arthroplasty. *J. Knee Surg.* **2019**, *32*, 596–599. [CrossRef] [PubMed]
43. Chan, J.Y.; Giori, N.J. Uncemented Metal-Backed Tantalum Patellar Components in Total Knee Arthroplasty Have a High Fracture Rate at Midterm Follow-Up. *J. Arthroplast.* **2017**, *32*, 2427–2430. [CrossRef]
44. Grassi, A.; Compagnoni, R.; Ferrua, P.; Zaffagnini, S.; Berruto, M.; Samuelsson, K.; Svantesson, E.; Randelli, P. Patellar resurfacing versus patellar retention in primary total knee arthroplasty: A systematic review of overlapping meta-analyses. *Knee Surg. Sports Traumatol. Arthrosc.* **2018**, *26*, 3206–3218. [CrossRef] [PubMed]
45. Sabatini, L.; Barberis, L.; Camazzola, D.; Centola, M.; Capella, M.; Bistolfi, A.; Schiraldi, M.; Massè, A. Bicruciate-retaining total knee arthroplasty: What's new? *World J. Orthop.* **2021**, *12*, 732–742. [CrossRef]
46. Victor, J.; Vermue, H. Custom TKA: What to expect and where do we stand today? *Arch. Orthop. Trauma. Surg.* **2021**, *141*, 2195–2203. [CrossRef] [PubMed]
47. Jamari, J.; Ammarullah, M.I.; Santoso, G.; Sugiharto, S.; Supriyono, T.; Prakoso, A.T.; Basri, H.; van der Heide, E. Computational Contact Pressure Prediction of CoCrMo, SS 316L and Ti6Al4V Femoral Head against UHMWPE Acetabular Cup under Gait Cycle. *J. Funct. Biomater.* **2022**, *13*, 64. [CrossRef]

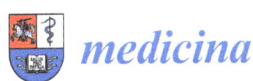

Article

Spacer Block Technique Was Superior to Intramedullary Guide Technique in Coronal Alignment of Femoral Component after Fixed-Bearing Medial Unicompartmental Knee Arthroplasty: A Case–Control Study

O-Sung Lee [1], Myung Chul Lee [2], Chung Yeob Shin [2] and Hyuk-Soo Han [2,*]

1. Department of Orthopedic Surgery, Eulji University School of Medicine, Uijeongbu-si 11759, Republic of Korea
2. Department of Orthopedic Surgery, Seoul National University College of Medicine, Seoul 03080, Republic of Korea
* Correspondence: oshawks7@snu.ac.kr; Tel.: +82-2-2072-4060

Abstract: *Backgrounds and Objectives*: The spacer block technique in unicompartmental knee arthroplasty (UKA) has still a concern related to the precise position of the component in the coronal and sagittal planes compared to intramedullary guide technique. The purposes of this study were to explore whether the spacer block technique would improve the radiological alignment of implants and clinical outcomes compared with the outcomes of the intramedullary guide technique in fixed-bearing medial UKA. *Materials and Methods*: In total, 115 patients who underwent unilateral, fixed-bearing medial UKA were retrospectively reviewed and divided into group IM (intramedullary guides; n = 39) and group SB (spacer blocks; n = 76). Clinical assessment included range-of-motion and patient-reported outcomes. Radiological assessment included the mechanical femorotibial angle, coronal and sagittal alignments of the femoral and tibial components, and coronal femorotibial congruence angle. *Results*: All clinical outcomes showed no significant differences between groups. The coronal femoral component angle was valgus 2.4° ± 4.9° in IM group and varus 1.1° ± 3.2° ($p < 0.001$). In group IM, the number of outlier in coronal femoral component angle (<−10° or 10°<) was 3 cases, while in group SB, there was no outlier ($p = 0.014$). The coronal femorotibial congruence angle was significantly less in group SB (mean 1.9°, range, −3.2°~8.2°) than in group IM (mean 3.4°, range, −9.6°~16.5°) ($p = 0.028$). *Conclusions*: In the group SB, the coronal alignment of femoral component was closer to neutral, and outlier was less frequent than in the group IM. The spacer block technique was more beneficial in achieving proper coronal alignment of the femoral component and congruence of femorotibial components compared to the intramedullary guide technique in fixed-bearing medial UKAs.

Keywords: spacer block; intramedullary rod; femorotibial congruence; unicompartmental arthroplasty

1. Introduction

Unicompartmental knee arthroplasty (UKA) is a more attractive treatment option than total knee arthroplasty (TKA) for patients with unicompartmental knee osteoarthritis; it is associated with less postoperative morbidity, more rapid recovery, more physiological kinematics, and greater patient satisfaction [1–4]. However, the national registries of Europe and Oceania consistently report inferior long-term survivorship of UKAs compared to TKAs [5]. It has been suggested that both implantation and ligament balancing during UKA may be rather inaccurate. Inappropriate component alignment may trigger edge loading, early polyethylene wear, and a high revision rate [6,7]. Mobile-bearing UKA features a round-on-round interface and provided that the orientation of knee components is within a tolerable range, any effect on knee mechanics may be negligible [8,9]. However, fixed-bearing UKA features a round-on-flat interface; thus, it exhibits relatively narrower tolerance in terms of component-to-component malpositioning [10]. These characteristics of fixed-bearing UKA are associated with risks of edge loading and rapid wear [11,12].

Although new patient-specific instrument and navigation techniques are under development, conventional UKA techniques using intramedullary guides or spacer blocks remain widely used. In the context of mobile-bearing UKA, it remains unclear whether new intramedullary rod guides improve radiological alignment and clinical outcomes [13,14]. During fixed-bearing UKA, intramedullary rods have been widely used to align the femoral component. However, given the unsatisfactory accuracy of intramedullary alignment, extramedullary alignment using a spacer block or a tensor device is becoming popular [15–18]. Gap creation using a spacer block aligns the distal femoral resection parallel to the tibial resection in extension; the component gap can be predicted prior to femoral osteotomy. However, it is difficult to define a gap that reflects the physiologically relevant soft tissue balance; a surgeon's technical proficiency and subjective assessment of gap balancing are contributing factors.

In contrast to a TKA, coronal alignment of the components of a UKA is independent of the axis of the lower leg. Rather, the femoral and tibial component have an effect on each other especially in their coronal positioning in knee extension [19]. Although the spacer block technique shows promise in terms of reconstructing physiological joint tension, limited data are available regarding optimal femoral component positions in the coronal and sagittal planes. This technique produces the alignment of the femoral component according to positioning of the spacer introduced after cutting the tibia. Surgeon connects the block to this spacer for cutting the distal femur parallel to the tibial cutting surface on the coronal plane.

The purposes of the present study were to explore whether the spacer block technique improved implant radiological alignment and clinical outcomes, compared to use of an intramedullary guide, in patients undergoing fixed-bearing medial UKAs. It was hypothesized that the use of a spacer block would improve postoperative femoral component positioning and the congruence of femorotibial (FT) components.

2. Materials and Methods

In total, 129 consecutive patients who underwent unilateral, fixed-bearing medial UKA from February 2010 to May 2018 were eligible for inclusion. Fourteen were excluded for the following reasons: fewer than 2 years of follow-up (n = 4), postoperative complications including an infection (n = 1) and loosening (n = 3), and missing clinical data or radiographs (n = 6). Finally, 115 patients who were available for clinical and radiographic evaluation with minimum 2-year follow-up were divided into two groups according to the surgical instrument and implant used: group IM (intramedullary rod guide; n = 39) (MIS Miller/Galante, Zimmer, Warsaw, IN, USA) and group SB (spacer block; n = 76) (Sigma High Performance Partial Knee, DePuy Synthes, Warsaw, IN, USA). The study was approved by the institutional review board (approval no. H-2005-180-1126). The indications for UKA were identical in both groups: A clinical and radiographic diagnosis of isolated medial compartmental osteoarthritis, passive knee flexion contracture <10°, active maximal flexion >100°, and varus deformity <10°. Patient demographics were collected from medical records; these data are summarized in Table 1. There were no significant differences in demographic characteristics between the groups.

Table 1. Demographic and preoperative clinical and radiological data of patients in the intramedullary guide and spacer block groups.

Variable	Intramedullary Guide Group	Spacer Block Group	p Value
No. of subjects	39	76	
Age (year)	64.9 ± 9.1	66.4 ± 6.3	n.s †
Sex (male/female)	4/35	6/70	n.s *
BMI (kg/m^2)	26.0 ± 3.3	26.2 ± 3.2	n.s †
Clinical parameters			
Flexion contracture of knee (°)	2.6 ± 4.0	3.8 ± 6.2	n.s †
Maximal flexion angle of knee (°)	136.7 ± 8.4	132.4 ± 11.4	n.s †
Hospital for Special Surgery score	64.0 ± 12.1	59.7 ± 19.8	n.s †
Knee Society Knee Score	54.1 ± 20.8	48.4 ± 21.0	n.s †
Knee Society Function Score	41.8 ± 17.9	37.6 ± 16.1	n.s †
Pain visual analog scale (0–10)	6.5 ± 2.0	7.2 + 1.9	n.s †
WOMAC	48.0 ± 12.2	48.5 ± 11.3	n.s †
Radiological parameters			
Mechanical femorotibial angle (°)	−6.6 ± 4.1	−5.3 ± 2.9	0.05 †
Medial proximal tibial angle (°)	−3.5 ± 2.6	−3.3 ± 2.2	n.s †
Tibial posterior slope (°)	9.9 ± 2.8	9.7 ± 3.0	n.s †

BMI, body-mass index; WOMAC, Western Ontario and McMaster Universities Arthritis Index; n.s, not significant. Related to Mechanical femorotibial angle and Medial proximal tibial angle, varus alignment was designated as negative values, and valgus alignment was designated as positive values. * Derived with Pearson chi-square test. † Derived with Student's t-test.

3. Surgical Technique

All patients were operated upon by two experienced surgeons (HSH and MCL). A medial mini-parapatellar arthrotomy was performed through a skin incision of approximately 10 cm in length. After osteophyte resection, medial soft tissue release was confined to the deep medial collateral ligament. No further release to correct varus alignment was performed. The tibia was first cut using extramedullary guides to ensure coronal alignment between the native medial proximal tibial angle (MPTA) and 0° varus/valgus to the mechanical tibial axis. The sagittal alignment was aimed to be similar to the native medial posterior tibial slope. For femoral preparation, in group IM, a hole was created for insertion of the intramedullary guide (using an 8 mm drill), 1 cm anterior to the origin of the posterior cruciate ligament and immediately anterior to the femoral intercondylar notch. The intramedullary rod was inserted, and a distal femoral resection guide was then attached with the valgus angle measured on preoperative standing whole lower extremity radiographs. In group SB, a spacer block of the appropriate size (thickness) was placed; the gap from full extension to full flexion was checked. The goal was to ensure that the flexion and extension gaps were balanced with the spacer blocks in various sizes. A distal femoral cutting guide of the same thickness was inserted and pinned in place with the knee in extension. In both groups, femoral component rotation was performed to create a rectangular flexion gap. For confirmation of proper gap, the flexion gap is measured in about 100° flexion using the gap checking device that matches the spacer block thickness used for cutting the distal femur. Additionally, then, the extension gap is measured with this device. The correct gap indicating natural tension was assessed subjectively by checking whether the gap was loose with a thinner gap checker and tight with a thicker one (Figure 1). All components were cemented in both groups. All patients followed the same postoperative rehabilitation protocol, and full weight-bearing (as tolerated) the day after surgery.

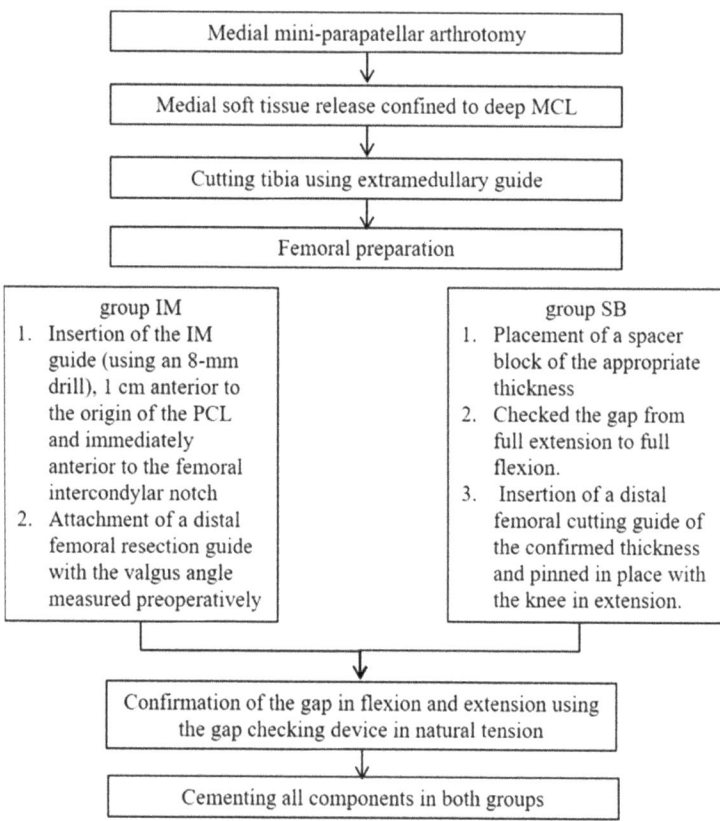

Figure 1. Schematic diagram of surgical procedure in UKA. MCL; medial collateral ligament, IM; intramedullary, SB; space block.

4. Clinical and Radiological Assessment

Clinical and radiological evaluations were performed preoperatively, at 6 weeks and 3 months postoperatively, and annually thereafter. Information was retrieved from the clinical data repository regarding the pre- and post-operative ranges of motion, as well as clinical scores including the Hospital for Special Surgery score, the Knee Society Knee and Function Scores, the pain visual analog scale score, and the Western Ontario McMaster Universities Osteoarthritis Index.

Standardized anteroposterior and lateral radiographs of the knee, whole lower extremity standing anteroposterior (AP) radiographs were obtained for radiologic assessment. All radiological parameters were measured twice at a 2-week interval using a Picture Archiving and Communication System by two orthopedic surgeons who were not members of the surgical team. The preoperative mechanical FT varus angle, MPTA, and posterior tibial slope angle were measured. Postoperatively, the mechanical FT varus angle, coronal femoral component (α) angle and coronal tibial component (β) were determined by measuring varus ($-$)/valgus ($+$) alignment of each component relative to the long axis of the tibia on AP radiograph [11,20]. Sagittal femoral component angle was determined as the angle between a line perpendicular to the component part placed on distal femur cut and a long axis of the femur [21]. Sagittal tibial component angle was determined as the angle between a line perpendicular to the long axis of the tibia and a line tangential to the tibial component on a lateral radiograph (Figure 2). The coronal FT component congruence angle was defined as the angle of tilt between the line perpendicular to the long axis of the femoral component surface and the clearly visible lower margin of the tibial component in the AP view; lateral convergences between these two lines were assigned positive values. Clinical and radiological results achieved at 2 years postoperatively were used for comparison between the groups.

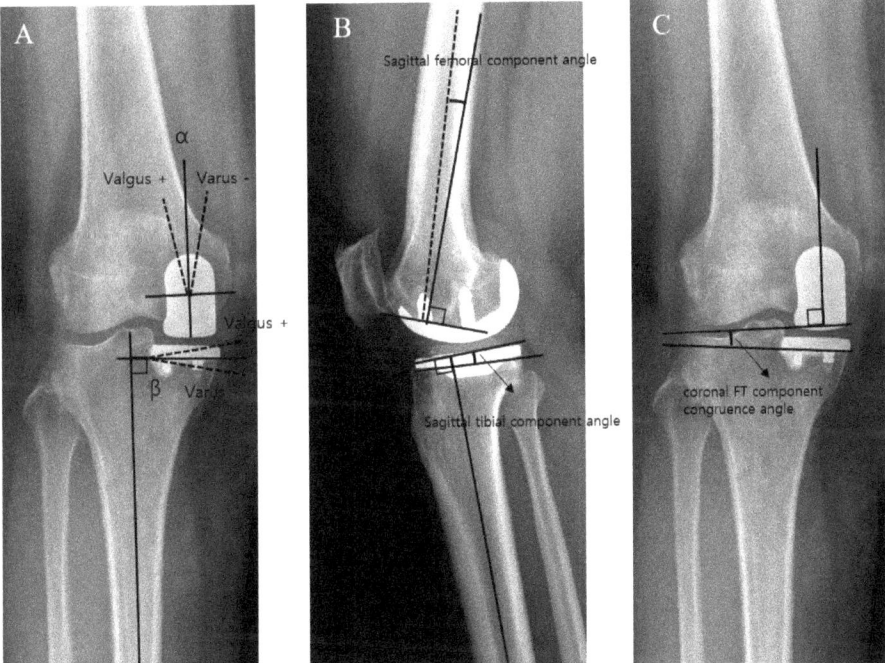

Figure 2. Measurement of alignments of the femoral and tibial components on postoperative radiographs. (**A**) Coronal femoral component angle (α) and coronal tibial component angle (β). (**B**) Sagittal femoral component angle and sagittal tibial component angle. (**C**) Coronal FT component congruence angle.

5. Statistical Analysis

Continuous variables are presented as means with standard deviations; categorical variables are presented as frequencies with percentages. The Kolmogorov–Smirnov test was used to explore the normality of data distribution. Comparisons were performed using Pearson chi-square test and Student's t-test. Intraclass correlation coefficients were calculated to assess the inter- and intraobserver reliabilities of radiological measurements. To reveal the sample size of this study sufficient for adequate power, the statistical software G*Power (Erdfelder, Faul, Lang and Buchner, 2014) was used for power analysis. A post hoc power analysis was performed and showed a sufficient sample size for this retrospective study with an alpha of 0.05 and a power > 0.8.) All statistical analyses were performed using SPSS software (ver. 25.0.0). A p-value < 0.05 was considered to indicate statistical significance.

6. Results

Neither demographic nor preoperative clinical and radiological data differed significantly between the two groups, with the exception of the mechanical FT varus angle (group IM, 6.6° vs. group SB 5.3°; p = 0.05) (Table 1). No intraoperative complications or instrument-related problems were encountered in either group. The postoperative clinical and radiological data of both groups are summarized in Table 2. The clinical outcomes (except the maximal knee flexion angle) improved significantly in both groups. No significant differences were found in any postoperative clinical parameter in either group.

Table 2. Comparison of postoperative clinical and radiological data between patients in the intramedullary guide and spacer block groups.

Variable	Intramedullary Guide Group (N = 39)	Spacer Block Group (N = 76)	p Value
Clinical parameters			
Flexion contracture of knee (°)	1.2 ± 2.6	0.3 ± 1.1	n.s
Maximal flexion angle of knee (°)	134.4 ± 8.8	135.7 ± 5.5	n.s
Hospital for Special Surgery score	95.6 ± 3.0	90.3 ± 9.0	n.s
Knee Society Knee Score	93.5 ± 4.5	92.5 ± 9.2	n.s
Knee Society Function Score	88.5 ± 8.4	91.7 ± 8.0	n..s
Pain visual analog scale (0–10)	1.0 ± 1.3	1.5 ± 1.7	n.s
WOMAC	8.9 ± 7.0	9.1 ± 13.3	n.s
Radiological parameters			
Mechanical FT angle (°)	−1.8 ± 3.7	−0.3 ± 3.2	0.025
Difference from preoperative value (°)	4.8 ± 3.5	5.0 ± 2.2	n.s
Coronal femoral component angle (α) (°)	2.4 ± 4.9	−1.1 ± 3.2	<0.001
Number of outlier in α angle (<−10 or 10<)	3	0	0.014
Coronal tibial component angle (β) (°)	−1.0 ± 4.3	−3.0 ± 2.4	0.001
Difference from preoperative MPTA (°)	2.4 ± 4.9	0.2 ± 2.8	0.003
Sagittal femoral component angle (°)	3.1 ± 8.7	5.0 ± 4.1	n.s
Sagittal tibial component angle (°)	7.2 ± 3.5	8.2 ± 2.7	n.s
Difference from preoperative tibial posterior slope (°)	−2.8 ± 4.0	−1.4 ± 3.4	n.s
Coronal FT component congruence angle (°)	3.4 ± 4.5	1.9 ± 2.6	0.028

FT, femorotibial; WOMAC, Western Ontario and McMaster Universities Arthritis Index; DFBA, distal femoral bowing angle; MPTA, medial proximal tibial angle; n.s, not significant. In representing mechanical FT angle, coronal femoral.

However, several radiological parameters differed significantly between the groups. Although the extent of correction of the mechanical FT angle did not differ between the groups, the postoperative mechanical FT varus angle was smaller in group SB than in group IM (−1.8° ± 3.7° vs. −0.3° ± 3.2°, $p = 0.025$), which was similar to the preoperative difference. The coronal femoral component angle (α) was valgus 2.4° ± 4.9° in group IM, and varus 1.1° ± 3.2° in group SB, respectively ($p < 0.001$) (Figure 3).

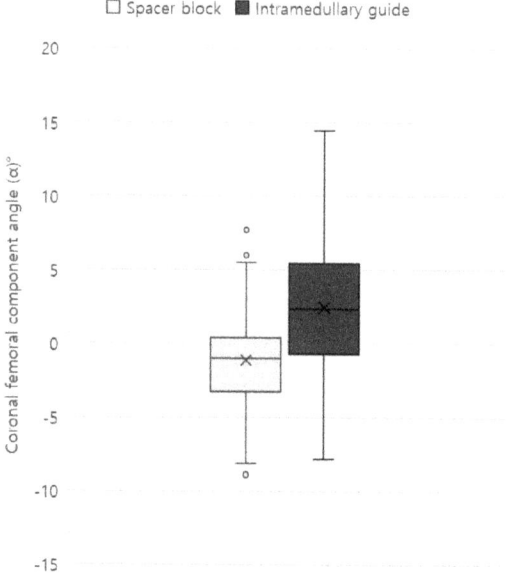

Figure 3. Boxplot of the distribution of the coronal femoral component angle in group SB and IM.

The number of outlier in α angle (<−10 or 10<) was 3 in group IM, and 0 in group SB, respectively (p = 0.014) [22]. The postoperative coronal tibial component angle (β) significantly differed between the two groups (group IM, varus 1° ± 4.3° vs. group SB, 3.0° ± 2.4°; p = 0.001), and MPTA change also significantly differed between the groups (group IM, 2.4° ± 4.9° vs. group SB, 0.2° ± 2.8°; p = 0.003). Sagittal femoral and tibial component angles showed no significant difference between the two groups. Finally, the coronal FT component congruence angle of group SB (mean, 1.9°; range, −3.2 to 8.2°) was less than that of group IM (mean, 3.4°; range, −9.6 to 16.5°) (p = 0.028) (Figure 4). All radiological measurements exhibited excellent intraclass correlation coefficients in terms of both intra- and interobserver reliabilities (0.81–0.92).

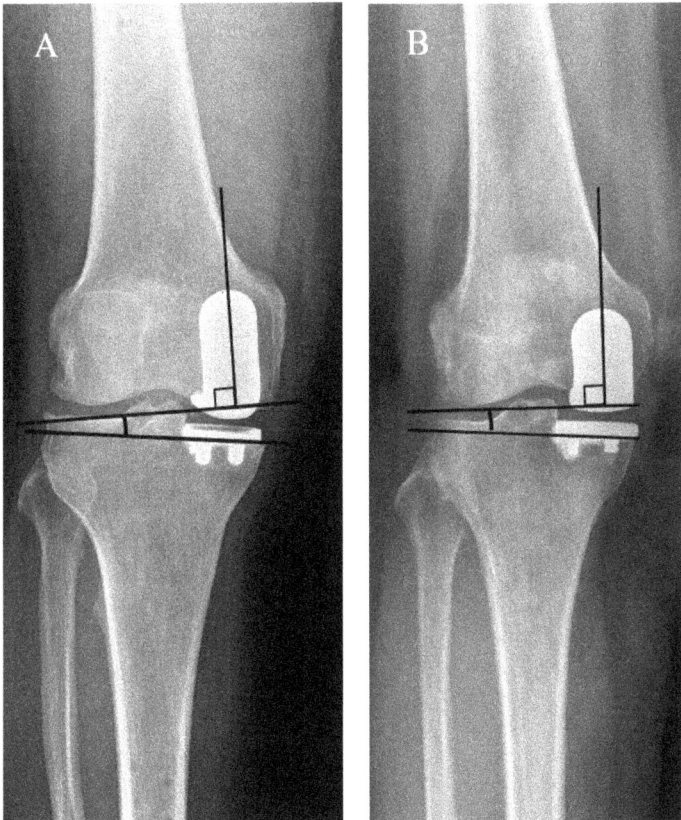

Figure 4. Radiographs showing that the coronal FT component congruence angle of group SB is smaller than that of group IM. (**A**). Showing the coronal FT component congruence angle of group IM, (**B**) Showing the coronal FT component congruence angle of group SB.

7. Discussion

The principle findings of the present study were as follows: (1) the femoral component implanted by the spacer block technique has more neutral alignment relative to the long axis of the tibia with less outliers (>±10° deviation from neutral) [22]. (2) the mean and variation of the coronal FT component congruence angle in patients for whom the spacer block technique was used were lower than the corresponding values in patients treated using the intramedullary guide technique after fixed-bearing medial UKA. However, there were no significant between-group differences in clinical outcomes on short-term follow-up.

The success of UKA relies on appropriate implant alignment and positioning, as well as correct soft tissue tensioning, to ensure a balanced flexion-extension gap and stability [1–4]. Good surgical technique and instruments that avoid edge loading attributable to component-to-component mal-positioning are essential. In contrast to TKA, coronal alignment of the femoral component during UKA does not affect the leg axis; however, it influences relative component positioning in extension [8]. During UKA, the appropriateness of intramedullary alignment of the femoral component has been questioned, given the limited precision of manipulation, as well as potential morbidity created by trochlear cartilage perforation and medullary canal opening [15–17]. The spacer block technique seeks to ensure a rectangular, medial extension gap, thereby achieving maximum possible contact between femoral and tibial components. In this technique, the femoral component is aligned with the tibial cut by introduction of a spacer in extension after cutting the tibia. The intraoperatively, symmetrically resected medial extension gap also ensures parallel positioning of implants in the coronal plane.

In terms of evaluation of postoperative implant alignment after TKA, many studies have indicated that proper alignment of implant has a beneficial impact on implant survival and functional outcomes after TKA [23–25]. However, in contrast of TKA, the impact of implant alignment on long-term survival and clinical outcomes after UKA is unclear. UKA is known to have a widely acceptable range of component alignment within $\pm 10°$ of coronal and sagittal alignment for the femoral component and $\pm 5°$ coronal and sagittal alignment for the tibial component [11,22]. Despite acceptable deviation of postoperative limb alignment from neutral alignment may not have an effect on outcomes, far outliers of deviation may lead to harmful effect on survival and clinical outcomes after UKA. In our study, although the mean values of the coronal femoral component angle in both groups were within varus/valgus 3 degrees, the femoral component in the SB group has more neutral alignment relative to the long axis of the tibia with less outliers ($> \pm 10°$ deviation from neutral). Additionally, the mean coronal FT component congruence angle in SB group was lower than that in IM group, which may be associated with a risk of accelerated wear in the components.

Studies of mobile-bearing UKA using spacer blocks demonstrated a range of femoral component coronal alignments (8–11° valgus and 8–13° varus) [8,11]. However, during mobile-bearing UKA, because of the spherical nature of the femoral component, femoral malalignment of 10° and tibial malalignment of 5° did not hinder good clinical outcomes [11]. One retrospective study evaluated 193 consecutive patients who had undergone fixed-bearing medial UKA using the spacer technique [19]. The clinical results were comparable to those afforded by the intramedullary guide technique. However, the precision was lower and outliers were more frequent. In the present study, femoral implants exhibited no differences in terms of coronal or sagittal plane accuracies between groups SB and IM; however, the component-to-component congruence was better in group SB. When using the spacer block technique, the position of the femoral component is determined in the planes of the tibial component. Because femoral alignment is thus dependent on tibial alignment, the femoral and tibial components lie parallel, with only $1.9 \pm 2.6°$ of asymmetry. This alignment is better than that of the intramedullary guide technique, where the femoral component position is independent of tibial component position. Given the narrower tolerable congruence between the femoral and tibial components of fixed-bearing UKA, compared to mobile-bearing UKA, the spacer block technique may be superior to the intramedullary guide technique.

When using the spacer block technique, care must be taken to avoid transference of any tibial malalignment to the femoral component; tibial resection must be very precise. However, no consensus has emerged regarding ideal positioning of the tibial component during UKA. In the present study, we first cut the tibia using extramedullary guides to achieve coronal alignment between the native MPTA and the 0° varus/valgus mechanical tibial axis; we also achieved sagittal alignment similar to that of the native medial posterior tibial slope. The mean coronal tibial component angle differed by 2° between groups IM and SB. Although the angle of group IM was more neutrally aligned to the mechanical tibial axis, compared to the angle of group SB (89° and 87°, respectively), the short-term clinical outcomes did not differ between the two groups. The significance of coronal tibial or femoral component alignment, and congruence between femoral and tibial components, should be explored over a longer follow-up period. Importantly, there is a need to address wear, aseptic loosening, and implant survival.

The optimal knee alignment during UKA remains controversial; few reports have addressed this aspect. The ideal component alignments and their effects on long-term UKA outcomes remain unknown. Overcorrection of a tibiofemoral deformity should be avoided to reduce the risk of degenerative change in the contralateral compartment; many authors have recommended that knee alignment should be relatively undercorrected during medial UKA [17,26]. However, undercorrection would increase the load on the medial compartment, which may accelerate polyethylene wear. In a retrospective case series (471 UKAs), more than 50% of failures occurred within 5 years of implantation [26]. The major cause of failure was development of other-compartment arthritis (39.5%), followed by aseptic loosening (25.4%). The FT angles tended to be greater in patients with contralateral arthritis. However, pre-medial UKA radiographs were not available for most patients. The use of a spacer block to determine femoral component position during UKA is associated with a risk of overcorrection [27]. However, the intramedullary guide technique is associated with risks of overstuffing and overcorrection when determining final polyethylene thickness. In the present study, we achieved a mean of 5° of correction and slight varus alignment in both groups. The correction was similar to that other studies (4° to 5°) [19,28].

The present study had several limitations. First, it was retrospective in nature and did not involve randomization; selection bias may have influenced the findings. The preoperative mechanical FT angles significantly differed between the two groups. Second, we compared two different kinds of implants; this might have caused other forms of undetected bias. However, in terms of evaluation of the coronal and sagittal alignments of the tibial component, it is reasonable that our measurement method provides constant results regardless of the design of the implant (Figure 1). Additionally, in terms of measurement of the sagittal alignment of femoral component, we used the distal femur cutting line in order to minimize the bias due to the difference of the implants. Additionally, in terms of the coronal alignment of femoral component, we tried to minimize the bias by using the measuring method introduced by Gulati et al. [11], which is based on long axis of the femoral component regardless of the type of implant and most widely used in the evaluation of component alignment after UKA. Third, postoperative coronal tibial component angle (β) significantly differed between the SB and IM groups, which could affect the coronal femoral component angle (α). However, the more varus the coronal tibial component angle was set, the larger the coronal FT component congruence angle would become in the IM group (Figure 5). Therefore, we could reduce the concern about errors caused by the difference in the coronal tibial component angle after surgery. Finally, all measurements were performed using simple radiographs alone. Accordingly, component rotational errors could not be assessed.

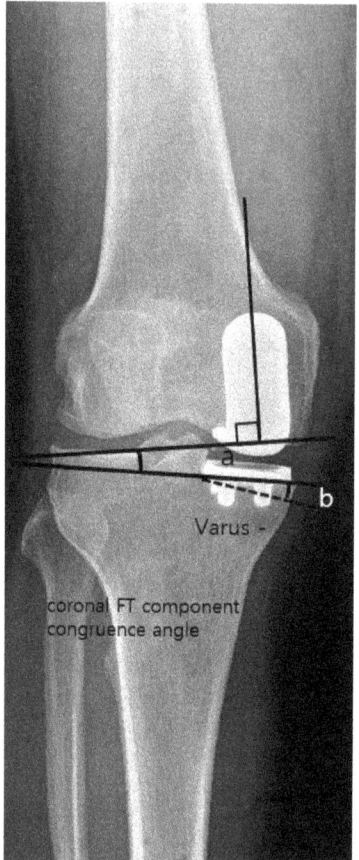

Figure 5. Figure that expresses the imaginary lines showing the coronal FT component congruence angle increases as the varus degree of coronal tibial component angle increases. The (**a**) indicates the coronal FT component congruence, and the (**b**) indicates the the varus degree of coronal tibial component angle.

8. Conclusions

The spacer block technique was more beneficial in achieving proper coronal alignment of the femoral component compared to the intramedullary guide technique in fixed-bearing medial UKAs. The coronal alignment of femoral component was closer to neutral, and outlier was less frequent. Moreover, the congruence of FT components afforded by the spacer block technique was superior to that of the intramedullary guide technique after fixed-bearing medial UKA. Bone resection using a spacer block ensured that the implants were parallel in the coronal plane and may reduce edge loading. However, there were no significant differences in clinical outcomes between the two techniques on short-term follow-up.

Author Contributions: Conceptualization, H.-S.H. and M.C.L.; Methodology, H.-S.H. and O.-S.L.; Formal Analysis, H.-S.H. and O.-S.L.; Investigation, O.-S.L.; Resources, H.-S.H. and M.C.L.; Data Curation, C.Y.S., H.-S.H. and O.-S.L.; Writing—Original Draft Preparation, O.-S.L.; Writing—Review and Editing, C.Y.S., H.-S.H. and O.-S.L.; Visualization, O.-S.L.; Supervision, H.-S.H. and M.C.L. All authors have read and agreed to the published version of the manuscript.

Funding: This research received no external funding.

Institutional Review Board Statement: This study was approved by Seoul National University College of Medicine/Seoul National University Hospital Institutional Review Board (IRB no.: H-2005-180-1126).

Informed Consent Statement: Patient consent was waived due to anonymity of the data used in the study. It was approved by the Institutional Review Board of Seoul National University Hospital.

Data Availability Statement: The data presented in this study are available on request from the corresponding author. The data are not publicly available due to privacy.

Conflicts of Interest: The authors declare that they have no competing interest.

References

1. Foran, J.R.H.; Brown, N.M.; Della Valle, C.J.; Berger, R.A.; Galante, J.O. Long-term Survivorship and Failure Modes of Unicompartmental Knee Arthroplasty. *Clin. Orthop. Relat. Res.* **2013**, *471*, 102–108. [CrossRef] [PubMed]
2. Friesenbichler, B.; Item-Glatthorn, J.F.; Wellauer, V.; von Knoch, F.; Casartelli, N.; Maffiuletti, N.A. Short-term functional advantages after medial unicompartmental versus total knee arthroplasty. *Knee* **2018**, *25*, 638–643. [CrossRef] [PubMed]
3. Matsumoto, T.; Muratsu, H.; Kubo, S.; Kuroda, R.; Kurosaka, M. Intra-operative joint gap kinematics in unicompartmental knee arthroplasty. *Clin. Biomech.* **2013**, *28*, 29–33. [CrossRef] [PubMed]
4. Al-Dadah, O.; Hawes, G.; Chapman-Sheath, P.J.; Tice, J.W.; Barrett, D.S. Unicompartmental vs. segmental bicompartmental vs. total knee replacement: Comparison of clinical outcomes. *Knee Surg. Relat. Res.* **2020**, *32*, 47. [CrossRef]
5. Niinimäki, T.; Eskelinen, A.; Mäkelä, K.; Ohtonen, P.; Puhto, A.-P.; Remes, V. Unicompartmental Knee Arthroplasty Survivorship is Lower Than TKA Survivorship: A 27-year Finnish Registry Study. *Clin. Orthop. Relat. Res.* **2014**, *472*, 1496–1501. [CrossRef]
6. Van Der List, J.P.; Zuiderbaan, H.A.; Pearle, A.D. Why Do Medial Unicompartmental Knee Arthroplasties Fail Today? *J. Arthroplast.* **2015**, *31*, 1016–1021. [CrossRef]
7. Epinette, J.-A.; Brunschweiler, B.; Mertl, P.; Mole, D.; Cazenave, A.; French Society for Hip and Knee. Unicompartmental knee arthroplasty modes of failure: Wear is not the main reason for failure: A multicentre study of 418 failed knees. *Orthop. Traumatol. Surg. Res.* **2012**, *98*, S124–S130. [CrossRef]
8. Kim, J.-G.; Kasat, N.S.; Bae, J.-H.; Kim, S.-J.; Oh, S.-M.; Lim, H.-C. The radiological parameters correlated with the alignment of the femoral component after Oxford Phase 3 unicompartmental knee replacement. *J. Bone Jt. Surgery. Br. Vol.* **2012**, *94*, 1499–1505. [CrossRef]
9. Zhu, G.-D.; Guo, W.-S.; Zhang, Q.-D.; Liu, Z.-H.; Cheng, L.-M. Finite Element Analysis of Mobile-bearing Unicompartmental Knee Arthroplasty: The Influence of Tibial Component Coronal Alignment. *Chin. Med. J.* **2015**, *128*, 2873–2878. [CrossRef]
10. Deschamps, G.; Chol, C. Fixed-bearing unicompartmental knee arthroplasty. Patients' selection and operative technique. *Orthop. Traumatol. Surg. Res.* **2011**, *97*, 648–661. [CrossRef]
11. Gulati, A.; Chau, R.; Simpson, D.; Dodd, C.; Gill, H.; Murray, D. Influence of component alignment on outcome for unicompartmental knee replacement. *Knee* **2009**, *16*, 196–199. [CrossRef] [PubMed]
12. Argenson, J.-N.A.; Parratte, S. The Unicompartmental Knee: Design and technical considerations in minimizing wear. *Clin. Orthop. Relat. Res.* **2006**, *452*, 137–142. [CrossRef] [PubMed]
13. Tuecking, L.-R.; Savov, P.; Richter, T.; Windhagen, H.; Ettinger, M. Clinical validation and accuracy testing of a radiographic decision aid for unicondylar knee arthroplasty patient selection in midterm follow-up. *Knee Surg. Sport. Traumatol. Arthrosc.* **2020**, *28*, 2082–2090. [CrossRef] [PubMed]
14. Jang, K.-M.; Lim, H.C.; Han, S.-B.; Jeong, C.; Kim, S.-G.; Bae, J.-H. Does new instrumentation improve radiologic alignment of the Oxford®medial unicompartmental knee arthroplasty? *Knee* **2017**, *24*, 641–650. [CrossRef] [PubMed]
15. Kort, N.; van Raay, J.; Thomassen, B. Alignment of the femoral component in a mobile-bearing unicompartmental knee arthroplasty: A study in 10 cadaver femora. *Knee* **2007**, *14*, 280–283. [CrossRef]
16. Ma, B.; Long, W.; Rudan, J.F.; Ellis, R.E. Three-Dimensional Analysis of Alignment Error in Using Femoral Intramedullary Guides in Unicompartmental Knee Arthroplasty. *J. Arthroplast.* **2006**, *21*, 271–278. [CrossRef]
17. Levine, B.; Rosenberg, A.G. The Simple Unicondylar Knee: Extramedullary Technique. *Clin. Sports Med.* **2014**, *33*, 77–85. [CrossRef]
18. Kim, T.K.; Mittal, A.; Meshram, P.; Kim, W.H.; Choi, S.M. Evidence-based surgical technique for medial unicompartmental knee arthroplasty. *Knee Surg. Relat. Res.* **2021**, *33*, 2. [CrossRef]
19. Matziolis, G.; Mueller, T.; Layher, F.; Wagner, A. The femoral component alignment resulting from spacer block technique is not worse than after intramedullary guided technique in medial unicompartmental knee arthroplasty. *Arch. Orthop. Trauma Surg.* **2018**, *138*, 865–870. [CrossRef]
20. Sarmah, S.S.; Patel, S.; Hossain, F.S.; Haddad, F.S. The radiological assessment of total and unicompartmental knee replacements. *J. Bone Jt. Surgery. Br. Vol.* **2012**, *94*, 1321–1329. [CrossRef]
21. Mittal, A.; Meshram, P.; Kim, W.H.; Kim, T.K. Unicompartmental knee arthroplasty, an enigma, and the ten enigmas of medial UKA. *J. Orthop. Traumatol.* **2020**, *21*, 15. [CrossRef] [PubMed]

22. Kazarian, G.S.; Barrack, T.N.; Okafor, L.; Barrack, R.L.; Nunley, R.M.; Lawrie, C.M. High Prevalence of Radiographic Outliers and Revisions with Unicompartmental Knee Arthroplasty. *J. Bone Jt. Surg.* **2020**, *102*, 1151–1159. [CrossRef] [PubMed]
23. Harvie, P.; Sloan, K.; Beaver, R.J. Three-Dimensional Component Alignment and Functional Outcome in Computer-Navigated Total Knee Arthroplasty: A Prospective, Randomized Study Comparing Two Navigation Systems. *J. Arthroplast.* **2011**, *26*, 1285–1290. [CrossRef]
24. Lad, D.G.; Thilak, J.; Thadi, M. Component alignment and functional outcome following computer assisted and jig based total knee arthroplasty. *Indian J. Orthop.* **2013**, *47*, 77–82. [CrossRef] [PubMed]
25. Huijbregts, H.J.T.A.M.; Khan, R.J.K.; Fick, D.P.; Hall, M.J.; Punwar, S.A.; Sorensen, E.; Reid, M.J.; Vedove, S.D.; Haebich, S. Component alignment and clinical outcome following total knee arthroplasty: A randomised controlled trial comparing an intramedullary alignment system with patient-specific instrumentation. *Bone Jt. J.* **2016**, *98*, 1043–1049. [CrossRef]
26. Citak, M.; Dersch, K.; Kamath, A.F.; Haasper, C.; Gehrke, T.; Kendoff, D. Common causes of failed unicompartmental knee arthroplasty: A single-centre analysis of four hundred and seventy one cases. *Int. Orthop.* **2014**, *38*, 961–965. [CrossRef] [PubMed]
27. Suzuki, T.; Ryu, K.; Kojima, K.; Iriuchishima, T.; Saito, S.; Nagaoka, M.; Tokuhashi, Y. Evaluation of spacer block technique using tensor device in unicompartmental knee arthroplasty. *Arch. Orthop. Trauma. Surg.* **2015**, *135*, 1011–1016. [CrossRef]
28. Kinsey, T.L.; Anderson, D.N.; Phillips, V.M.; Mahoney, O.M. Disease Progression After Lateral and Medial Unicondylar Knee Arthroplasty. *J. Arthroplast.* **2018**, *33*, 3441–3447. [CrossRef]

Disclaimer/Publisher's Note: The statements, opinions and data contained in all publications are solely those of the individual author(s) and contributor(s) and not of MDPI and/or the editor(s). MDPI and/or the editor(s) disclaim responsibility for any injury to people or property resulting from any ideas, methods, instructions or products referred to in the content.

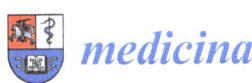

Article

Risk Factors and Preventive Strategies for Perioperative Distal Femoral Fracture in Patients Undergoing Total Knee Arthroplasty

Ki Ho Kang, Man Soo Kim, Jae Jung Kim and Yong In *

Department of Orthopaedic Surgery, Seoul St. Mary's Hospital, College of Medicine, The Catholic University of Korea, 222, Banpo-daero, Seocho-gu, Seoul 06591, Republic of Korea
* Correspondence: iy1000@catholic.ac.kr

Abstract: *Background and Objectives*: Perioperative distal femoral fracture is rare in patients undergoing total knee arthroplasty (TKA). In such rare cases, additional fixation might be required, and recovery can be delayed. Several studies have focused on perioperative distal femoral fractures in TKA, but there remains a lack of information on risk factors. The purpose of this study was to investigate risk factors for perioperative distal femoral fractures in patients undergoing TKA and suggest preventive strategies. *Materials and Methods*: This retrospective study included a total of 5364 TKA cases in a single institution from 2011 to 2022. Twenty-four distal femoral fractures occurred during TKA or within one month postoperatively (0.45%). Patient demographics, intraoperative findings, and postoperative progress were obtained from patient medical records and radiographs. Risk factors for fractures were analyzed using multivariate Firth logistic regression analysis. *Results*: Although all 24 distal femoral fractures occurred in female patients (24 of 4819 patients, 0.50%), the incidence rate of fracture between male and female patients was not significantly different ($p = 0.165$). The presence of osteoporosis and insertion of a polyethylene (PE) insert with knee dislocation were statistically significant risk factors ($p = 0.009$ and $p = 0.046$, respectively). However, multivariate logistic regression analysis showed that only osteoporosis with bone mineral density (BMD) < -2.8 (odds ratio 2.30, 95% CI (1.03–5.54), $p = 0.043$) was an independent risk factor for perioperative distal femoral fracture in TKA patients. *Conclusions*: Our results suggest that osteoporosis with BMD < -2.8 is a risk factor for distal femoral fractures in patients undergoing TKA. In these patients, careful bone cutting, adequate gap balancing, and especially the use of the sliding method for insertion of a PE insert are recommended as preventive strategies.

Keywords: total knee arthroplasty; femur fracture; polyethylene insert; osteoporosis; multivariate logistic analysis

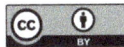

1. Introduction

Fracture of the distal femur during primary total knee arthroplasty (TKA) is a rare complication, with two previous studies reporting an overall incidence ranging from 0.39% to 2.2% [1,2]. These fractures can happen intraoperatively or be found during the postoperative rehabilitation period without definite fracture history [3]. Although the majority of studies report an incidence below 1%, if a distal femoral fracture does occur, it can affect postoperative recovery and outcomes [4]. In fractures with minimal displacement, conservative treatment without additional fixation can lead to good outcomes [2]. However, most fractures require additional fixation [5]. Some severe cases require revision TKA [1]. Clinical outcomes are generally good with proper management; however, non-weight bearing or partial weight bearing for a period of 6–8 weeks as well as limitation of range of motion (ROM) after TKA are common, even in minimally displaced cases [4,6].

There are several known risk factors in distal femoral fracture during TKA, including osteoporosis, rheumatoid arthritis (RA), advanced age, female gender, and posterior-stabilized (PS) implant design [1,5,7–11]. Studies have shown that the wide box cut is a risk factor for femoral fracture in PS TKA [8,9]. Recent PS TKA systems apply minimal box-cutting designs, and most PS surgeons would not change their main implant to a cruciate-retaining type in their practice. In other studies reporting on female sex, osteoporosis, and RA as risk factors for femoral fractures during TKA, fewer than 10 cases of femoral fracture were included in each study [5,10,11]. Recently, one study presented risk factors in the Asian population [6], including female sex, osteoporosis, and small femur size; however, objective evaluation of osteoporosis was inadequate because bone mineral density (BMD) measurement was not routinely conducted. There is a lack of research on risk factors for femoral fracture during TKA [1,7].

The purpose of this study was to investigate risk factors of perioperative distal femoral fracture in a TKA series using PS implants at a single institution. We hypothesized that certain patient demographics or surgical techniques might be associated with perioperative distal femoral fracture. We would like to suggest optimal surgical strategies to prevent distal femoral fracture based on risk factors during TKA.

2. Materials and Methods

2.1. Patient Selection

A total of 5402 primary TKAs was performed on 3922 patients at our institution between September 2011 and October 2022 by two surgeons. All patients were of Asian ethnicity. Patients who previously underwent unicompartmental knee arthroplasty (UKA) and osteotomy around the knee were excluded. A total of 31 fractures occurred during the TKA procedure or within one month after TKA. A patient was excluded if the fracture occurred anywhere other than the distal femur. Cases that had occurred more than one month prior or in which the fracture was caused by definite trauma were also excluded. The remaining 5340 primary TKAs and 24 distal femoral fracture cases were enrolled in this study (Figure 1). This study was approved by the institutional review board of our institution {KC22RASI0865, approved on 25 November 2022}.

2.2. Group Assessment

Patients were divided into two groups with or without perioperative distal femoral fracture. The following demographic and surgical factors were compared between the two groups: age, sex, side, body mass index (BMI), preoperative hip-knee-ankle angle (HKAA), preoperative femorotibial angle (FTA), bone mineral density (BMD), surgical interval, type of implant, and mode of polyethylene (PE) insert insertion. All patients underwent BMD evaluation using dual-energy X-ray absorptiometry (DXA, Hologic Inc., Marlborough, MA, USA) prior to surgery. The BMD value was determined as the lowest T-score value among the femur head, total femur, and average lumbar spine, excluding outliers. The surgical interval of TKA was divided into three categories: unilateral TKA, same-day bilateral TKA, and staggered bilateral TKA with a one-week interval. PS-type implants of various knee systems were used, including 2244 TKAs using Lospa (Corentec, Seoul, Republic of Korea), 964 TKAs using Vanguard (Zimmer Biomet, Warsaw, IN, USA), 664 TKAs using advanced coated system (ACS) (Implantcast GmbH, Buxtehude, Germany), 351 TKAs using Exult (Corentec, Seoul, Republic of Korea), 261 TKAs using PFC (DePuy Synthes, Warsaw, IN, USA), 150 TKAs using Persona (Zimmer Biomet, Warsaw, IN, USA), 116 TKAs using Journey II (Smith & Nephew, Memphis, TN, USA), 56 TKAs using Legion (Smith & Nephew, Memphis, TN, USA), and 34 TKAs using Attune (DePuy Synthes, Warsaw, IN, USA). A total of 14 TKAs with fewer than 10 of a particular knee system were not described separately.

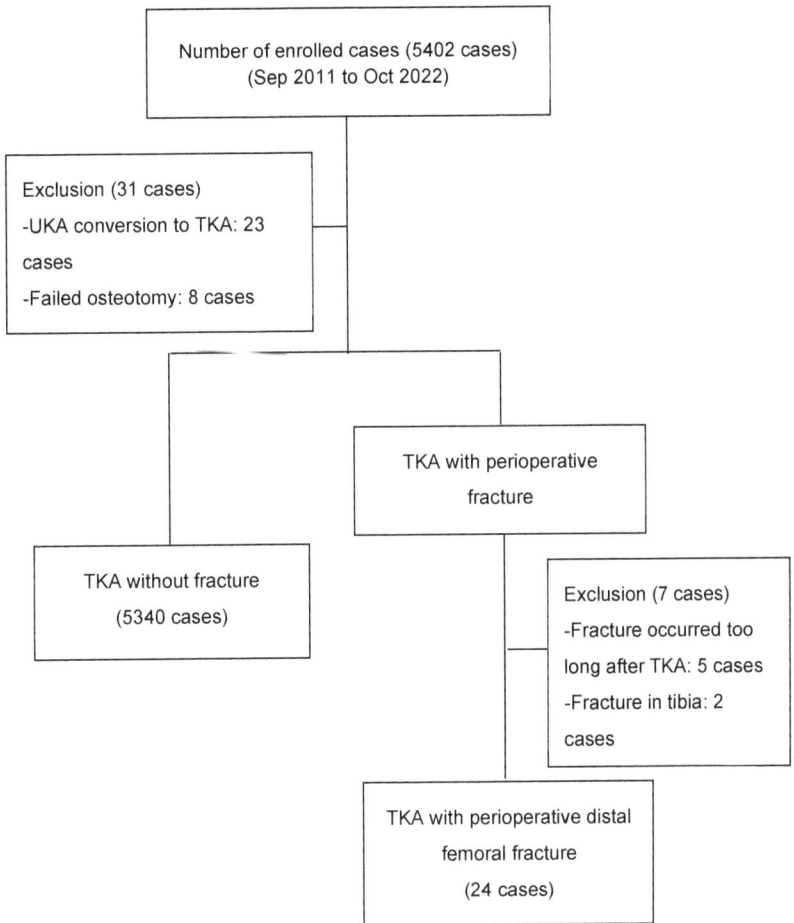

Figure 1. Participant flow diagram.

2.3. Surgical Procedure

All operations were performed by two surgeons in a standard fashion under general anesthesia with tourniquet inflation to 300 mmHg. A PS knee system with the subvastus approach was used in all cases. A measured resection technique was used for bone cutting. Proper gap balancing was applied after bone cutting. Extension and 90° flexion gaps were measured using a tensor device (B.Braun-Aesculap, Tuttlingen, Germany) and scaled forceps (B.Braun-Aesculap) with the application of a 200-N distraction force. In the case of a tight medial gap, multiple needling puncturing was performed with a standard 18-gauge needle based on digital palpation of taut medial collateral ligament (MCL) fibers [12]. All components were fixed using bone cement. Two PE insert insertion methods were used; the knee dislocation method and the sliding method (Figure 2). The PE insert insertion method was determined according to the design of the locking mechanism of the knee system or the status of soft tissue balance. Some knee systems required knee dislocation for secure PE insert insertion, and some allowed sliding insertion of PE insert without knee dislocation.

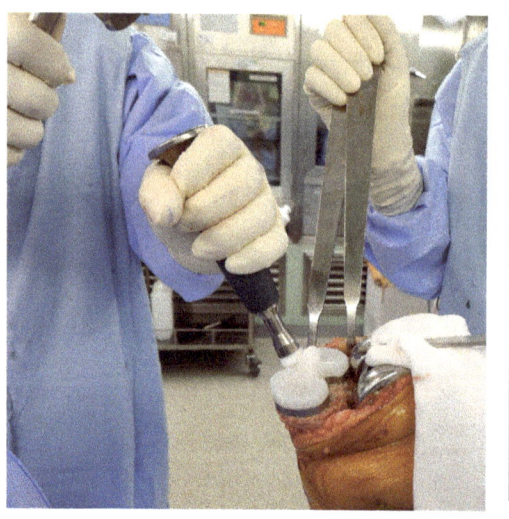 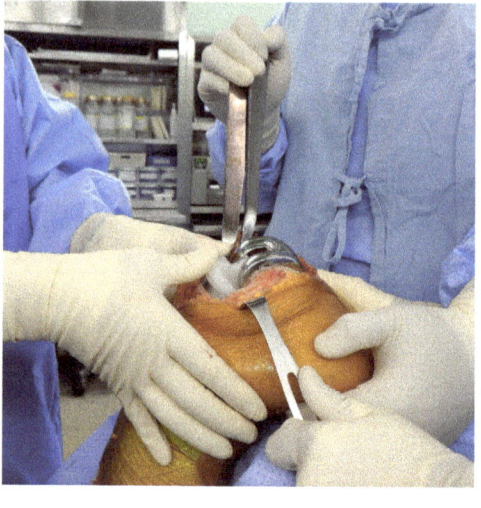

(a) (b)

Figure 2. Modes of polyethylene (PE) inert insertion. (**a**) Insertion of the PE insert with knee dislocation. (**b**) Insertion of the PE insert with the sliding method.

2.4. Statistical Methods

Descriptive analyses were based on means and standard deviations for continuous variables and frequencies and percentages for categorical variables. The chi-square or Fisher exact test for categorical variables was used to compare two groups according to demographic characteristics. In this study, Firth logistic regression analysis was used to estimate the odds ratio (OR) with a 95% confidence interval (CI) due to the small number of fracture cases (24 cases) [13]. Multivariate logistic regression analysis was carried out to identify risk factors significantly related to perioperative distal femoral fracture ($p < 0.1$). All statistical analyses were performed using the SPSS ver. 29.0 program (SPSS Inc., Chicago, IL, USA). A p-value < 0.05 was considered statistically significant. Data are expressed as mean values with standard error of the mean (SEM) unless otherwise stated.

3. Results

Periopcrative distal femoral fractures occurred with an incidence of 0.45% (24 cases) during TKA. Table 1 shows the demographics between patients that underwent TKA without fracture and those with perioperative distal femoral fracture. A total of 17 fractures occurred in 2701 Lospa (Corentec, Seoul, Republic of Korea) TKAs (0.63%) and 7 fractures in 717 ACS (Implantcast GmbH, Buxtehude, Germany) TKAs (0.98%). There were no significant differences between the without fracture group and with fracture group except for BMD value ($p = 0.009$), and mode of PE insert insertion ($p = 0.046$). Although all patients with fractures were female (0.50%), female sex was not a statistically significant factor ($p = 0.165$).

Among the 24 fractures, 22 (91.7%) had a varus knee deformity with an average HKAA of varus of 9.7°. Seventeen fractures (70.8%) happened on the medial femoral condyle of varus deformed knee with an average HKAA of 9.4° (Table 2). The 21 cases (87.5%) that occurred intraoperatively were performed with screw fixation alone. All intraoperative fracture cases but one case achieved bony union, which required revision TKA because subsidence had occurred one month after fixation (Patient B; Table 2). All three postoperative fracture cases occurred 10 to 14 days after the operation without definite trauma history and had a fracture in the lateral femoral condyle that required revision TKA. Among the total 24 fracture patients, 19 (79.2%) were diagnosed with osteoporosis with a

BMD value of −2.5 or less, of which 16 cases (66.7%) were identified as osteoporosis with a BMD value less than −2.8.

Table 1. Demographics of patients with a perioperative distal femoral fracture with TKA.

	TKA without Fracture (n = 5340)	TKA with Perioperative Distal Femoral Fracture (n = 24)	p-Value
Age	70.3 ± 6.6	72.4 ± 7.3	0.125
Sex			0.165
Female	4795 (89.8%)	24 (100%)	
Male	545 (10.2%)	0 (0%)	
Side			0.981
Right	2683 (50.2%)	12 (50%)	
Left	2657 (49.8%)	12 (50%)	
BMI	26.2 ± 6.8	26.3 ± 4.1	0.930
Preoperative HKAA (°)	8.1 ± 5.4 varus	8.4 ± 5.8 varus	0.788
Preoperative FTA (°)	2.9 ± 5.6 varus	2.6 ± 5.1 varus	0.799
BMD	−2.7 ± 1.0	−3.2 ± 0.9	0.009
Type of TKA			0.663
Unilateral TKA	2395 (44.9%)	9 (37.5%)	
Same-Day Bilateral TKA	1810 (33.9%)	10 (41.7%)	
Staggered Bilateral TKA	1135 (21.3%)	5 (20.8%)	
Implant			
Lospa	2684 (50.3%)	17 (70.8%)	
Vanguard	964 (18.1%)	0 (0%)	
ACS	710 (13.3%)	7 (29.2%)	
Exult	351 (6.6%)	0 (0%)	
PFC	261 (4.9%)	0 (0%)	
Persona	150 (2.8%)	0 (0%)	
Journey II	116 (2.2%)	0 (0%)	
Legion	56 (1.0%)	0 (0%)	
Attune	34 (0.6%)	0 (0%)	
Other	14 (0.3%)	0 (0%)	
Mode of PE insert insertion			0.046
Dislocation method	3662 (68.6%)	21 (87.5%)	
Sliding method	1678 (31.4%)	3 (12.5%)	

HKAA; hip-knee-ankle angle; FTA; femorotibial angle.

Based on univariate factor analysis, variables that were statistically different and may affect fracture as potential predictors were used for additional univariate logistic regression analysis. Among them, BMD less than −2.8 (odds ratio [2.30], 95% CI [1.03–5.54], p = 0.042) was the only factor that correlated with a risk of perioperative distal femoral fracture in TKA. The BMD value of −2.8 was arbitrarily set as the cut-off value because it was the most statistically significant BMD value among values less than −2.5. BMD value of −2.5 corresponding to osteoporosis was not statistically significant. The parameters included in the multivariate logistic regression model were variables with a p-value less than 0.1 and were the mode of PE insert insertion method and BMD less than −2.8. Only one risk factor remained statistically significant. Patients with a BMD value less than −2.8 increased the risk for distal femoral fracture (odds ratio [2.30], 95% CI [1.03–5.54], p = 0.043) (Table 3).

Table 2. Summary of perioperative distal femoral fracture with TKA.

Patient	Sex	Age	Side	BMI	ASA	BMD	Pre FTA (+: Varus, −: Valgus)	Pre HKAA (+: Varus, −: Valgus)	Surgeon	Implant	Mode of PE Insert Insertion	Site of Fracture	Time Discovered	Management
A	F	53	Lt.	25.8	1	−2.7	0.7	7.8	Senior	Lospa	Dislocation	lateral condyle	Intraoperative	Screw fixation
B	F	55	Lt. (Staggered)	22.6	1	−3.6	−10.2	−3.9	Senior	Lospa	Dislocation	medial condyle	Intraoperative	Screw fixation
C	F	69	Rt. (Same-day)	24.2	2	−3.6	5.9	8.2	Senior	Lospa	Dislocation	medial condyle	Intraoperative	Revision TKA
D	F	75	Rt. (Staggered)	24.8	2	−2.9	3.9	9.9	Senior	Lospa	Dislocation	medial condyle	Intraoperative	Screw fixation
E	F	80	Rt.	19.7	2	−3.4	−10.8	−7.5	Senior	Lospa	Dislocation	medial condyle	Intraoperative	Screw fixation
F	F	79	Lt. (Staggered)	30.0	2	−4.4	4.7	12.9	Senior	ACS	Dislocation	medial condyle	Intraoperative	Screw fixation
G	F	74	Lt. (Same-day)	18.7	1	−4.6	9.3	15.5	Senior	Lospa	Dislocation	medial condyle	Intraoperative	Screw fixation
H	F	72	Rt. (Same-day)	25.6	2	−1.9	0.4	2.8	Senior	Lospa	Dislocation	medial condyle	Intraoperative	Screw fixation
I	F	73	Rt.	27.7	2	−3.8	3.1	7.4	Senior	ACS	Dislocation	medial condyle	Intraoperative	Screw fixation
J	F	76	Rt.	23.7	3	−4.1	2.2	10.5	Senior	ACS	Dislocation	medial condyle	Intraoperative	Screw fixation
K	F	73	Rt.	26.7	2	−3.7	0.3	6.1	Senior	ACS	Dislocation	medial condyle	Intraoperative	Screw fixation
L	F	69	Lt. (Same-day)	29.3	2	−2.8	−1.9	5.4	Senior	Lospa	Dislocation	lateral condyle	Postoperative 10 days	Revision TKA
M	F	71	Rt. (Staggered)	35.3	2	−2.2	8.9	16.8	Junior	Lospa	Dislocation	medial condyle	Intraoperative	Screw fixation
N	F	81	Lt.	23.2	3	−3.6	5.1	8.7	Junior	Lospa	Dislocation	medial condyle	Intraoperative	Screw fixation
O	F	65	Lt. (Same-day)	25.2	2	−1.6	8.9	15.1	Senior	ACS	Dislocation	lateral condyle	Intraoperative	Screw fixation
P	F	70	Lt. (Same-day)	33.3	2	−3.7	3.8	12.7	Senior	Lospa	Dislocation	lateral condyle	Postoperative 14 days	Revision TKA
Q	F	66	Lt. (Same-day)	34.6	2	−2.6	8.7	14.1	Senior	Lospa	Dislocation	medial condyle	Intraoperative	Screw fixation
R	F	78	Rt.	26.7	2	−3.1	5.0	6.9	Junior	Lospa	Sliding	medial condyle	Intraoperative	Screw fixation
S	F	78	Rt. (Staggered)	25.5	2	−5.0	2.8	8.2	Senior	ACS	Dislocation	medial condyle	Intraoperative	Screw fixation
T	F	75	Lt. (Same-day)	27.7	2	−2.9	1.1	6.4	Junior	ACS	Dislocation	medial condyle	Intraoperative	Screw fixation
U	F	83	Rt.	25.9	3	−2.1	3.7	14.3	Junior	Lospa	Sliding	medial condyle	Intraoperative	Screw fixation
V	F	77	Lt.	22.6	2	−4.4	5.9	11.5	Senior	Lospa	Dislocation	lateral condyle	Postoperative 14 days	Revision TKA
W	F	74	Rt. (Same-day)	28.8	2	−1.3	0.2	5.2	Junior	Lospa	Sliding	medial condyle	Intraoperative	Screw fixation
X	F	71	Lt. (Same-day)	24.4	2	−2.9	1.1	6.0	Senior	Lospa	Dislocation	medial condyle	Intraoperative	Screw fixation

FASA; American Society of Anesthesiologists, FTA; femorotibial angle, HKAA; hip-knee-ankle angle, F; female, Lt.; left, Rt.; right.

Table 3. Multivariate logistic regression analysis of perioperative distal femoral fracture risk factors with TKA.

	Univariate			Multivariate		
	Odds Ratio	95% CI	p-Value	Adjusted Odds Ratio	95% CI	p-Value
Age	1.05	0.99–1.12	0.127			
Sex (Female)	5.57	0.78–707.69	0.104			
Side (Rt.)	0.99	0.45–2.19	0.981			
Type of TKA						
Unilateral TKA	reference					
Same-Day Bilateral TKA	1.59	0.65–3.96	0.302			
Staggered Bilateral TKA	1.17	0.38–3.27	0.775			
Mode of PE insert insertion (Knee Dislocation)	2.73	0.99–10.25	0.052	1.87	0.68–7.04	0.244
BMD ≤ −2.5 (Osteoporosis)	1.99	0.82–5.71	0.132			
BMD < −2.8	2.30	1.03–5.54	0.042	2.30	1.03–5.54	0.043
Preoperative HKAA	1.01	0.94–1.09	0.800			

HKAA; hip-knee-ankle angle.

4. Discussion

This study evaluated the risk factors associated with perioperative distal femoral fractures in primary TKA. Among 5364 TKAs, 24 fractures occurred. The BMD value and mode of PE insert insertion (dislocation method) were the significant risk factors. In multivariate logistic regression analysis of risk factors, only BMD less than −2.8 showed a 2.30-fold increase in fracture risk.

Perioperative distal femoral fracture in TKA is uncommon, and there is a paucity of studies on this topic. Because some fractures that are not clinically important may be missed, the reported incidence might be underestimated [8]. In our study, there was a 0.45% incidence of perioperative femoral fracture with 5364 TKAs, similar to the incidence observed in previous studies (0.39% to 2.2%) [1,2]. According to a recently published systematic review, the overall incidence was from 0.2% to 4.4% [4]. Thus far, prospective studies have not been possible due to the small sample size and lack of predictability of fractures.

The risk factors for distal femoral fracture have been addressed in several previous studies. Osteoporosis is a well-known risk factor, but there is a lack of studies suggesting the cut-off value of osteoporosis. In our institution, DXA was included as a part of the routine preoperative workup for TKA candidates. Most of the patients with fractures were shown to have a low BMD value. In our study, BMD less than −2.8 was the only significant risk factor in multivariate logistic regression analysis. These patients should be informed about their low bone quality and associated risks preoperatively [14]. Then, the surgery should be performed with consent. McClung et al. reported that BMD value is important but emphasized that it was not the only determinant for fracture risk and assessment with individual patient risk [15]. However, according to our study, special attention should be given to patients with a BMD value less than −2.8 during surgery based on the 2.30-fold increase in fracture risk. In our practice, even in patients with osteoporosis, the same rehabilitation program was applied if there was no intraoperative fracture. However, medical treatment for osteoporosis was started or continued depending on the patient's situation [16].

Alden et al. reported that fracture occurs more commonly in female patients [1]. In our results, the fracture group was all female, which is consistent with previous studies. However, being female was not a significant risk factor in our analysis. According to large population-based cohort studies, an increased risk of symptomatic knee OA was associated with being female, particularly in the Asian population [17]. Although no fracture cases occurred in male patients, since there were more female patients undergoing TKA, the risk of fracture in females was not significantly different in our study.

PS design of TKA has been associated with fracture. Lombardi et al. reported 40 distal femoral intercondylar fractures in 898 PS TKAs (4.4%) [9]. Alden et al. also reported a relative risk of 4.74 for femoral fracture with PS femoral components. In our study, all patients underwent the PS type TKA. Therefore, it was not possible to compare the sample with other types. The wider box cut in the PS type and inappropriate medial or lateral placement to a thin column of bone might result in a high incidence of fracture, which can be reduced by box design improvement and careful resection technique [1,9]. It was expected that advanced age would be a risk factor for fracture, but our results showed no relationship with age. A previous study showed that same-day bilateral TKA was a risk factor, but there was no such correlation in our study based on univariate logistic regression analysis [6]. Other known risk factors, such as chronic use of corticosteroids, RA, or neurological abnormalities, were not included in this analysis because there were few or no corresponding patients [18].

Perioperative distal femoral fractures can occur at various stages of the TKA procedure. It was reported that most fractures occurred during exposure and bone preparation of the femur and impaction of the femoral implants [1,2]. During the removal of a large osteophyte, inadequate box cut, thin column of the medial and lateral condyle, wrong hammering direction, and/or excessive force could cause fracture at this stage [6,10]. In our study, we found that distal femoral fracture, especially medial femoral condylar fracture, was more likely to occur at a certain stage of TKA. In patients with osteoporosis, we technically focused on soft tissue balancing, especially medial gap, and the PE insert insertion method. A tight medial gap in varus-deformed osteoporotic patients was the most common scenario for distal femoral fracture during TKA at the reduction stage of the knee joint after inserting PE insert with the knee dislocation. Depending on the knee systems, due to the design of the dovetail mechanism, knee dislocation is required to secure the insertion of the PE insert. Greater tension is applied to the MCL with the varus-deformed knee. If the medial gap balancing in the flexion position is not appropriate in these patients, the medial femoral condylar fracture risk is elevated during the knee reduction stage. There were only three cases (12.5%) of fractures among the implants using the sliding method in our study. Although this factor was not significant in our study, it reduced the risk of fracture by 2.73-fold in univariate logistic regression analysis. Alden et al. reported that performing a proper medial release prior to flexing the knee decreased tension on the MCL in the varus knee [1]. Extra attention should be paid to achieving the adequate medial gap, especially when inserting PE insert insertion using the knee dislocation method. After experiencing the fractures, the pie-crusting technique using multiple needle puncturing was applied to obtain the appropriate medial gap for the varus knee in our practice (Figure 3). The pie-crusting technique was reported to be effective and safe for both valgus and varus deformities during TKA [19,20]. In addition, multiple needle puncturing of the MCL is a more effective and safer technique relative to the blade knife technique [12,21].

Management options for perioperative distal femoral fracture are based on stable fixation and on surgeon preference. Huang et al. reported that screw fixation is more appropriate than plate fixation because the reduction of fracture fragments is easy, the plate could have affected the femoral component position, and the cement provides an additional stable force for the fracture fragment [11]. In our study, all fractures found intraoperatively were fixed with a screw alone. Among these cases, only one case of subsidence occurred after one month, and revision TKA was performed in that case. In the three cases of postoperative fractures, revision TKA was also required. These three cases occurred without any definite trauma and were different from previously reported periarticular fractures. The previously published periarticular fracture occurred on average two to four years after TKA with low-energy trauma [22]. It is thought that the perioperative fracture occurred during surgery, but that could not be verified. Shahi et al. reported 15 cases similar to our postoperative fracture cases in fracture patterns, and all of them underwent revision

TKA [23]. With the recent development of three-dimensional technology, a clinical workflow for personalized surgical treatment can be developed in postoperative fracture cases [24]. After screw fixation, non-weight bearing or partial weight bearing was recommended to patients for 4–6 weeks, depending on the status of stability. Full weight bearing and full ROM exercise immediately after surgery were allowed in cases of revision TKA.

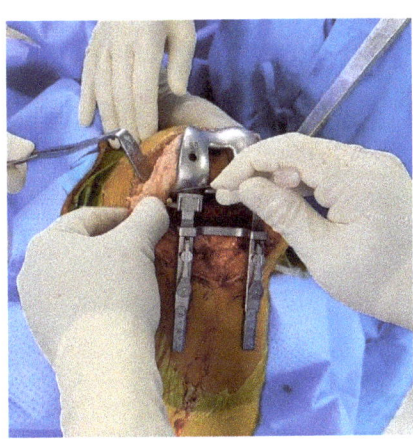 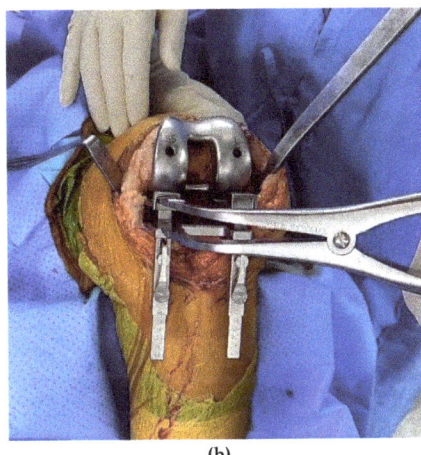

(a) (b)

Figure 3. Ease of tension on the medial collateral ligament. (**a**) Pie-crusting with multiple needle puncturing. (**b**) Spreading medial flexion gap using a tensor device.

There exist limitations in our study. First, this study is a retrospective analysis. As mentioned earlier, the low incidence of perioperative fractures with TKA precludes a prospective study. Second, this study was carried out in a single hospital. If the study had included patients from several hospitals, the results would be more relevant, at least at the national level. Third, other known risk factors for distal femoral fracture, such as chronic use of corticosteroids, RA, and neurological abnormalities, could not be included in this analysis because there were few or no corresponding patients. In addition, clinical results confirmed by imaging studies were good in patients with appropriate treatment after a fracture. However, the clinical outcomes were not compared using patient-reported outcome measures (PROMs).

5. Conclusions

Perioperative distal femoral fractures during primary TKA are rare, but patients with osteoporotic bone and BMD values less than −2.8 need extra care during the TKA procedure. When inserting the PE insert, the sliding method can reduce the risk of distal femoral fracture. When using the knee dislocation method for insertion of PE insert, the medial and lateral gaps should be sufficiently balanced.

Author Contributions: Conceptualization, K.H.K. and Y.I.; methodology, K.H.K., M.S.K. and Y.I.; software, K.H.K. and J.J.K.; validation, K.H.K., M.S.K. and Y.I.; formal analysis, K.H.K. and J.J.K.; investigation, K.H.K. and M.S.K.; resources, K.H.K. and J.J.K.; data curation, J.J.K.; writing—original draft preparation, K.H.K.; writing—review and editing, K.H.K., M.S.K., J.J.K. and Y.I.; visualization, J.J.K.; supervision, M.S.K. and Y.I.; project administration, K.H.K. and Y.I. All authors have read and agreed to the published version of the manuscript.

Funding: This research received no external funding.

Institutional Review Board Statement: The study was conducted in accordance with the Declaration of Helsinki and approved by the Institutional Review Board of Seoul St. Mary's Hospital (KC22RASI0865 and 25 November 2022).

Informed Consent Statement: Informed consent was obtained from all subjects involved in the study.

Data Availability Statement: The data published in this research are available on request from the first author (K.H.K).

Conflicts of Interest: The authors declare no conflict of interest.

References

1. Alden, K.J.; Duncan, W.H.; Trousdale, R.T.; Pagnano, M.W.; Haidukewych, G.J. Intraoperative fracture during primary total knee arthroplasty. *Clin. Orthop. Relat. Res.* **2010**, *468*, 90–95. [CrossRef] [PubMed]
2. Pinaroli, A.; Piedade, S.R.; Servien, E.; Neyret, P. Intraoperative fractures and ligament tears during total knee arthroplasty. A 1795 posterostabilized TKA continuous series. *Orthop. Traumatol. Surg. Res.* **2009**, *95*, 183–189. [CrossRef] [PubMed]
3. Abdelaal, A.M.; Khalifa, A.A. Nonsurgical management of atraumatic early distal femoral periprosthetic insufficiency fracture after primary total knee arthroplasty, a report of two cases. *Trauma Case Rep.* **2022**, *42*, 100704. [CrossRef] [PubMed]
4. Purudappa, P.P.; Ramanan, S.P.; Tripathy, S.K.; Varatharaj, S.; Mounasamy, V.; Sambandam, S.N. Intra-operative fractures in primary total knee arthroplasty—A systematic review. *Knee Surg. Relat. Res.* **2020**, *32*, 40. [CrossRef] [PubMed]
5. Agarwala, S.; Bajwa, S.; Vijayvargiya, M. Intra-operative fractures in primary Total Knee Arthroplasty. *J. Clin. Orthop. Trauma* **2019**, *10*, 571–575. [CrossRef]
6. Mak, Y.F.; Lee, Q.J.; Chang, W.E.; Wong, Y.C. Intraoperative femoral condyle fracture in primary total knee arthroplasty—A case-control study in Asian population. *Knee Surg. Relat. Res.* **2020**, *32*, 31. [CrossRef]
7. Hernigou, P.; Mathieu, G.; Filippini, P.; Demoura, A. Intra-and postoperative fractures of the femur in total knee arthroplasty: Risk factors in 32 cases. *Rev. Chir. Orthop. Reparatrice Appar. Mot.* **2006**, *92*, 140–147. [CrossRef]
8. Delasotta, L.A.; Orozco, F.; Miller, A.G.; Post, Z.; Ong, A. Distal femoral fracture during primary total knee arthroplasty. *J. Orthop. Surg.* **2015**, *23*, 202–204. [CrossRef]
9. Lombardi, A.V., Jr.; Mallory, T.H.; Waterman, R.A.; Eberle, R.W. Intercondylar distal femoral fracture. An unreported complication of posterior-stabilized total knee arthroplasty. *J. Arthroplast.* **1995**, *10*, 643–650. [CrossRef]
10. Pun, A.H.; Pun, W.K.; Storey, P. Intra-operative fracture in posterior-stabilised total knee arthroplasty. *J. Orthop. Surg.* **2015**, *23*, 205–208. [CrossRef]
11. Huang, Z.Y.; Ma, J.; Shen, B.; Pei, F.X. Intraoperative Femoral Condylar Fracture during Primary Total Knee Arthroplasty: Report of Two Cases. *Orthop. Surg.* **2015**, *7*, 180–184. [CrossRef]
12. Koh, I.J.; Kwak, D.S.; Kim, T.K.; Park, I.J.; In, Y. How effective is multiple needle puncturing for medial soft tissue balancing during total knee arthroplasty? A cadaveric study. *J. Arthroplast.* **2014**, *29*, 2478–2483. [CrossRef]
13. Firth, D. Bias Reduction of Maximum-Likelihood-Estimates. *Biometrika* **1993**, *80*, 27–38. [CrossRef]
14. Lewiecki, E.M.; Binkley, N.; Bilezikian, J.P. Treated Osteoporosis Is Still Osteoporosis. *J. Bone. Miner. Res.* **2019**, *34*, 605–606. [CrossRef]
15. McClung, M.R. The relationship between bone mineral density and fracture risk. *Curr. Osteoporos. Rep.* **2005**, *3*, 57–63. [CrossRef]
16. LeBoff, M.S.; Greenspan, S.L.; Insogna, K.L.; Lewiecki, E.M.; Saag, K.G.; Singer, A.J.; Siris, E.S. The clinician's guide to prevention and treatment of osteoporosis. *Osteoporos. Int.* **2022**, *33*, 2049–2102. [CrossRef]
17. Fransen, M.; Bridgett, L.; March, L.; Hoy, D.; Penserga, E.; Brooks, P. The epidemiology of osteoarthritis in Asia. *Int. J. Rheum. Dis.* **2011**, *14*, 113–121. [CrossRef]
18. Kim, K.I.; Egol, K.A.; Hozack, W.J.; Parvizi, J. Periprosthetic fractures after total knee arthroplasties. *Clin. Orthop. Relat. Res.* **2006**, *446*, 167–175. [CrossRef]
19. Aglietti, P.; Lup, D.; Cuomo, P.; Baldini, A.; De Luca, L. Total knee arthroplasty using a pie-crusting technique for valgus deformity. *Clin. Orthop. Relat. Res.* **2007**, *464*, 73–77. [CrossRef]
20. Bellemans, J.; Vandenneucker, H.; Van Lauwe, J.; Victor, J. A new surgical technique for medial collateral ligament balancing: Multiple needle puncturing. *J. Arthroplast.* **2010**, *25*, 1151–1156. [CrossRef]
21. Kwak, D.S.; In, Y.; Kim, T.K.; Cho, H.S.; Koh, I.J. The pie-crusting technique using a blade knife for medial collateral ligament release is unreliable in varus total knee arthroplasty. *Knee Surg. Sports Traumatol. Arthrosc.* **2016**, *24*, 188–194. [CrossRef] [PubMed]
22. Chmell, M.J.; Moran, M.C.; Scott, R.D. Periarticular Fractures after Total Knee Arthroplasty: Principles of Management. *J. Am. Acad. Orthop. Surg.* **1996**, *4*, 109–116. [CrossRef] [PubMed]
23. Shahi, A.; Saleh, U.H.; Tan, T.L.; Elfekky, M.; Tarabichi, S. A Unique Pattern of Peri-Prosthetic Fracture Following Total Knee Arthroplasty: The Insufficiency Fracture. *J. Arthroplast.* **2015**, *30*, 1054–1057. [CrossRef] [PubMed]
24. Moldovan, F.; Gligor, A.; Bataga, T. Structured Integration and Alignment Algorithm: A Tool for Personalized Surgical Treatment of Tibial Plateau Fractures. *J. Pers. Med.* **2021**, *11*, 190. [CrossRef]

Disclaimer/Publisher's Note: The statements, opinions and data contained in all publications are solely those of the individual author(s) and contributor(s) and not of MDPI and/or the editor(s). MDPI and/or the editor(s) disclaim responsibility for any injury to people or property resulting from any ideas, methods, instructions or products referred to in the content.

Review

Detection of Prosthetic Loosening in Hip and Knee Arthroplasty Using Machine Learning: A Systematic Review and Meta-Analysis

Man-Soo Kim, Jae-Jung Kim, Ki-Ho Kang, Jeong-Han Lee and Yong In *

Department of Orthopaedic Surgery, Seoul St. Mary's Hospital, College of Medicine, The Catholic University of Korea, 222, Banpo-daero, Seocho-gu, Seoul 06591, Republic of Korea
* Correspondence: iy1000@catholic.ac.kr; Tel.: +82-2-2258-2838

Abstract: *Background*: prosthetic loosening after hip and knee arthroplasty is one of the most common causes of joint arthroplasty failure and revision surgery. Diagnosis of prosthetic loosening is a difficult problem and, in many cases, loosening is not clearly diagnosed until accurately confirmed during surgery. The purpose of this study is to conduct a systematic review and meta-analysis to demonstrate the analysis and performance of machine learning in diagnosing prosthetic loosening after total hip arthroplasty (THA) and total knee arthroplasty (TKA). *Materials and Methods*: three comprehensive databases, including MEDLINE, EMBASE, and the Cochrane Library, were searched for studies that evaluated the detection accuracy of loosening around arthroplasty implants using machine learning. Data extraction, risk of bias assessment, and meta-analysis were performed. *Results*: five studies were included in the meta-analysis. All studies were retrospective studies. In total, data from 2013 patients with 3236 images were assessed; these data involved 2442 cases (75.5%) with THAs and 794 cases (24.5%) with TKAs. The most common and best-performing machine learning algorithm was DenseNet. In one study, a novel stacking approach using a random forest showed similar performance to DenseNet. The pooled sensitivity across studies was 0.92 (95% CI 0.84–0.97), the pooled specificity was 0.95 (95% CI 0.93–0.96), and the pooled diagnostic odds ratio was 194.09 (95% CI 61.60–611.57). The I2 statistics for sensitivity and specificity were 96% and 62%, respectively, showing that there was significant heterogeneity. The summary receiver operating characteristics curve indicated the sensitivity and specificity, as did the prediction regions, with an AUC of 0.9853. *Conclusions*: the performance of machine learning using plain radiography showed promising results with good accuracy, sensitivity, and specificity in the detection of loosening around THAs and TKAs. Machine learning can be incorporated into prosthetic loosening screening programs.

Keywords: loosening; arthroplasty; machine learning; transfer learning; review; prosthesis

1. Introduction

Total hip arthroplasty (THA) and total knee arthroplasty (TKA) are effective procedures that significantly improve quality of life and functional recovery in orthopedic surgery [1–8]. THA and TKA show sufficient survival rates [9,10], with 95% survivorship over 15 years in the case of TKA [10] and over 90% survivorship over 10 years in the case of THA, with continuous technological advancement [9]. Due to these successful results, the use of THAs and TKAs is continuously increasing. However, the ratio of revision THA and TKA is also expected to continue increasing because of continuous increases in total joint arthroplasty surgery and average life expectancy [11–15]. In the United States, revision TKA is expected to increase by 601% between 2005 and 2030; revision THA is expected to increase by 137% [13].

As revision THAs and TKAs increase, the associated economic burden is expected to gradually increase [16,17]. Therefore, understanding the causes and risk factors of revision THA and TKA to improve the durability of revision surgery is increasingly important [16,17]. The most common causes of revision TKA are infection and aseptic loosening; the rate of aseptic loosening has increased recently [16–19]. In revision THA, infection and aseptic loosening also account for the largest proportion of revision surgeries [20–22]. As the diagnosis of prosthetic loosening is still challenging, various imaging tools are used for diagnosis, including plain radiographs, scintigraphy, arthrograms, fluorodeoxyglucose-positron emission tomography (FDG-PET) scans, and MRI [23,24]. However, except for plain radiography, these tools are invasive and expensive; therefore, plain radiography is the most cost effective method [25]. In addition, there is diversity in terms of concordance rates among the expert physicians assessing the cases [26,27].

Due to recent developments, machine learning has begun to be used widely in orthopedic surgery [28,29]. In particular, machine learning shows excellent performance in the field of diagnosis through images [28,29]. In fact, various techniques using machine learning are being used to diagnose lung disease [30] and breast cancer using radiographs [31]; these techniques are actually used as auxiliary diagnostic devices to assist doctors in diagnosis in hospitals [30,31]. Studies using machine learning to detect prosthetic loosening after arthroplasty surgery in orthopedic surgery are also continuously increasing in number [32–36]. Therefore, the purpose of this study is to conduct a systematic review and meta-analysis to demonstrate the analysis and performance of machine learning in diagnosing prosthetic loosening after total hip arthroplasty (THA) and total knee arthroplasty (TKA). We hypothesized that the model using machine learning is useful and can be incorporated into screening programs in diagnosing prosthetic loosening of THAs and TKAs.

2. Materials and Methods

This study was performed following the guidelines of the Preferred Reporting Items for Systematic Reviews and Meta-Analysis (PRISMA) statement (S1 PRISMA Checklist) [37].

2.1. Data and Literature Sources

The study design was performed according to the Cochrane Review Methods. Multiple comprehensive databases, including MEDLINE, EMBASE, and the Cochrane Library, were searched in September 2022 for studies in English that detected the loosening of implants using machine learning (S1 Search Strategy). There were no restrictions on publication year. Search terms included mesh "Arthroplasty" and key words "replacement" "joint replacement" "alloarthroplasty", mesh "machine learning" and key words "transfer learning", "artificial intelligence", "deep learning", "neural network", "decision trees", and mesh "osteolysis" and key words "bone loss", "bone resorption", "loosening", "failure". After the initial electronic search, manual searches of the reference lists and the bibliographies of identified articles, including relevant reviews and meta-analyses, were conducted to identify trials that the electronic search may have missed. Identified articles were individually assessed for inclusion.

2.2. Study Selection

Two reviewers independently determined study inclusion according to the pre-defined selection criteria. Titles and abstracts were screened for relevance. In cases of uncertainty, the full article was evaluated to determine eligibility. Discrepancies were resolved through discussion. Studies included met these criteria: (1) used a machine learning algorithm as an index for the diagnosis of prosthetic loosening or osteolysis; and (2) the integrated data (true positive, false negative, false positive, and true negative) were provided directly or indirectly. The exclusion criteria included: (1) animal studies; (2) studies with incomplete data; and (3) reviews, comments, letters, and research for which full text cannot be obtained.

2.3. Data Extraction

Two reviewers independently extracted data from each study using a standardized data extraction form. Disagreements were resolved by discussion; those unresolved through discussion were reviewed by a third reviewer. The following variables were included: first author, publication year, country, study type, index test, eligibility criteria, reference standard, type of arthroplasty, sample size, machine learning algorithm, preprocessing, augmentation, model structure, the calculated area under the curve (AUC), accuracy, sensitivity, and specificity. We attempted to contact the study authors for supplementary information when there were insufficient or missing data in the articles. The third senior investigator was consulted to resolve any disagreement during data extraction.

The quality of all literature was evaluated by two researchers using the Quality Assessment of Diagnostic Accuracy Studies (QUADAS-2) [38], which is composed of patient selection, index test, reference standard, and flow and timing. If there is any disagreement in this process, the third author was responsible for making the decision.

2.4. Statistical Analyses

All extracted data analyses and picture production were performed with the R language using R studio. A bivariate random effect model was selected to analyze the true positive, false negative, false positive, and true negative values of 2×2 tables recorded in the sheet and test the heterogeneity. The sensitivity, specificity, positive likelihood ratio (PLR), negative likelihood ratio (NLR), diagnostic score, and diagnostic odds ratio (DOR) were calculated after integration. In addition, by drawing the summary receiver operating characteristics (SROC) through the Midas command, AUC discriminated the diagnostic ability of machine learning [39].

Heterogeneity was determined using the I2 statistic, with values of 25%, 50%, and 75% considered as indicating low, moderate and high heterogeneity, respectively. Due to the high levels of heterogeneity, a random-effects model was used to combine available data by meta-analysis. Random-effect DerSimonian and Laird models were used to calculate weighted averages of the transformed values, which were then back-transformed to produce final pooled rates [40]. Pre-planned sub-groups were designed according to the type of arthroplasty. Publication bias determination was usually only performed when the number of included articles was 10 or more; however, we used a funnel plot to evaluate publication bias.

3. Results

3.1. Identification of Studies

A study-flow diagram shows the process for study identification, inclusion, and exclusion (Figure 1). An initial electronic search yielded 1306 studies. Three additional publications were obtained through manual searching. In total, 82 potentially eligible studies were assessed for inclusion after screening titles and abstracts. After we reviewed the full texts, an additional 77 studies were excluded. Finally, five studies were included in the meta-analysis.

3.2. Study Characteristics and Quality of Included Studies

The study characteristics are summarized in Table 1. All studies were published from 2019 to 2022. All studies were retrospective studies. In total, 2013 patients with 3236 images were assessed, involving 2442 cases (75.5%) with THAs and 794 cases (24.5%) with TKAs. Among THAs, loosening occurred in 1136 cases (46.5%). Loosening occurred in 343 TKA cases (43.2%). Three studies included only THAs, one study included only TKAs, and one study included both THAs and TKAs. All five studies of these studies were retrospective studies and used the transfer learning method. The most common and best-performing machine learning algorithm was DenseNet; in one study, a novel stacking approach using a random forest showed similar performance to DenseNet. The characteristics of the included studies are summarized in Tables 1 and 2.

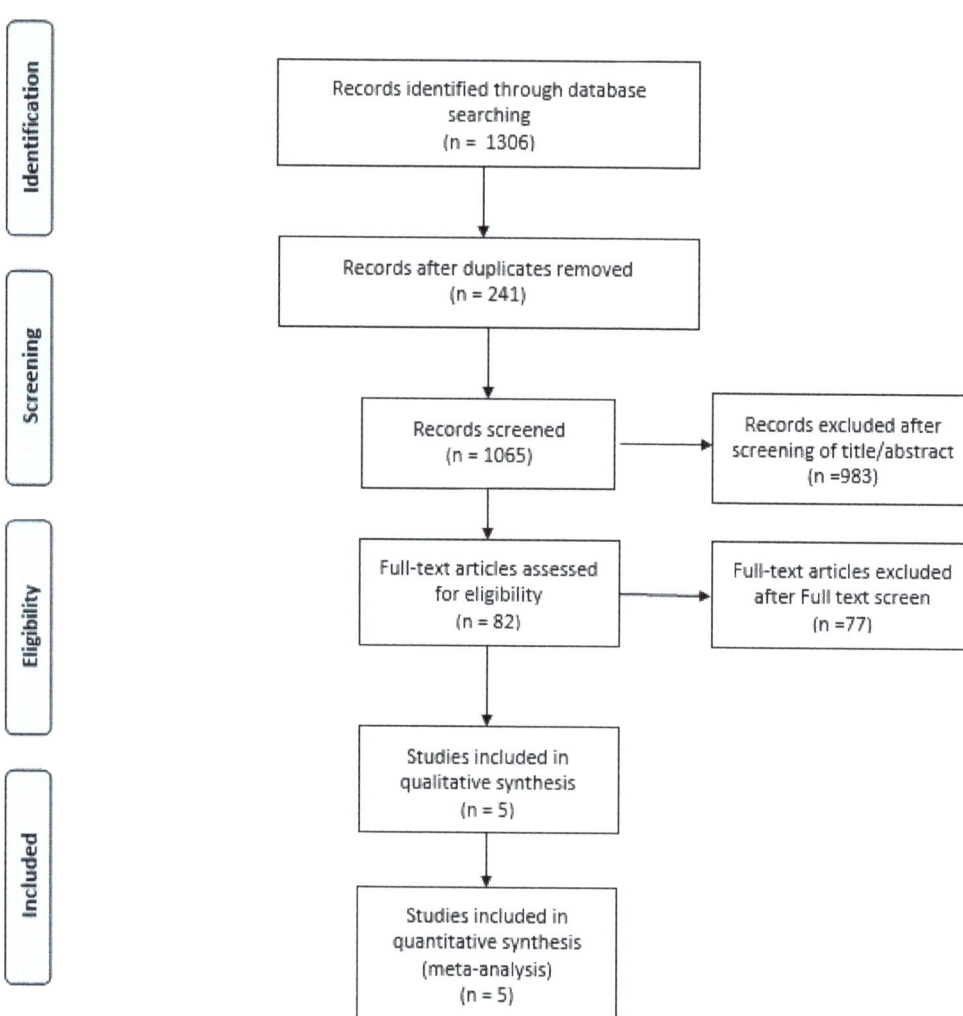

Figure 1. PRISMA flow diagram for systematic review.

3.3. Descriptive Statistics

The study with the highest accuracy was performed by Loppini et al. [34] in 2022 (96.8%), while the study carried out by Borjali et al. [32] in 2019 had the lowest accuracy (77.0%). The specificity and sensitivity values of each machine learning model are presented in Figure 2. Sensitivity values for machine learning models in this study ranged between 0.71 (95% CI: 0.60–0.80) and 0.97 (95% CI: 0.95–0.98) in THA. The pooled sensitivity across studies was 0.93 (95% CI: 0.81–0.98) in THA. Sensitivity values for machine learning models ranged between 0.70 (95% CI: 0.61–0.78) and 0.96 (95% CI: 0.93–0.98) in TKA. The pooled sensitivity across studies was 0.88 (95% CI: 0.81–0.98) in TKA. Specificity values for machine learning models in this study ranged between 0.95 (95% CI: 0.91–0.97) and 0.97 (95% CI: 0.95–0.98) in THA. The pooled sensitivity across studies was 0.96 (95% CI: 0.95–0.97) in THA. Specificity values for machine learning models ranged between 0.91 (95% CI: 0.87–0.94) and 0.95 (95% CI: 0.91–0.97) in TKA. The pooled specificity across studies was 0.93 (95% CI: 0.90–0.95) in TKA. The pooled sensitivity across studies was 0.92 (95% CI: 0.84–0.97), the pooled specificity was 0.95 (95% CI: 0.93–0.96) (Figure 2).

Table 1. Summary of general study characteristics.

Study	Country	Design	Pre-Processing	Index Test	Eligibility Criteria	Reference Standard	Arthroplasty Type	Failure Detection	Number of Loosening vs. Non-Loosening	Type of Validation	Data Source
Borjali et al., 2019 [32]	USA	Retrospective study		X-ray	Yes	Operation record	THA	Loosening	17 THAs vs. 23 THAs	Five-fold cross validation	Single center
Shah et al., 2020 [36]	USA	Retrospective study		X-ray Demographic & comorbidity data	Yes	Operation record	THA TKA	Loosening	137 TKAs, 85 THAs vs. 217 TKAs, 258 THAs	Training 60% Validation 20% Test 20%	Single center from 2012–2018
Loppini et al., 2022 [34]	Italy	Retrospective study		X-ray	Yes	Operation record	THA	Loosening malposition wear infection	420 failed THA vs. 210 normal THA 922 failed images vs. 931 non-failed images	Training 63% Validation 27% Test 10%	Single center from 2009–2019
Lau et al., 2022 [33]	Hong Kong	Retrospective study		X-ray Clinical information	Yes	Operation record	TKA	Loosening	206 TKAs vs. 234 TKAs	Test 75% (345 images) Validation 25% (95 images)	Single center
Rahman et al., 2022 [35]	Qatar	Retrospective study		X-ray	Yes	Research results	THA	Loosening	112 THAs vs. 94 THAs	Five-fold cross validation Training 70% Validation 10% Test 20%	Images from published article

THA: total hip arthroplasty; TKA: total knee arthroplasty.

Table 2. Artificial intelligence-based prediction model characteristics described in included studies.

Study	AI Method	Pre-Processing	Augmentations	Model Structure	AUC	Accuracy	Sensitivity	Specificity	AI vs. Expert Doctor
Borjali et al., 2019 [32]	DL	Transfer learning	Reorientation, magnification	DenseNet Re-trained CNN Pre-trained CNN	Pre-trained 0.950 Re-trained 0.800	Pre-trained 0.950	Pre-trained 0.940	Pre-trained 0.960	Orthopaedic surgeon: accuracy 0.770 sensitivity 0.530 specificity 0.960

Table 2. Cont.

Study	AI Method	Pre-Processing	Augmentations	Model Structure	AUC	Accuracy	Sensitivity	Specificity	AI vs. Expert Doctor
Shah et al., 2020 [36]	DL	Resize segmentation Transfer learning	None	ResNet AlexNet Inception DenseNet		Resnet 0.882 Alexnet 0.901 Inception 0.922 DenseNet 0.953 Best-model overall 0.883 TKA 0.858 THA 0.901	Best model overall 0.702 TKA 0.698 THA 0.703	Best model overall 0.956 TKA 0.952 THA 0.946	None
Loppini et al., 2022 [34]	DL	Resize transfer learning	Transformation Horizontal flip Rotation Zoom	DenseNet	0.993	Training 0.990 Validation 0.975 Test 0.968	0.968	0.968	None
Lau et al., 2022 [33]	DL	Transfer learning	None	Xception	Pre-trained test 0.935	0.963	0.961	0.909	Two senior orthopaedic specialists with 15–20 years' experience; accuracy 0.921
Rahman et al., 2022 [35]	DL	Cropping resize normalization transfer-learning	Rotation Scaling translation	Resnet18 Resnet50 Resnet101 InceptionV3 DenseNet161 DenseNet201 Mobilenetv2 Googlenet Staking approach	DenseNet201 Staking approach using Random forest	DenseNet 0.947 Random forest 0.961	DenseNet 0.9467 Random forest 0.964	DenseNet 0.945 Random forest 0.964	None

AI: artificial intelligence, AUC: area under the curve, DL: deep learning, CNN: convolutional neural networks, THA: total hip arthroplasty, TKA: total knee arthroplasty.

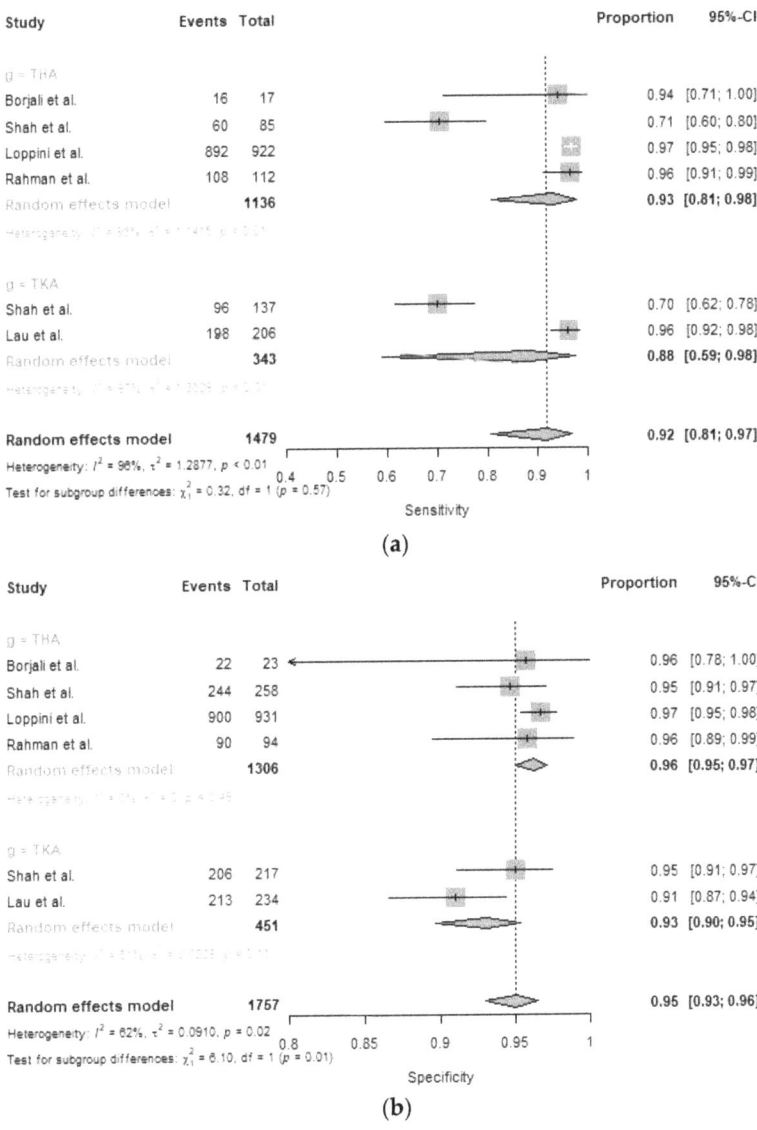

Figure 2. Forest plots for sensitivity (**a**) and specificity (**b**). GLMM: generalized linear mixed model, CI: confidence interval, THA: total hip arthroplasty, TKA: total knee arthroplasty [32–36].

The pooled positive LR was 16.63 (95% CI: 10.55–26.20), while the pooled negative LR was 0.09 (95% CI: 0.03–0.27). The DOR values in this study ranged between 41.83 (95% CI: 20.51–85.30) and 863.23 (95% CI: 518.14–1438.14) in THA. The pooled DOR across studies was 282.93 (95% CI: 59.31–1349.64) in THA. The DOR values for machine learning models ranged between 43.85 (95% CI: 21.60–89.03) and 251.04 (95% CI: 108.70–579.74) in TKA. The pooled DOR across studies was 103.37 (95% CI: 18.70–571.35) in TKA. The pooled DOR was 194.09 (95% CI: 61.60–611.57) (Figure 3). The I2 statistics for sensitivity and specificity were 96.0% and 62.0%, showing that there was significant heterogeneity. The SROC curve indicated the sensitivity and specificity, as well as the prediction regions, with an AUC of 0.9853 (Figure 4).

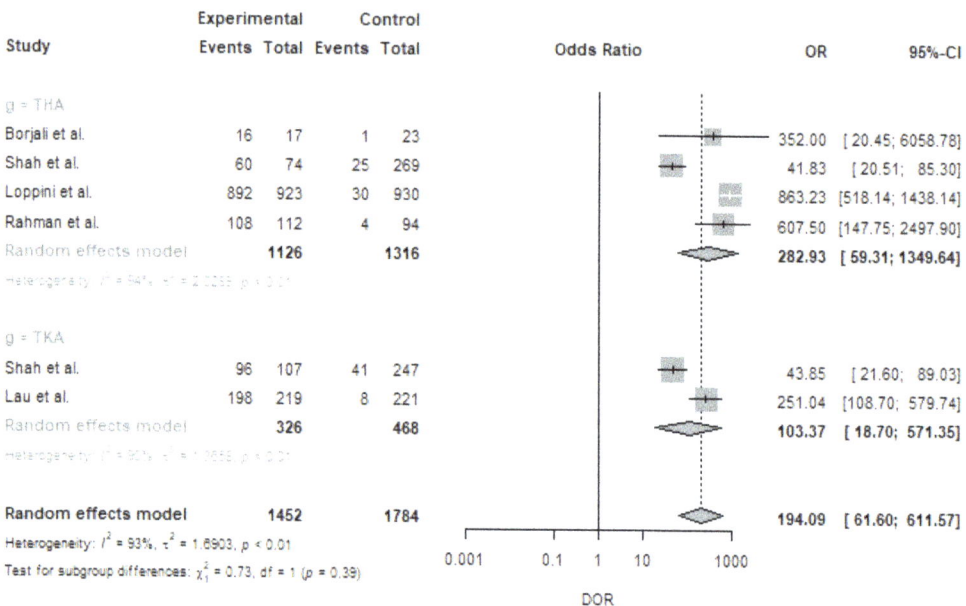

Figure 3. Forest plots diagnostic odds ratio. IV: interval variance; CI: confidence interval, THA: total hip arthroplasty; TKA: total knee arthroplasty; DOR: diagnostic odds ratio [32–36].

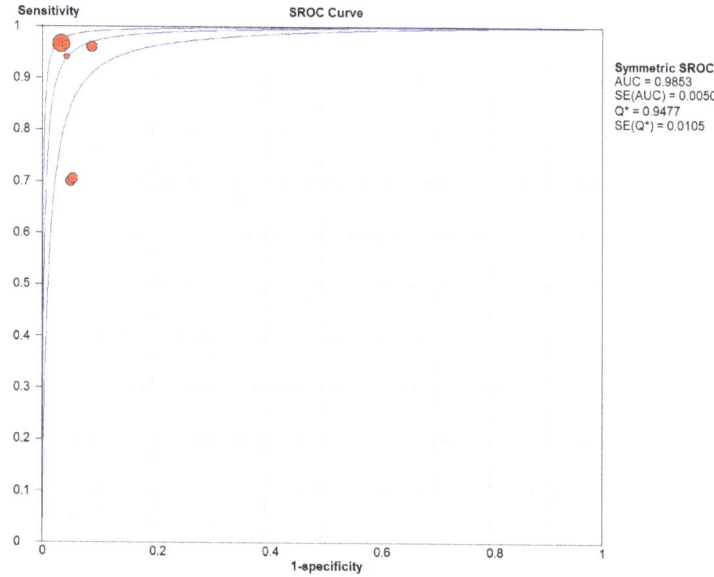

Figure 4. Summary receiver operating characteristics (sROC) curve, the calculated area under the curve (AUC) = 0.985. SROC: summary receiver operating characteristics; SE: standard error; AUC: Area under the curve.

3.4. Quality Assessment and Publication Biases

The quality assessment results of five studies performed using the QUADAS-2 scale are indicated in Figure 2. The figure shows that the overall quality of the included studies was good; all studies were "unclear" or "low risk" with no study including "high risks".

Although the sample size of the included literature was relatively small, the quality of the research was persuasive. (Figure 5) In addition, the funnel plot was asymmetrical, indicating the tendency of publication bias in this meta-analysis. (Figure 6).

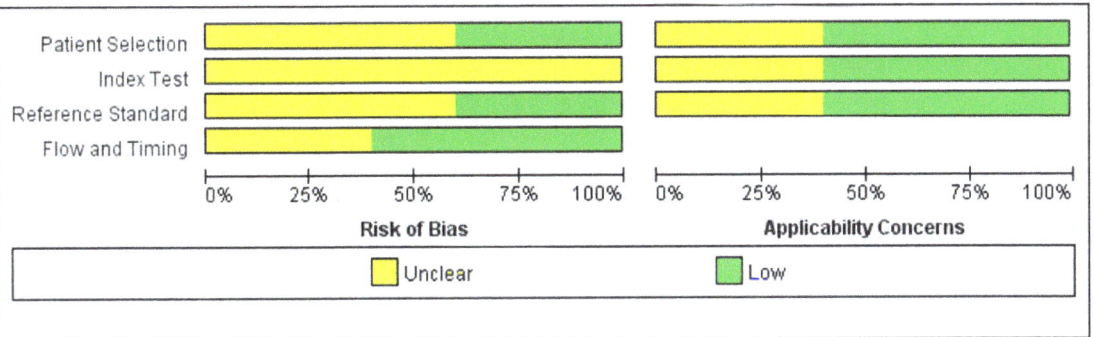

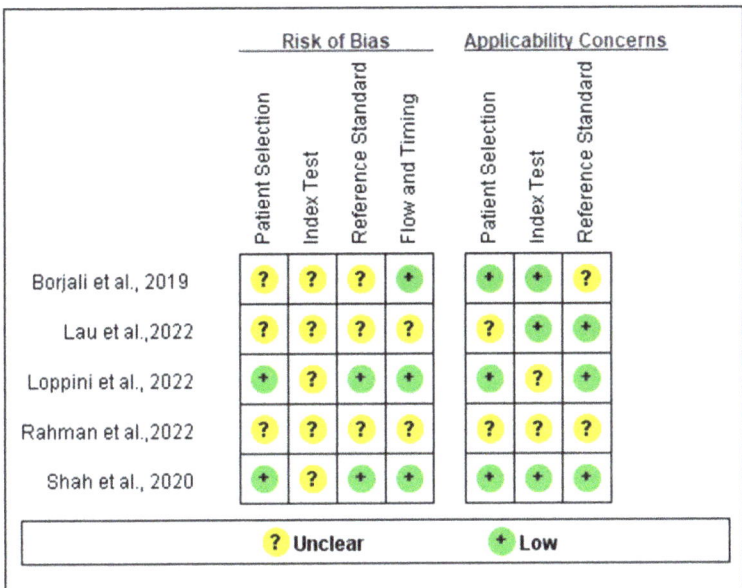

Figure 5. Methodological assessment by QUADAS-2 [32–36].

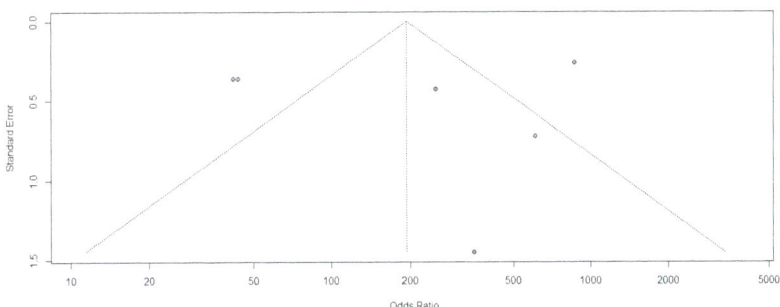

Figure 6. Funnel plot.

4. Discussion

As a result of this systematic review, the diagnostic accuracy of the simple radiographic image-based artificial intelligence (AI) model for discriminating relaxation around implants after THA and TKA was over 0.9 in combined sensitivity, specificity, and AUC. As the machine learning for this purpose is in its immature stage, sufficient research results have not been secured. AI model studies using this imaging have not provided clear conclusions about clinical implementation and widespread use.

In the field of orthopedic surgery, THA and TKA are well known as the most effective and satisfactory surgical treatments [7,8]. In addition, long-term follow-up results have shown excellent survival rates [9,10]. The development of materials and technologies related to THA and TKA has contributed to the increase in the number of THA and TKA worldwide [41,42]. However, artificial joints inevitably have the risk of revision operation; thus, the most common cause of revision operation is loosening due to osteolysis [16,17]. Therefore, there has been a continuous demand for the early detection of prosthetic loosening around the implant. However, the accuracy of detection of prosthetic loosening in practice has not been as high as expected [43,44]. Temmerman et al. [44] analyzed the accuracy using radiography to diagnose cementless femoral component loosening; the sensitivity was 50% and the specificity was 89.5%. Cheung et al. [43] reported sensitivity and specificity of 83% and 82%, respectively. In addition to this, the inter-observer agreement between observers evaluating prosthetic loosening was also surprisingly poor [44]. Therefore, there has been a growing interest in tools that can have constant and high sensitivity, specificity, and accuracy in evaluating prosthetic loosening in THA and TKA [32,33]. Machine learning (ML) is on the rise as an alternative [32,33].

ML is a branch of AI that uses data to learn and improve tasks using various systems and algorithms [45,46]. Deep learning (DL) is a type of ML that allows complex tasks to be learned using large amounts of training information [47]. DL uses artificial neural networks (ANNs) made up of neurons arranged in a hierarchical structure. Convolutional neural networks (CNNs) are a subtype of DL that are effective and excellent at image processing. [48] A CNN uses a complex set of layers through which data is passed with a filter that can be trained to create a final or output layer [48]. The studies investigated in this review all have a common feature of using one of the various CNN algorithms [32–36]. This study is significant in its being the first to review studies that differentiate loosening around artificial joints using a CNN model. That model demonstrates excellent ability for image discrimination through plain radiographic images in the field of orthopedics [32–36].

Studies using AI in relation to arthroplasty in orthopedic surgery are gradually increasing in number [28,29]. These studies involve prediction of arthroplasty component size [49], length of stay and costs before primary arthroplasty [50], transfusion after arthroplasty [51], patient dissatisfaction following primary arthroplasty [52], and automated detection and classification of arthroplasty implant from knee radiograph [53]. In studies related to images, CNN models are generally most common; all the studies in this review detected prosthetic loosening using widely used CNN models learned through Imagenet. A further two studies used DenseNet [32,34] and one study used Exception [33]. The other two studies analyzed various CNN models and selected the model with the highest accuracy, which was DenseNet [35,36]. One study had limitations in accuracy with only images [36] while increasing the accuracy to more than 90% by providing additional patient data [36]. The remaining studies achieved satisfactory accuracy without additional patient data [32–35]. CNN models have been and are continuing to be developed. Additional research using the new CNN models will be needed in the future.

All five studies showed satisfactory results in terms of accuracy, sensitivity and specificity [32–36]. Accuracy, sensitivity, and specificity all showed high values of 0.9 or more [32–36]. The accuracy shown using simple plain radiographs, rather than more advanced imaging, shows similar or superior results compared to studies conducted only with imaging in other medical fields [28]. In a study by Adams et al., deep CNN was used for diagnosing femur neck fractures. The studies in this review showed excellent results with accuracy, specificity, and sensitivity of about 0.9 [54]. In a study by Urakawa et al., hip intertrochanteric fracture was diagnosed using a deep CNN model; the results of that study also showed a similar 95% accuracy [55]. In fact, two studies in this review compared diagnosis rates with orthopedic surgeons and showed higher accuracy than orthopedic surgeons [32,33]. Lau et al. reported that the accuracy of the machine learning model was 96.3%, while the average of the two orthopedic surgeons was 92% [33]. Borjali et al. demonstrated that the orthopedic surgeons' accuracy were 77%, which was lower than that of the machine learning model [32]. In particular, the specificity was similar; however, the sensitivity was poor in that study, indicating that loosening was not well differentiated [32].

Even when examining THA and TKA separately by sub-group analysis, the machine learning model showed high accuracy, sensitivity, and specificity in discriminating loosening around THAs and TKAs [32–36]. In the case of THA, four studies were included and showed excellent results, with accuracy, sensitivity, and specificity above 90% [32,34–36]. In the case of TKA, there are limitations as only data from two studies were included; however, this result also showed over 90% accuracy, sensitivity, and specificity [33,36]. Since the number of TKA samples was too small to perform sub-group analysis according to the type of joint arthroplasty, clear results require additional future TKA studies [33,36].

In the results of the meta-analysis, the heterogeneity among studies was particularly high at over 90% in sensitivity and, except in some cases, high in specificity [32–36]. Although difficulty arises in clearly explaining such high heterogeneity, potential reasons for heterogeneity include the diversity of CNN models used in this study, differences in patients' demographic data, differences in processes in creating CNN models, and the number of images used in the study [32–36]. This can be inferred from differences in quality. In this study, a random effect model was used due to high heterogeneity; this model was high in all values, including sensitivity and specificity.

There were some limitations in our research. Firstly, this study only included five articles; thus, the sample size was relatively small with only 1000 cases in the loosening group and 1500 cases in the non-loosening group [32–36]. Secondly, though four of the five studies contained data collected by the researchers at the hospital [32–34,36], one study contained image data collected from published papers available on the Internet [35]. Therefore, future research should focus on using high-quality data collected from hospitals or research centers in a broader population of patients with periprosthetic osteolysis or loosening with various clinical symptoms. Furthermore, future studies should explicitly describe the role of machine learning tools being developed as screening, diagnostic, or prognostic tools. A third limitation is that publication bias may exist. One possible cause is that there may be unpublished studies using underperforming models. In addition, the overall model of this study was highly heterogeneous and included a significant number of studies that could contribute to both the occurrence of publication bias and the high statistical power of the asymmetric test. Future meta-analyses should ensure conduct that includes pre-print articles that can reduce publication bias. Fourthly, the language restrictions in the included studies may have increased the risk of bias in the study results. Fifthly, there are many different machine learning models available with different variants and parameters. However, we were unable to compare each variant of the model due to the insufficient sample size of individual models. Lastly, most studies developed new models for TKA loosening detection but did not perform external validation using other data sources. One common concern is that the local data sets used for validation may not be representative of the target population on a global scale. In future studies, external validation requires improvement.

This meta-analysis is of substantial significance in that this is the first method to quantitatively combine and interpret data examining prosthetic loosening from different studies, potentially providing key clues for clinical application and further research. This study provided an opportunity to examine the accuracy of the method using ML in the detection of prosthetic loosening in THA and TKA. In addition, it was confirmed that the model using ML could be used as an auxiliary aid device in detecting prosthetic loosening in clinical practice. However, additional large-scale analysis studies and more research would be needed.

5. Conclusions

The performance of machine learning on plain radiographs showed promising results with good accuracy, sensitivity, and specificity in the detection of loosening around THAs and TKAs. Machine learning can be incorporated into prosthetic loosening screening programs. However, more research results are needed to clearly judge the ability of the machine learning model to discriminate loosening around the joint arthroplasty.

Author Contributions: Y.I. had full access to all the data in the study and takes responsibility for the integrity of the data and the accuracy of the data analysis. Concept and design: M.-S.K. and Y.I.; Acquisition, analysis, or interpretation of data: M.-S.K., J.-J.K., K.-H.K. and J.-H.L.; Drafting of the manuscript: M.-S.K. and Y.I.; Critical revision of the manuscript for important intellectual content: All authors; Administrative, technical, or material support: M.-S.K., J.-J.K., K.-H.K. and J.-H.L.; Supervision: Y.I. All authors have read and agreed to the published version of the manuscript.

Funding: This research was supported by Basic Science Research Program through the National Research Foundation of Korea (NRF) and funded by the Ministry of Education (2021R1I1A1A01059558).

Institutional Review Board Statement: Not applicable.

Informed Consent Statement: Not applicable.

Data Availability Statement: The data presented in this study are available in the main article.

Conflicts of Interest: The authors declare no conflict of interest.

References

1. Carr, A.J.; Robertsson, O.; Graves, S.; Price, A.J.; Arden, N.K.; Judge, A.; Beard, D.J. Knee replacement. *Lancet* **2012**, *379*, 1331–1340.
2. Jang, S.; Shin, W.C.; Song, M.K.; Han, H.S.; Lee, M.C.; Ro, D.H. Which orally administered antithrombotic agent is most effective for preventing venous thromboembolism after total knee arthroplasty? A propensity score-matching analysis. *Knee Surg. Relat. Res.* **2021**, *33*, 10.
3. Kulshrestha, V.; Sood, M.; Kumar, S.; Sood, N.; Kumar, P.; Padhi, P.P. Does Risk Mitigation Reduce 90-Day Complications in Patients Undergoing Total Knee Arthroplasty?: A Cohort Study. *Clin. Orthop. Surg.* **2022**, *14*, 56–68.
4. Lee, J.K.; Lee, K.B.; Kim, J.I.; Park, G.T.; Cho, Y.C. Risk factors for deep vein thrombosis even using low-molecular-weight heparin after total knee arthroplasty. *Knee Surg. Relat. Res.* **2021**, *33*, 29.
5. Lee, J.M.; Ha, C.; Jung, K.; Choi, W. Clinical Results after Design Modification of Lospa Total Knee Arthroplasty System: Comparison between Posterior-Stabilized (PS) and PS Plus Types. *Clin. Orthop. Surg.* **2022**, *14*, 236–243.
6. Patrick, N.J.; Man, L.L.C.; Wai-Wang, C.; Tim-Yun, O.M.; Wing, C.K.; Hing, C.K.; Yin, C.K.; Ki-Wai, H.K. No difference in long-term functional outcomes or survivorship after total knee arthroplasty with or without computer navigation: A 17-year survivorship analysis. *Knee Surg. Relat. Res.* **2021**, *33*, 30. [CrossRef]
7. Song, S.J.; Kim, K.I.; Suh, D.U.; Park, C.H. Comparison of Patellofemoral-Specific Clinical and Radiographic Results after Total Knee Arthroplasty Using a Patellofemoral Design-Modified Prosthesis and Its Predecessor. *Clin. Orthop. Surg.* **2021**, *13*, 175–184. [CrossRef]
8. Takamura, D.; Iwata, K.; Sueyoshi, T.; Yasuda, T.; Moriyama, H. Relationship between early physical activity after total knee arthroplasty and postoperative physical function: Are these related? *Knee Surg. Relat. Res.* **2021**, *33*, 35. [CrossRef]
9. Clohisy, J.C.; Calvert, G.; Tull, F.; McDonald, D.; Maloney, W.J. Reasons for revision hip surgery: A retrospective review. *Clin. Orthop. Relat. Res.* **2004**, *429*, 188–192. [CrossRef]
10. Ranawat, C.S.; Flynn, W.F., Jr.; Deshmukh, R.G. Impact of modern technique on long-term results of total condylar knee arthroplasty. *Clin. Orthop. Relat. Res.* **1994**, *309*, 131–135.
11. Bozic, K.J.; Kurtz, S.M.; Lau, E.; Ong, K.; Chiu, V.; Vail, T.P.; Rubash, H.E.; Berry, D.J. The epidemiology of revision total knee arthroplasty in the United States. *Clin. Orthop. Relat. Res.* **2010**, *468*, 45–51. [CrossRef]
12. Cram, P.; Lu, X.; Kates, S.L.; Singh, J.A.; Li, Y.; Wolf, B.R. Total knee arthroplasty volume, utilization, and outcomes among Medicare beneficiaries, 1991–2010. *JAMA* **2012**, *308*, 1227–1236. [CrossRef]
13. Kurtz, S.; Ong, K.; Lau, E.; Mowat, F.; Halpern, M. Projections of primary and revision hip and knee arthroplasty in the United States from 2005 to 2030. *J. Bone Joint Surg. Am.* **2007**, *89*, 780–785. [CrossRef]
14. Malviya, A.; Abdul, N.; Khanduja, V. Outcomes Following Total Hip Arthroplasty: A Review of the Registry Data. *Indian J. Orthop.* **2017**, *51*, 405–413. [CrossRef]

15. Weber, M.; Renkawitz, T.; Voellner, F.; Craiovan, B.; Greimel, F.; Worlicek, M.; Grifka, J.; Benditz, A. Revision Surgery in Total Joint Replacement Is Cost-Intensive. *Biomed. Res. Int.* **2018**, *2018*, 8987104. [CrossRef]
16. Geary, M.B.; Macknet, D.M.; Ransone, M.P.; Odum, S.D.; Springer, B.D. Why Do Revision Total Knee Arthroplasties Fail? A Single-Center Review of 1632 Revision Total Knees Comparing Historic and Modern Cohorts. *J. Arthroplast.* **2020**, *35*, 2938–2943. [CrossRef]
17. Na, B.-R.; Kwak, W.-K.; Lee, N.-H.; Song, E.-K.; Seon, J.-K. Trend Shift in the Cause of Revision Total Knee Arthroplasty over 17 Years. *Clin. Orthop. Surg.* **2023**, *15*, 219–226. [CrossRef]
18. Bosco, F.; Cacciola, G.; Giustra, F.; Risitano, S.; Capella, M.; Vezza, D.; Barberis, L.; Cavaliere, P.; Massè, A.; Sabatini, L. Characterizing recurrent infections after one-stage revision for periprosthetic joint infection of the knee: A systematic review of the literature. *Eur. J. Orthop. Surg. Traumatol.* **2023**, *Online ahead of print*.
19. Giustra, F.; Bistolfi, A.; Bosco, F.; Fresia, N.; Sabatini, L.; Berchialla, P.; Sciannameo, V.; Massè, A. Highly cross-linked polyethylene versus conventional polyethylene in primary total knee arthroplasty: Comparable clinical and radiological results at a 10-year follow-up. *Knee Surg. Sports Traumatol. Arthrosc.* **2023**, *31*, 1082–1088. [CrossRef]
20. Kenney, C.; Dick, S.; Lea, J.; Liu, J.; Ebraheim, N.A. A systematic review of the causes of failure of Revision Total Hip Arthroplasty. *J. Orthop.* **2019**, *16*, 393–395. [CrossRef]
21. Mponponsuo, K.; Leal, J.; Puloski, S.; Chew, D.; Chavda, S.; Ismail, A.; Au, F.; Rennert-May, E. Economic Burden of Surgical Management of Prosthetic Joint Infections Following Hip and Knee Replacements in Alberta, Canada: An analysis and comparison of two major urban centers. *J. Hosp. Infect.* **2022**. [CrossRef]
22. Ng, M.K.; Kobryn, A.; Emara, A.K.; Krebs, V.E.; Mont, M.A.; Piuzzi, N.S. Decreasing trend of inpatient mortality rates of aseptic versus septic revision total hip arthroplasty: An analysis of 681,034 cases. *Hip. Int.* **2022**. [CrossRef] [PubMed]
23. French, T.H.; Russell, N.; Pillai, A. The diagnostic accuracy of radionuclide arthrography for prosthetic loosening in hip and knee arthroplasty. *Biomed. Res. Int.* **2013**, *2013*, 693436. [CrossRef] [PubMed]
24. Signore, A.; Sconfienza, L.M.; Borens, O.; Glaudemans, A.; Cassar-Pullicino, V.; Trampuz, A.; Winkler, H.; Gheysens, O.; Vanhoenacker, F.; Petrosillo, N.; et al. Consensus document for the diagnosis of prosthetic joint infections: A joint paper by the EANM, EBJIS, and ESR (with ESCMID endorsement). *Eur. J. Nucl. Med. Mol. Imaging* **2019**, *46*, 971–988. [CrossRef] [PubMed]
25. Barnsley, L.; Barnsley, L. Detection of aseptic loosening in total knee replacements: A systematic review and meta-analysis. *Skeletal. Radiol.* **2019**, *48*, 1565–1572. [CrossRef] [PubMed]
26. Khalily, C.; Whiteside, L.A. Predictive value of early radiographic findings in cementless total hip arthroplasty femoral components: An 8- to 12-year follow-up. *J. Arthroplast.* **1998**, *13*, 768–773. [CrossRef]
27. Smith, T.O.; Williams, T.H.; Samuel, A.; Ogonda, L.; Wimhurst, J.A. Reliability of the radiological assessments of radiolucency and loosening in total hip arthroplasty using PACS. *Hip. Int.* **2011**, *21*, 577–582. [CrossRef]
28. Jamshidi, A.; Pelletier, J.P.; Martel-Pelletier, J. Machine-learning-based patient-specific prediction models for knee osteoarthritis. *Nat. Rev. Rheumatol.* **2019**, *15*, 49–60.
29. Rodríguez-Merchán, E.C. The current role of the virtual elements of artificial intelligence in total knee arthroplasty. *EFORT Open Rev.* **2022**, *7*, 491–497.
30. Kuo, K.M.; Talley, P.C.; Chang, C.S. The accuracy of machine learning approaches using non-image data for the prediction of COVID-19: A meta-analysis. *Int. J. Med. Inform.* **2022**, *164*, 104791. [CrossRef]
31. Hanis, T.M.; Islam, M.A.; Musa, K.I. Diagnostic Accuracy of Machine Learning Models on Mammography in Breast Cancer Classification: A Meta-Analysis. *Diagnostics* **2022**, *12*, 1643. [CrossRef]
32. Borjali, A.; Chen, A.F.; Muratoglu, O.K.; Morid, M.A.; Varadarajan, K.M. Detecting mechanical loosening of total hip replacement implant from plain radiograph using deep convolutional neural network. *arXiv* **2019**, arXiv:1912.00943.
33. Lau, L.C.M.; Chui, E.C.S.; Man, G.C.W.; Xin, Y.; Ho, K.K.W.; Mak, K.K.K.; Ong, M.T.Y.; Law, S.W.; Cheung, W.H.; Yung, P.S.H. A novel image-based machine learning model with superior accuracy and predictability for knee arthroplasty loosening detection and clinical decision making. *J. Orthop. Translat.* **2022**, *36*, 177–183. [PubMed]
34. Loppini, M.; Gambaro, F.M.; Chiappetta, K.; Grappiolo, G.; Bianchi, A.M.; Corino, V.D.A. Automatic Identification of Failure in Hip Replacement: An Artificial Intelligence Approach. *Bioengineering* **2022**, *9*, 288. [CrossRef]
35. Rahman, T.; Khandakar, A.; Islam, K.R.; Soliman, M.M.; Islam, M.T.; Elsayed, A.; Qiblawey, Y.; Mahmud, S.; Rahman, A.; Musharavati, F. HipXNet: Deep Learning Approaches to Detect Aseptic Loos-Ening of Hip Implants Using X-Ray Images. *IEEE Access* **2022**, *10*, 53359–53373.
36. Shah, R.F.; Bini, S.A.; Martinez, A.M.; Pedoia, V.; Vail, T.P. Incremental inputs improve the automated detection of implant loosening using machine-learning algorithms. *Bone Joint J.* **2020**, *102-b*, 101–106. [CrossRef]
37. Liberati, A.; Altman, D.G.; Tetzlaff, J.; Mulrow, C.; Gøtzsche, P.C.; Ioannidis, J.P.; Clarke, M.; Devereaux, P.J.; Kleijnen, J.; Moher, D. The PRISMA statement for reporting systematic reviews and meta-analyses of studies that evaluate healthcare interventions: Explanation and elaboration. *BMJ* **2009**, *339*, b2700. [CrossRef]
38. Whiting, P.F.; Rutjes, A.W.; Westwood, M.E.; Mallett, S.; Deeks, J.J.; Reitsma, J.B.; Leeflang, M.M.; Sterne, J.A.; Bossuyt, P.M. QUADAS-2: A revised tool for the quality assessment of diagnostic accuracy studies. *Ann. Intern. Med.* **2011**, *155*, 529–536. [CrossRef]

39. Jaeschke, R.; Guyatt, G.H.; Sackett, D.L. Users' guides to the medical literature. III. How to use an article about a diagnostic test. B. What are the results and will they help me in caring for my patients? The Evidence-Based Medicine Working Group. *JAMA* **1994**, *271*, 703–707. [CrossRef]
40. Reitsma, J.B.; Glas, A.S.; Rutjes, A.W.; Scholten, R.J.; Bossuyt, P.M.; Zwinderman, A.H. Bivariate analysis of sensitivity and specificity produces informative summary measures in diagnostic reviews. *J. Clin. Epidemiol.* **2005**, *58*, 982–990.
41. Gupta, P.; Czerwonka, N.; Desai, S.S.; deMeireles, A.J.; Trofa, D.P.; Neuwirth, A.L. The current utilization of the patient-reported outcome measurement information system (PROMIS) in isolated or combined total knee arthroplasty populations. *Knee Surg. Relat. Res.* **2023**, *35*, 3.
42. Wong, S.Y.W.; Ler, F.L.S.; Sultana, R.; Bin Abd Razak, H.R. What is the best prophylaxis against venous thromboembolism in Asians following total knee arthroplasty? A systematic review and network meta-analysis. *Knee Surg. Relat. Res.* **2022**, *34*, 37. [PubMed]
43. Chang, C.Y.; Huang, A.J.; Palmer, W.E. Radiographic evaluation of hip implants. *Semin Musculoskelet. Radiol.* **2015**, *19*, 12–20. [PubMed]
44. Temmerman, O.P.; Raijmakers, P.G.; Berkhof, J.; David, E.F.; Pijpers, R.; Molenaar, M.A.; Hoekstra, O.S.; Teule, G.J.; Heyligers, I.C. Diagnostic accuracy and interobserver variability of plain radiography, subtraction arthrography, nuclear arthrography, and bone scintigraphy in the assessment of aseptic femoral component loosening. *Arch. Orthop. Trauma Surg.* **2006**, *126*, 316–323. [PubMed]
45. Deo, R.C. Machine learning in medicine. *Circulation* **2015**, *132*, 1920–1930. [CrossRef]
46. Entezari, B.; Koucheki, R.; Abbas, A.; Toor, J.; Wolfstadt, J.I.; Ravi, B.; Whyne, C.; Lex, J.R. Improving Resource Utilization for Arthroplasty Care by Leveraging Machine Learning and Optimization: A Systematic Review. *Arthroplast. Today* **2023**, *20*, 101116.
47. Suzuki, K. Overview of deep learning in medical imaging. *Radiol. Phys. Technol.* **2017**, *10*, 257–273.
48. Soffer, S.; Ben-Cohen, A.; Shimon, O.; Amitai, M.M.; Greenspan, H.; Klang, E. Convolutional neural networks for radiologic images: A radiologist's guide. *Radiology* **2019**, *290*, 590–606. [CrossRef]
49. Kunze, K.N.; Polce, E.M.; Patel, A.; Courtney, P.M.; Levine, B.R. Validation and performance of a machine-learning derived prediction guide for total knee arthroplasty component sizing. *Arch. Orthop. Trauma Surg.* **2021**, *141*, 2235–2244. [PubMed]
50. Navarro, S.M.; Wang, E.Y.; Haeberle, H.S.; Mont, M.A.; Krebs, V.E.; Patterson, B.M.; Ramkumar, P.N. Machine Learning and Primary Total Knee Arthroplasty: Patient Forecasting for a Patient-Specific Payment Model. *J. Arthroplast.* **2018**, *33*, 3617–3623. [CrossRef]
51. Jo, C.; Ko, S.; Shin, W.C.; Han, H.S.; Lee, M.C.; Ko, T.; Ro, D.H. Transfusion after total knee arthroplasty can be predicted using the machine learning algorithm. *Knee Surg. Sport. Traumatol. Arthrosc.* **2020**, *28*, 1757–1764. [CrossRef]
52. Kunze, K.N.; Polce, E.M.; Sadauskas, A.J.; Levine, B.R. Development of Machine Learning Algorithms to Predict Patient Dissatisfaction After Primary Total Knee Arthroplasty. *J. Arthroplast.* **2020**, *35*, 3117–3122. [CrossRef] [PubMed]
53. Karnuta, J.M.; Luu, B.C.; Roth, A.L.; Haeberle, H.S.; Chen, A.F.; Iorio, R.; Schaffer, J.L.; Mont, M.A.; Patterson, B.M.; Krebs, V.E.; et al. Artificial Intelligence to Identify Arthroplasty Implants From Radiographs of the Knee. *J. Arthroplast.* **2021**, *36*, 935–940. [CrossRef] [PubMed]
54. Adams, M.; Chen, W.; Holcdorf, D.; McCusker, M.W.; Howe, P.D.; Gaillard, F. Computer vs human: Deep learning versus perceptual training for the detection of neck of femur fractures. *J. Med. Imaging Radiat. Oncol.* **2019**, *63*, 27–32. [CrossRef] [PubMed]
55. Urakawa, T.; Tanaka, Y.; Goto, S.; Matsuzawa, H.; Watanabe, K.; Endo, N. Detecting intertrochanteric hip fractures with orthopedist-level accuracy using a deep convolutional neural network. *Skeletal. Radiol.* **2019**, *48*, 239–244. [CrossRef] [PubMed]

Disclaimer/Publisher's Note: The statements, opinions and data contained in all publications are solely those of the individual author(s) and contributor(s) and not of MDPI and/or the editor(s). MDPI and/or the editor(s) disclaim responsibility for any injury to people or property resulting from any ideas, methods, instructions or products referred to in the content.

MDPI
St. Alban-Anlage 66
4052 Basel
Switzerland
www.mdpi.com

Medicina Editorial Office
E-mail: medicina@mdpi.com
www.mdpi.com/journal/medicina

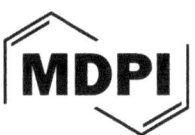

Disclaimer/Publisher's Note: The statements, opinions and data contained in all publications are solely those of the individual author(s) and contributor(s) and not of MDPI and/or the editor(s). MDPI and/or the editor(s) disclaim responsibility for any injury to people or property resulting from any ideas, methods, instructions or products referred to in the content.

www.ingramcontent.com/pod-product-compliance
Lightning Source LLC
LaVergne TN
LVHW070145100526
838202LV00015B/1893

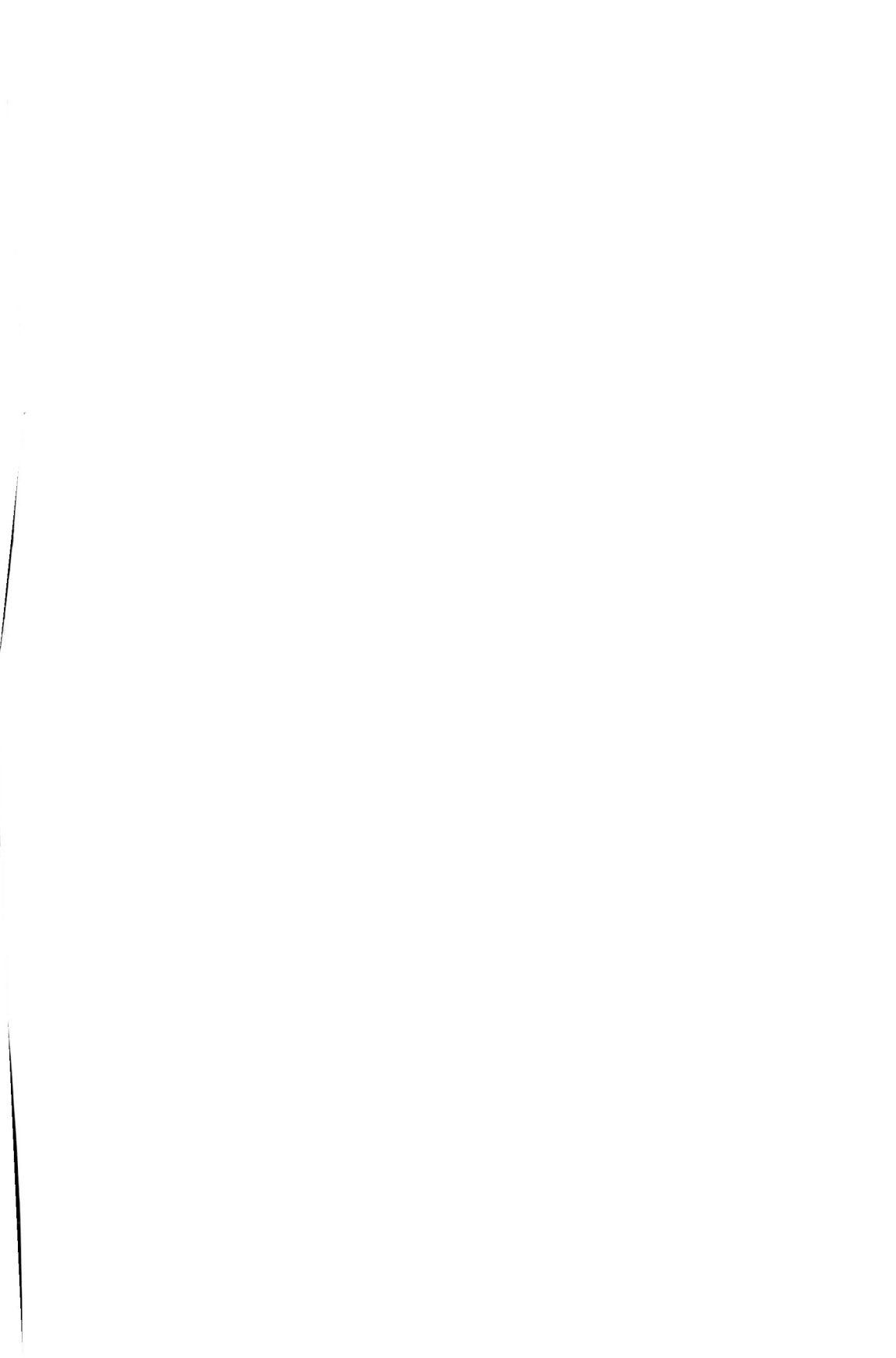